Nanotherapeutic Strategies and New Pharmaceuticals
(Part 1)

Edited By

Shahid Ali Khan
Department of Chemistry
University of Swabi, Swabi Anbar-23561
Khyber Pakhtunkhwa
Pakistan

Saad Salman
The University of Lahore
Islamabad Campus
Islamabad-44000
Pakistan

&

Youssef O. Al-Ghamdi
Department of Chemistry
College of Science Al-Zulfi, Majmaah University
Al-Majmaah 11952
Saudi Arabia

Nanotherapeutic Strategies and New Pharmaceuticals (Part I)

Editors: Shahid Ali Khan, Saad Salman and Youssef O. Al-Ghamdi

ISBN (Online): 978-981-5036-69-4

ISBN (Print): 978-981-5036-70-1

ISBN (Paperback): 978-981-5036-71-8

need for a court order if at any point you breach any terms of this License Agreement. In no event will any delay or failure by Bentham Science Publishers in enforcing your compliance with this License Agreement constitute a waiver of any of its rights.

3. You acknowledge that you have read this License Agreement, and agree to be bound by its terms and conditions. To the extent that any other terms and conditions presented on any website of Bentham Science Publishers conflict with, or are inconsistent with, the terms and conditions set out in this License Agreement, you acknowledge that the terms and conditions set out in this License Agreement shall prevail.

Bentham Science Publishers Pte. Ltd.
80 Robinson Road #02-00
Singapore 068898
Singapore
Email: subscriptions@benthamscience.net

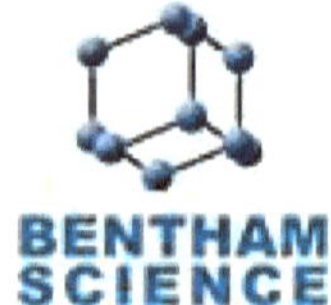

CONTENTS

PREFACE

Therapeutic agents have an impressive history in drug discovery and development which led to the identification of numerous phenomenal lead drug candidates. The current therapeutic regimens are allied with several inverse biological effects. Therefore, there is an urgent need for innovative and technological strategies to help in medical diagnosis and management. With the advancement of new technologies in medicinal chemistry, several highly specific, biocompatible, and non-toxic therapeutic agents are discovered and successfully applied for diverse clinical applications. Nanotechnology has perceived historic progress in the last few decades and recently proved its efficacy in every field of science and technology. Nanotechnology-based pharmaceuticals offered multifaceted and alternative methodologies to an overwhelmed conventional limitation of clinical therapies. Expertise in designing and developing nanoformulation helped in targeted drug delivery. Recently, the use of innovative therapeutic agents, particularly in nanomedicine, has accounted for a significant portion of the global pharmaceutical market and is predicted to continue to grow rapidly in the near future.

Dr. Shahid has worked on a variety of scientific platforms over the years. He has authored multiple research publications and is well-known for his scientific knowledge. In 2019, he envisioned creating a comprehensive book on nanotherapeutics in the biological sector, which had previously been spread across the literature. Dr. Saad Salman and Dr. Youssef O. Al-Ghamdi, the co-editors, later joined hands in this scientific voyage. This book is the result of over ten years of research and the diverse contributions of more than 50 fertile brains. Many well-known scientists from various countries, including the United States, the United Kingdom, Italy, Pakistan, Malaysia, India, and Bangladesh, contributed numerous book chapters to the premises of the book titled "Nanotherapeutic strategies and new pharmaceuticals" in this book, which resulted in part I and part II. For instance, COVID-19: an outbreak, application of nanotherapeutics agents in disease control, wound healing, surgery, stem cell, central nervous, haematology, cancer therapy, Gene therapy/editing and many more. Volume-I contains 9 chapters and each chapter has a minimum of 6,000 words. This indicates that each chapter has been meticulously detailed and structured.

Furthermore, each chapter is written by specialists in respective fields, and it was made mandatory to keep it as easy as possible to make it accessible to both beginners and experts. As a result, this book is one of the best for a wide range of readers. Furthermore, this book is structured to address a wide range of topics relevant to chemists, biologists, pharmacists, and material scientists.

We are very thankful to all the authors who spare time from their busy schedules and contributed their ideas and knowledge to this book. In addition, we also pay our sincerest gratitude to the team of Bentham Science, who made great efforts to make this book series possible.

Shahid Ali Khan
Department of Chemistry
University of Swabi, Swabi Anbar-23561
Khyber Pakhtunkhwa
Pakistan

Saad Salman
The University of Lahore
Islamabad Campus
Islamabad-44000
Pakistan

&

Youssef O. Al-Ghamdi
Department of Chemistry
College of Science Al-Zulfi, Majmaah University
Al-Majmaah 11952
Saudi Arabia

About the Editors

Shahid Ali Khan (Editor)

Dr. Shahid Ali Khan did his master of science (MSC) in 2010 in organic chemistry from Kohat University of Science and Technology, and Master of Philosophy (MPhil) in Natural Product and Medicinal Chemistry in 2014 from ICCBS Karachi and Ph.D. in Nanocatalysis in 2017 from King Abdulaziz University, Saudi Arabia. Dr. Khan got the best Ph.D. thesis award. Dr. Khan joined the University of Swabi as Assistant Professor in Feb. 2018 and still working in the same University. During his stay at the University of Swabi, Dr. Khan has supervised 7 MSC students and Co-supervised 8 Mphil students. Currently, many students of Dr. Khan's research group are involved in the synthesis and designing of nanocatalyst and hydrogels for various technological applications. During this period, Dr. Khan have completed 2 projects as a PI and 4 projects as a Co-PI, while many projects are under progress.

Moreover, Dr. Khan is working on multi-dimensional projects including Natural product chemistry, medicinal chemistry, Nanocatalysis and self-assembled hydrogels for diverse applications. Dr. Khan is also involved in the designing and synthesis of thin films as solid support for the stabilization of zero-valent metal nanoparticles for functional group transformation. Dr. Khan teaches various courses in Organic Chemistry, Physical chemistry, and spectroscopy to BS, MS, and Ph.D. students.

In brief, Dr. Khan has published 62 publications with a cumulative impact factor of 255 and has published 8 book chapters in various international journals of high repute.

Saad Salman (Co-Editor)

Dr. Saad Salman is a Lecturer at the Department of Pharmacy, The University of Lahore (Islamabad Campus), teaching Undergraduate and Postgraduate students. He is a Certified Health Researcher from NIH, USA. He has over twenty-one International publications, two International books, two book chapters, and thirty abstracts published. He is the founder and CEO of Research and Publication Inc.,which provides solutions to research students. He had received numerous awards at various conferences. He is an active member of the American Society of Pharmacology and Experimental Therapeutics (ASPET), the American Pharmacist Association, and the American Society of Consultant Pharmacists.

Youssef O. Al-Ghamdi (Co-Editor)

Youssef O. Al-Ghamdi received a bachelor's degree in Chemistry from Umm AL-Qura University, Makkah, Saudi Arabia, in 2008. Dr. Alghamdi received his master's degree in Organic Chemistry from King Khalid University, Abha, Saudi Arabia, in 2012, and the Ph.D. degree in Organic Chemistry, Polymers King Abdulaziz University, Jeddah, Saudi Arabia in 2018. He joined the College of Science at Al-Zulfi branch, Majmaah University, and currently chair the department of chemistry. Dr. Alghamdi is heading several units such as Planning and Development and Unit of Scientific Affairs. He is a member of the College Council, College of Science, Al-Zulfi, Majmaah University and a member of Labs and Facilities. **Dr. Youssef O. Al-Ghamdi** is involved in teaching various courses in Organic Chemistry, to BS and he has published 20 publications.

List of Contributors

Abid Mehmood Yousaf	Department of Pharmacy, COMSATS University Islamabad Lahore Campus, Lahore, Pakistan
Adeel Hassan	The University of Lahore, Islamabad Campus, Islamabad, Pakistan
Amin Ullah	Department of English, City University of Science and Technology, Peshawar, Pakistan
Arpan Dey	Delhi Public School, West Bengal, India
Ayesha Sajjad	The University of Lahore, Islamabad Campus, Islamabad, Pakistan
Fabeha Shafaat	Bolton School, Bolton, United Kingdom
Fahad Hassan Shah	Department of Biological Sciences, College of Natural Sciences, Kongju National University, Gongju, Republic of Korea
Fakhar ud Din	Department of Pharmacy, Faculty of Biological Sciences, Quaid-i-Azam University, Islamabad, Pakistan
Fayaz Ali	School of Pharmacy and State Key Laboratory of Quality Research in Chinese Medicine, Macau University of Science and Technology, Macao, China
Han Gon Choi	College of Pharmacy & Institute of Pharmaceutical Science and Technology, Hanyang University, Seoul, South Korea
Junaid Dar	The University of Lahore, Islamabad Campus, Islamabad, Pakistan
Kashif Iqbal	The University of Lahore, Islamabad Campus, Islamabad, Pakistan
Laiba Zakir	The University of Lahore, Islamabad Campus, Islamabad, Pakistan
Mahjoub Jabli	Department of Chemistry, College of Science Al-Zulfi, Majmaah University, Saudi Arabia
Maryam Bibi	Department of Pharmacy, Faculty of Biological Sciences, Quaid-i-Azam University, Islamabad, Pakistan
Muhammad Bilal	The University of Lahore, Islamabad Campus, Islamabad, Pakistan
Muhammad Tayyab Noor Khattak	Department of Chemistry, Govt Postgraduate College, Nowshera, Pakistan
Nipun Gorantla	Marvin Ridge High School, North Carolina, United States
Niyati H. Patel	Middlesex County Academy of Allied Health and Biomedical Sciences, New Jersey, United States
Robaica Khan	The University of Lahore, Islamabad Campus, Islamabad, Pakistan
Roberto Parisi	Department of Medicine, Surgery and Dentistry, University of Salerno, Salerno, Italy
Saad Salman	The University of Lahore, Islamabad Campus, Islamabad, Pakistan
Sakina Munir	The University of Lahore, Islamabad Campus, Islamabad, Pakistan
Sami G. Almalki	Department of Medical laboratory sciences, College of Applied Medical Sciences, Majmaah University, Al Majma'ah, Saudi Arabia
Sawara Sajal	The University of Lahore, Islamabad Campus, Islamabad, Pakistan

Shah Hussain	Department of Chemistry, Govt Postgraduate College, Nowshera, Pakistan
Sher Ali Shah	Department of Chemistry, University of Swabi, Khyber Pakhtunkhwa, Pakistan
Shahid Ali Khan	Department of Chemistry, University of Swabi, Swabi, Khyber Pakhtunkhwa, Pakistan
Shah Hussain	Department of Chemistry, Govt Postgraduate College Nowshera, Khyber Pakhtunkhwa, Pakistan
Sibgha Batool	Department of Pharmacy, Faculty of Biological Sciences, Quaid-i-Azam University, Islamabad, Pakistan
Sifeng Lucy Chen	Department of Life Sciences, Imperial College, London, United Kingdom
Song Ja Kim	Department of Biological Sciences, College of Natural Sciences, Kongju National University, Gongju, Republic of Korea
Veena Ganti	William Mason High School, Mason, United States
Waseeq Ur Rehman	Department of Chemistry, Govt Postgraduate College Nowshera, Khyber Pakhtunkhwa, Pakistan
Yasir Anwar	Department of Biological, Sciences, Faculty of Science, King Abdulaziz University, Jeddah, Kingdom of Saudi Arabia
Yi Zhun Zhu	School of Pharmacy and State Key Laboratory of Quality Research in Chinese Medicine, Macau University of Science and Technology, Macau, China
Yinghuai Zhu	School of Pharmacy and State Key Laboratory of Quality Research in Chinese Medicine, Macau University of Science and Technology, Macau, China
Youssef O. Al-Ghamdi	Department of Chemistry, College of Science Al-zulfi, Majmaah University, Al Majma'ah, Saudi Arabia
Zubair Ahmad	Department of Chemistry, University of Swabi, Swabi, Khyber Pakhtunkhwa, Pakistan

CHAPTER 1

Advances in Nanotherapeutic Agents

Waseeq Ur Rehman[1], Shahid Ali Khan[2,*], Zubair Ahmad[2], Muhammad Tayyab Noor Khattak[1], Shah Hussain[1], Youssef O. Al-Ghamdi[3], Mahjoub Jabli[3] and **Yasir Anwar[4]**

[1] *Department of Chemistry, Govt Postgraduate College, Nowshera 24100, Khyber Pakhtunkhwa, Pakistan*

[2] *Department of Chemistry, University of Swabi, Anbar-23561, Khyber Pakhtunkhwa, Pakistan*

[3] *Department of Chemistry, College of Science Al-Zulfi, Majmaah University, Al-Majmaah, 11952, Saudi Arabia*

[4] *Department of Biological Sciences, Faculty of Science, King Abdulaziz University, P. O, Box 80203, Jeddah, 21589, Kingdom of Saudi Arabia*

Abstract: Nanotechnology is an emerging field of science covering all the technological fields. Likewise all other fields, the medical field is also encountered by nanotechnology. In this regard, nanopharmaceuticals has gained the attention of researchers, leading to the development of nanomedicines. Nanopharmaceuticals are biologicals active molecules used for the effectiveness of drug therapies on the nanoscale. Nanomedicines in the fast-developing area have shown very fruitful results. Nanomedicines offer varieties of properties, for example, it has the capability to cross the cell barriers in order to reach the targeted organelles. It also overcomes the multidrug-resistant and prevents the effect on healthy cells. Drug delivery based on nanoparticles has many applications. Nanoparticles-based drug delivery system delivers the specified drug to the cells of the targeted tissue by controlled release. Thus, it has overcome the limitations of conventional therapies. The anti-cancer drug delivery to the cancerous cells is one of the examples of nanocarriers-based therapy. Nanoshells are used in this regard. Nanoshells load the specified anticancer pharmaceuticals, penetrate the cells and attack the targeted organelles within cells. The main and important properties of this therapy are the prevention of healthy cells from the drug effect. Nanotechnology is also used in diagnosis. It is used in the diagnosis of bone fractures, cardiovascular diseases, cancerous cells identification, and the detection of tumors in the brain. Nanolaser-based surgery is also the emerging field of nanotechnology. For this purpose, nano microscopy was used. In nano microscopy, surgery nano-based tools are used in which have the ability to penetrate the cells and remove/ kill the infected organelles. In this chapter, almost all the aspects of nanotechnology have been discussed, with a special focus on nanocarriers.

---

* **Corresponding author Shahid Ali Khan:** Department of Chemistry, University of Swabi, Swabi Anbar-23561, Khyber Pakhtunkhwa, Pakistan; E-mail: skhan@uoswabi.edu.pk

Keywords: Nanoscience, Nanomedicines, Nanobots, Nanoendoscopes, Nanolasers, Nanotechnology in Radiology.

1. OVERVIEW OF NANOSCIENCE

The study of natural, synthetic, or semisynthetic substances at the submicroscopic level is called nanoscience. At the nano level, the features of various elements vary significantly as compared with the outdated microscale [1]. Nanostructured substances exhibit extraordinary features due to their high surface capacity and hence, are used in every field of science and medicine. Even in daily life, they are most liked by the public due to two distinctive features, *i.e* small size, and big function. This science is so broad that a particular worldwide accepted description, but generally, they are defined from the size of the particles they possess. According to IUPAC and EU, the nanoparticles have a size that ranges from one nanometer to 100 nanometers [2]. On the other hand, the size of medical nanomaterials is about 20-200 nm or maybe more than that [3]. Pokropivny, V. *et al.*, taxonomized nanostructured materials as zero-dimensional things (nanospheres), one-dimensional (nanotubes), two dimensional (nanosheets), and three-dimensional (structures made out of individual squares in the nanometer scale, or mass materials) [4]. Early Egyptian peoples of 9th century BC made use of artificial stain to decorate utensils, and the stain was formulated from nanosized gold or silver. Another example is "Egyptian blue" which was used in the 3rd century BC [5].

In the modern age, the field of nanoparticles was developed by Michael Faraday (1875). He made gold at the nanoscale from aurum chloride through electrolysis [6]. In 1959 Richard Feynman established the foundation of current nanotechnology through his well-known speech, "There is plenty of room at the bottom [7]. In the 1980s, Buckminster fullerenes (by Buckminster) were introduced that further strengthen the field of nanotechnology. Carbon nanotubes were also developed in this period [8]. For the observation of nanoparticles, various techniques were developed at the beginning of the 20th century. These techniques include TEM, SEM, scanning tunneling microscope, and atomic force microscopy [9 - 11].

1.1. Nanomedicine–A Chronological Perception and Functions

Now a day's nanotechnology is applied in medical fields where nanomedicine exhibit higher therapeutic value than ordinary medicine. Due to the improved therapeutic value, nano-sized medicine has very high efficacy as compared to traditional medicine. Furthermore, nanosized drug delivery systems, nanosized imaging, and diagnostic systems are also introduced with the same properties i-e small size and high efficacy. In 1909, Paul Ehrlich introduced the concept of "magic bullet", for drugs, launched the current therapeutic investigation [12]. Variation of the pharmacokinetics of a drug (which is necessary for its biological action) *via* its structural reformation is constrained by the structural requirement. Nanotechnology offers the likelihood to bypass this restriction by controlling the pharmacokinetics (increased absorption rate of the drugs). In 1960 Horne and Bangham reported the self-assembling properties of phospholipids. They self-assemble their structure like a plasma membrane. They can form vesicular masses of nano-size and the nanovesicles were called "liposomes" [13]. In the 1970s that drug designers employed nanocarriers for drug delivery.

In 1976 a nano-pharmaceutical scientist, Peter Speiser, studied the polyacrylamide (PAAM) based nanoparticles for vaccination and were adjuvants in nature [14]. These NP's were spherical with a size of fewer than 80 nanometers which form real colloidal aqueous solutions. The NP's were compatible to deliver antigenic material (tetanus vaccine and human intravenous immunoglobulin G) and administered parenterally. These preparations show intact biological activity and high antibody production in animals.

In 1979, Couvreur *et al.*, shown the highly lipophilic characteristics of nanosized polyalkylcyanoacrylate and built up the first decomposable nanocapsules for anticancer drug delivery, and displayed successful endocytic application in calf serum [15].

Papahadjopoulos, along with Bangham, independently in 1967, studied the characterization of smectic mesophases, worked on the methods of water-soluble materials into phospholipidic vesicles, and Gregory Gregoriadis in 1971 showed that liposomes could deliver enzymes for therapeutic purposes [16].

With the expanded exploration in clinical, intra-and intercellular cycles, and huge developments in fundamental natural sciences and nanotechnology, it became clear that control of articles at the nanoscale level could take into consideration huge in the clinical field. Various materials and bodies may act as nanocarriers. Medications or proteinous drugs (*e.g.*, Denileukin diftitox or hormones or enzymes) can be securely conveyed with the assistance of nanocarriers. Besides, the nanocarriers ars more efficient for drug delivery. As a result of these extensive researches, different nano antibiotics were introduced in the market, for instance, (i) AmBisome® (combination of liposomes encapsulating amphotericin B) for fungal diseases, (ii) Liposomal doxorubicin (combination of liposomes encapsulating doxorubicin) for treatment of mammary gland cancer [17], (iii) DOX/ICG Coencapsulated Liposome-Coated Thermosensitive Nanogels for

NIR-Triggered Simultaneous Drug Release a combination of 100-nm PEGylated DOX hydrochloride coated by liposomes designed for the cure of refractory Kaposi's sarcoma in humans with AIDs virus [17]. Furthermore, it was testified that liposome-coated drugs possess a less toxic effect on the heart as compared to non-coated drugs [18 - 21]. The capacity and power of nanotherapeutics were largely discovered, but only a few clinically approved medications reached the market. All these studies have highlighted the value of nanotherapeutics as a product of nanotechnology so that they can be used for drug delivery with numerous benefits.

1.1.1. Beating the Limitations of Common Medications with Nanomedications

Nanomedicines offer a high surface volume ratio, thus they provide greater active sites, which results in fast chemical reactions. The nanomedicines have the characteristic to reach the targeted sites by bypassing the cell membranes. Due to this characteristic, the selectivity problem resolves. In conventional therapies, the therapeutic agents cannot reach inside the cell resulting the selectivity problems followed by the affecting of healthy cells. The nanomedicines solved these limitations [22, 23].

2. NANOTECHNOLOGY-BASED GADGETS FOR DIAGNOSIS AND TREATMENTS

2.1. Nanoelectronics in Radioscopy and Radiology

In hospitals, X-ray emission is frequently applied to detect fractures in bones, diagnose tumors, and diagnosis of other fatal diseases like TB, cancer, *etc.* In 2005 J. Zhang *et al.* reported about a field discharge x-rays generating machine that can deliver scanning x-rays, and picture anything from various positions deprived of automated movement. The principal module of the gadget was a gated carbon nanotube (CNT) field discharge (that acts as a negative electrode) with an assortment of electrons producing picture elements that are discretely addressable by means of a metal–oxide–semiconductor field impact semiconductor-based electronic course. They assessed the various physiognomies of that x-ray track and confirmed its imaging proficiency. The device can be used for tomography, laminography, mammography, and tomosynthesis with a simple laboratory system, fast processing and requires less energy. Tomosynthesis is an X-ray setup that can be applied as a preliminary test for early signs of breast carcinoma in women with no warning sign.

The X-ray strength of the device was adequate to be used as a medical device. The gated carbon nanotube-based cold cathode X-ray equipment is a portable machine to be used in operations theaters or hospitals [24]. The X-ray machine is less expensive, energy-efficient requires less support with good imaging features.

2.2. Nanolasers in Surgery

Surgical Blade and needle are perhaps the traditional tools for surgery or dissection, but the launch of lasers in surgery has further developed the field of surgeons in operations and investigational biological techniques. Laser microsurgery can be applied for removal as well as an overhaul of tissues [25]. With the help of nanolasers, a researcher can focus on a particular organelle inside a solitary cell also, slaughter it without upsetting the remainder of the cell, only a few hundred nanometers away. It is promising to cut conduits to some degree more modest measure of than 1 micron wide inside a cell's distance across 10 to 20 microns. Applying a laser shoot for just 10 to 15 femtoseconds in 1 micron wide, the total of photons grouped into each burst possesses 100 quadrillion watts for every square meter, fourteen times of greatness exceptional than outdoors daylight. The shooting power constructs an electric field sufficiently intense to focus electrons on the concentration and make a miniature emission. The cell receives the energy from a few nanojoules because the laser shoot is so flitting. It is sufficient energy to kill a cell.

This technology gives the idea about the function of the cytoskeleton in giving shape and support to the cell. Independent functions of cell organelles can find out using this technique. The technology might be advanced to do surgical procedures devoid of damaging other neighboring tissues. Near IR 10-15 second laser shoots are nowadays used in microscopy and nanosurgery of active cells [26]. For corneal surgical procedures, femtolasers are used. Regeneration of motor nerves or other nerves is an emerging therapy for neurological problems, but the therapy is fruitful only for mice and zebrafish without using accurate methods for cutting axons (axotomy). Axotomy is applied in *Caenorhabditis elegans* (roundworm) and the degenerated nerves were successfully recovered after the laser therapy [27].

Femtolaser has function like a microscopic "nano-blade or nanosissors" that is fit for cutting nerve axons or other nanostructured parts. The wavelength of the pulse is very short or in other words, highly energetic, allowing all the photons in the beam amass around there. They possess high energy but do not destroy neighboring tissues. The laser-cut axons vanished by vaporization and no further tissue is affected. This study promotes nerve regeneration *in-vivo*.

2.3. Nanorobotics

Nanorobots are very useful in certain cases while performing surgical operations. Such robots are called nanobots and they are so small and flexible that they can be introduced into the animal or human body *via* body openings or through a small operation. A working nanobot, programmed by a specialist, could go about as a free specialist inside of the human body. It can perform various functions like diagnosis, evacuation, or remedy of the injury and is controlled by an onboard PC. Such ideas, when sci-fi, are presently viewed as inside the domain of plausibility. Nanorobots will be fit for doing the exact and refined intracellular medical procedures, which are past the capacity of controls by the human hand. A gadget was produced for helping insignificantly intrusive thumping heart intrapericardial mediations [28]. This is based on the hypothesis of an endoscopic mechanical gadget that adheres to the epicardium by attractions and explores by crawling like a worm to any situation on the outside heavily influenced by a specialist. This technique hinders cardiovascular adjustment, lung decrease, differential lung air circulation, and reinsertion of laparoscopic apparatuses for saving different treatment places, accordingly paying the opportunity of diminished problem to the patient. The framework has a functioning station through which different apparatuses can be presented for treatment. This modern pattern validated fruitful spinning and movement on beating heart in an inadequate amount of trials in pigs.

2.3.1. Design of Nanorobots

The technology NCD (nanorobot controls design) is a methodology used to operate as a test platform for nanorobot 3-dimensional system development, as well as a rapid prototyping system for medical nanorobots. The NCD simulations show how to interrelate and regulate a nanorobotic within the body. For nanorobot task-based presenting, a progressive nano mechatronics system provides physical and numerical results. The nanorobot project involves advanced microchip technologies as well as biologically inspired elements such as "molecular sorting rotors" and a robot arm (telescoping deceiver). The external form of the nanorobot is composed of diamonded material, to which an engineered glycocalyx sheet can be added, which decreases fibrinogen (and other blood proteins) adsorption and bioactivity while ensuring adequate biocompatibility to avoid immunity invasion. A series of chemotactic sensors, each of whose receptors have a different affinity for each kind of particle, is well-versed in a variety of molecule types. Difficulties detected by these sensors may necessarily require a new trajectory planning. Sensor capabilities and layout are dependent on the context and task specifics. As a result, the nanorobot needs transducer specifications as well as useful detectors that are closely connected to the specific biomedical function. The nanorobot in this review can perceive obstacles over a spectrum of almost 1 mm and with an angular resolution equal to a diameter of 100 nm. Since the biological molecules are too small to detect accurately, the automaton must depend on chemicals touch sensors. This description of interaction capabilities enables a comparison of various nanotechnological sensor-based behavior [29].

2.3.2. Nanorobots in Gene Therapy

Medical nanorobots will willingly handle genetic diseases by analyzing the microstructures of both DNA and proteins present in the cell to recognized or desired reference structures. Such errors will either be fixed, or desired improvements could be made in place. In certain cases, chromosomal replacement treatment is more effective at overhauling than CY. An assembler-built fix ewer floats within the nucleus of a human cell, achieving some genome servicing. The nanotechnology slowly brings an unwound strand into a gap in its prow for inspection, stretching a mega coil of DNA between its lower pair of robot arms. Meanwhile, upper arms separate regulatory proteins from the chains and store them in an intake terminal [30, 31]. Internal medicine will take on new significance with trillions of nanorobots coursing through a bloodstream. Cancer, bacterial infectious diseases, and coronary artery disease could all be eradicated if the disease was attacked at the microscopic level.

2.3.3. Various Possible Uses of Nanorobots in Dentistry

2.3.3.1. Major Tooth Repair

Epigenetic technology, tissue regeneration, and tissue renewal approaches are also examples of nanodental technologies for tooth restoration. Biologically autologous entire replacement teeth with both synthetic and biological elements are often manufactured and installed by nanorobotics, resulting in full dentition auxiliary treatment [32, 33].

2.3.3.2. Tooth Durability and Appearance

Nano-dentistry has established azure, a nanostructured composite that improves tooth toughness and access. Upper varnish surfaces are replaced with sapphire, a covalently bonded artificial stone. Cerulean is sensitive to acid oxidation in the same way as a coating does. Cerulean offers the best regular whitening coating, as well as a beautification option [33].

2.3.3.3. Maintenance of Oral Hygiene

However, a gargle full of clever nano-robots could detect & kill pathogens, enabling the mouth's harmless vegetation to thrive in a clean environment. Besides that, the systems can detect food, residue, or parmesan particles on the teeth and propel them away to be washed away. Tools that are submerged in liquid and willing to float around will be able to penetrate exteriors that are beyond the reach of toothbrush spines or floss fibers. Dentifrice-delivered sub-occlusally abode nano-robots patrol both supra- and subgingival exteriors, metabolizing stuck organic matter and completing continuous calculus regeneration. They prevent tooth decay and act as a constant buffer against bad breath [34, 35].

2.3.3.4. Orthodontic Treatment

A frictional type of force opposes this effort when a tooth is sliding across an arch-cable. The use of excessive orthodontic force can result in root desorption and anchorage injury. In research published by Katz, the strength of orthodontic wires was reduced by covering them with synthetic fullerene-like tungsten disulphide nanoparticles (IFeWS2), which have outstanding dry lubrication properties. In the future, orthodontic nanorobots could be able to work specifically on periodontal tissues, allowing for quick and painless teeth straightening, gyrating, and vertical repositioning in minutes to hours [36].

2.3.4. Nanorobot for Brain Aneurysm

The nanorobot, which operating system biotechnology for medical device development and testing, is used to diagnose aneurysms. Device methodology, the established process, and inside-body transduction are the three main features. Instruments prototyping is a quantitative nanotechnology technique that aids in the analysis of main characteristics in medical instrumentation and system prototyping. The industry has historically used a similar approach to develop race vehicles, aircraft, submarines, integrated circuits, and medical equipment [37]. The same principle can now be applied to the production and testing of medical nanorobots [38 - 40]. The nanorobot manufacturing technology should be integrated into a biochip system. As a result, new materials, photonics, and nano bioelectronics are discussed alongside a description of the nanorobot design. Often used as criteria for nanorobot morphology and inside-body activity are cell morphology, microbiology, and proteomics. Medical diagnosis is dependent on changes in chemical gradients and telemetric instrumentation, with nanorobots, enabled focused on proteomic over presentation [41]. Biomolecules are too rare to be easily identified: Instead, the robot detects them using chemical nano biosensor interaction [42]. The key morphologic features associated with a brain aneurysm are used to design the study of nanorobots detecting and interacting inside a disfigured blood vessel [43]. NOS (nitric oxide synthase) amounts in the brain are low, though certain false - positive can take place due to the progressive character of N-oxide roles with semi-carbazone (pNOS). As the fluid flow, nanorobots and blood cells constantly approach one end of the partition. The nanorobots should recognize proteins overexpression, and the configuration for sensing and control activation, such as controlling the identification borderlines, can be changed for various values. Any nanorobots that do not react when within the workspace are treated as though they have not detected any signal, and they flow with the fluid as it exists. If the nanorobot's electrochemical sensor senses NOS in small amounts or within a typical range, it produces a weak signal of less than 50 nA [44 - 46]. In this situation, the nanorobot disregards the NOS amount, believing that it is below appropriate intracranial NOS levels. Every time the cell phone receives at least a total of 100 nanorobots higher proteomic signal transduction, the model considers this as a good indication of the intracranial aneurysm as a functional verge for medical diagnosis, to avoid noise distortions and succeed a higher resolution.

3. NANOENDOSCOPES

PillCam was invented by Gavriel Iddan and fabricated by Given Imaging Ltd. in 2001. Its parts include a led light source, lens, battery, antenna, radio waves transmitter, and a micro-sized camera for capturing photos or videos. PillCam capsule endoscopy was produced to openly observe the gastrointestinal (GI) organization while maintaining patient comfort. Videocassette recorder tablet endoscopy is a key advancement that can foster superior quality imaging or video of the gut in its immaculateness [47]. After a few years, pill endoscopy was confirmed. Until now, it is used as a first-line assessment in quite a while with an indistinct gastrointestinal drain after a negative esophagogastroduodenoscopy and colonoscopy outcomes. Video case endoscopy is likewise significant in the evaluation of provocative and neoplastic disorders of the little bowel [48]. Changing the situating and development of a nanoscale will significantly improve the exactness of this strategy.

Various methodologies are being examined for the association of microcapsules, containing commonly dried out and moist hold just as force-driven methodologies like appendages with stick-on bases. A basic model with physical features like the alimentary canal can be used for such approaches [49]. Unequivocally situated microcapsules would facilitate the doctors to see any piece of within coating of the stomach or gut. Furthermore, these pill cams or nanobots could be changed to incorporate treatment systems too, like the arrival of medication or compound almost an unusual region such that they could be used for drugs delivery at abnormal sites. Comparative nanorobots will be developed for other organs of the body [48].

4. NANOPHARMACEUTICALS AND NANOMEDICINE

Nanomedicines and nanomedical devices play a significant role in the enhancement of diagnosis, treatment, and transport vehicles for drugs and in surgery. Liposomes nanoparticles as drug delivery are most valuable, which are already discussed.

Nanoparticles are used as nanocarriers in drug delivery to deliver the chemotropic and cytotoxic drug to the actually targeted tissues [50]. Nanomedicines offer handsome strategies to overcome the drawback of conventional methods. The nanomedicines have the capability to enhance selectivity thus, it prevents the affecting of healthy cells. Nanoparticles are used as nanocarriers to bypass the cell membrane to enter to the targeted organelles. Nanoparticles loaded drugs reduce the multidrug resistance and target only infected cells [51].

5. NANOMEDICINE:FUTURE OF CANCER TREATMENT

Malignant cells are the result of abnormal and uncontrolled cell division, having the ability to spread to other parts. As a result, the tumor is developed with abnormal growth [52 - 54]. There are many conventional therapies used for the treatment of cancer. These conventional therapies include chemotherapy, radiation and are surgical treatment. These typical medications are associated with long-term adverse effects. These adverse effects are the limitations of conventional therapies. Conventional methods have several limitations like lack of selectivity, which affects other cells and tissue. Conventional chemotherapeutics are unable to be solubilized in an aqueous medium. Another drawback of these therapies is the multidrug resistance, which leads to further complications [55 - 62].

For this purpose, new strategies have been developed to treat cancer with a minimum side effect on other cells. One of them is the drug delivery to reach the drug at the targeted site (cancerous cells and tissues) and does not affect the other cells. Nanotechnology and nanotherapy are emerging and developing fields having unlimited application in every field. Nanomedicine is one of the real applications of nanotherapy. Nanomedicines in cancer research get the attention of scientists due to a large number of positive effects. Nanomedicines reach the targeted site and protect other healthy cells from damage (Fig. **1**). It also overcomes the chemoselectivity problems. Chemotherapeutics are hydrophobic and can't dissolve in an aqueous medium, this limitation is also overcome through nanomedicines using nanocrystals and chitosan-based nanoparticles. It also solves the multidrug-resistant issue. In this regard, magnetic nanoparticles, lipids-based nanoparticles, and polymeric nanoparticles are used [63 - 68].

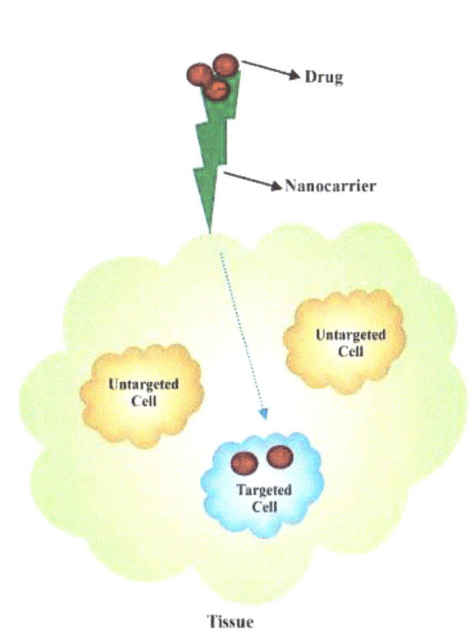

Fig. (1). Targeted drug delivery using nanocarriers.

The conventional drug possessing large particles and cant cross the cell boundary. Therefore it can't reach the specified site, results in the affecting of other cells [69]. As the cells of capillaries have a very low diameter therefore only nanoparticles can cross this barrier to enter into the cell. Nanoparticles have the ability to reach the targeted site; therefore, they completely get consumed in the cell. Nanoshells are nanoparticles that destroyed the cancerous cell from inside by temperature. Nanoshells have the ability to get absorbed different frequencies of light, due to which the temperature increases, which results in the destruction of cancerous cells from inside. Mechanistically when the nanoshells are entered into cells, infrared rays are applied, which get absorbed by these nanoshells. The temperature started giving up, resulting in the effective damage of cancerous affected cells only. The healthy cells near the canorous cells remain unaffected during this process [70, 71]. Gold nanoshells (nanoparticles) play a significant role in this regard. Gold nanoshells entered the cancerous cell and started destroying the host cell preventing the spare cells.

CONCLUSION

Nanotechnology is a fast-developing field of science. Nanotechnology deals with the tools on the nanoscale. Nanotechnology covers all the fields of science and has varieties of applications, especially in the field of medicines. Nano-scale medicines have the capability to reach inside the cell. In this regard, nanocarriers are used. Nanocarriers loaded the drug and dropped it to the targeted site, even inside the cell organelles. Nanomedicines overcome the limitations of conventional treatments by resolving selectivity problems, multidrug-resistant, and targeting. Similarly, nano-based tools are used for the treatment of and diagnosis of verities of disorders. This chapter covers the nanomedicines their application and advantages as well as the role of nanotechnology in biomedical fields.

CONSENT FOR PUBLICATION

Not applicable.

CONFLICT OF INTEREST

The author declares no conflict of interest, financial or otherwise.

ACKNOWLEDGMENT

The authors acknowledged the joint collaboration work between the Department of Chemistry, Post Graduate College, Nowshera, Pakistan, Department of Chemistry, University of Swabi, Pakistan, and College of Science Al-Zulfi, Majmaah University.

REFERENCES

[1]   Jain K. A Handbook of Nanomedicine Tatowa. NJ: Springer Bioscience/Humana Press 2007.

[2]   Vert M, Doi Y, Hellwich K-H, Hess M, Hodge P, Kubisa P, *et al.* Terminology for biorelated polymers and applications (IUPAC Recommendations 2012). Pure Appl Chem 2012; 84(2): 377-410.
        [http://dx.doi.org/10.1351/PAC-REC-10-12-04]

[3]   Saji VS, Choe HC, Yeung KW. Nanotechnology in biomedical applications: a review. Int J Nano Biomater 2010; 3(2): 119-39.
        [http://dx.doi.org/10.1504/IJNBM.2010.037801]

[4]   Pokropivny V, Skorokhod V. Classification of nanostructures by dimensionality and concept of

surface forms engineering in nanomaterial science. Mater Sci Eng C 2007; 27(5-8): 990-3.
[http://dx.doi.org/10.1016/j.msec.2006.09.023]

[5]　Johnson-McDaniel D, Barrett CA, Sharafi A, Salguero TT. Nanoscience of an ancient pigment. J Am Chem Soc 2013; 135(5): 1677-9.
[http://dx.doi.org/10.1021/ja310587c] [PMID: 23215240]

[6]　M. Farady. The Bakerian Lecture. Experimental relations of gold (and other metals) to light. Philos Trans Royal Soc London 1857; 147: 145-81.

[7]　Feynman RPJCIoT. Engineering, magazine S. There's plenty of room at the bottom 1960.

[8]　Endo M, Kroto H. Formation of carbon nanofibers. J Phys Chem 1992; 96(17): 6941-4.
[http://dx.doi.org/10.1021/j100196a017]

[9]　Binnig G, Quate CF, Gerber C. Atomic force microscope. Phys Rev Lett 1986; 56(9): 930-3.
[http://dx.doi.org/10.1103/PhysRevLett.56.930] [PMID: 10033323]

[10]　Stevenson A. Interactions of nanoparticles with cells for nanomedical applications. UK: Oxford University 2014.

[11]　Stirling DA. Nanotechnology Applications. The Nanotechnology Revolution: Pan Stanford. 2018; pp. 281-434.
[http://dx.doi.org/10.1201/9781315110837-9]

[12]　Strebhardt K, Ullrich A. Paul Ehrlich's magic bullet concept: 100 years of progress. Nat Rev Cancer 2008; 8(6): 473-80.
[http://dx.doi.org/10.1038/nrc2394] [PMID: 18469827]

[13]　Bangham AD, Standish MM, Weissmann G. The action of steroids and streptolysin S on the permeability of phospholipid structures to cations. J Mol Biol 1965; 13(1): 253-9.
[http://dx.doi.org/10.1016/S0022-2836(65)80094-8] [PMID: 5859040]

[14]　Birrenbach G, Speiser PP. Polymerized micelles and their use as adjuvants in immunology. J Pharm Sci 1976; 65(12): 1763-6.
[http://dx.doi.org/10.1002/jps.2600651217] [PMID: 1036442]

[15]　Couvreur P, Kante B, Roland M. Speiser PJJops. J Pharm Sci Adsorption of antineoplastic drugs to polyalkylcyanoacrylate nanoparticles and their release in calf serum. J Pharm Sci 1979; 68(12): 1521-4.

[16]　Connor J, Sullivan S, Huang L. Monoclonal antibody and liposomes. Pharmacol Ther 1985; 28(3): 341-65.
[http://dx.doi.org/10.1016/0163-7258(85)90058-0] [PMID: 3911220]

[17]　Yu L, Dong A, Guo R, Yang M, Deng L, Zhang JJABS, *et al.* DOX/ICG coencapsulated liposome-coated thermosensitive nanogels for NIR-triggered simultaneous drug release and photothermal effect. ACS Biomater Sci Eng 2018; 4(7): 2424-34.

[18]　Barenholz Y. Doxil®--the first FDA-approved nano-drug: lessons learned. J Control Release 2012; 160(2): 117-34.
[http://dx.doi.org/10.1016/j.jconrel.2012.03.020] [PMID: 22484195]

[19]　Gabizon A, Shmeeda H, Barenholz Y. Pharmacokinetics of pegylated liposomal Doxorubicin: review of animal and human studies. Clin Pharmacokinet 2003; 42(5): 419-36.
[http://dx.doi.org/10.2165/00003088-200342050-00002] [PMID: 12739982]

[20]　Gabizon A, Horowitz AT, Goren D, Tzemach D, Shmeeda H, Zalipsky S. *In vivo* fate of folate-targeted polyethylene-glycol liposomes in tumor-bearing mice. Clin Cancer Res 2003; 9(17): 6551-9.
[PMID: 14695160]

[21]　Soloman R, Gabizon AA. Clinical pharmacology of liposomal anthracyclines: focus on pegylated liposomal Doxorubicin. Clin Lymphoma Myeloma 2008; 8(1): 21-32.
[http://dx.doi.org/10.3816/CLM.2008.n.001] [PMID: 18501085]

[22]   Bar-Zeev M, Livney YD, Assaraf YG. Targeted nanomedicine for cancer therapeutics: Towards precision medicine overcoming drug resistance. Drug Resist Updat 2017; 31: 15-30.
[http://dx.doi.org/10.1016/j.drup.2017.05.002] [PMID: 28867241]

[23]   Shapira A, Livney YD, Broxterman HJ, Assaraf YG. Nanomedicine for targeted cancer therapy: towards the overcoming of drug resistance. Drug Resist Updat 2011; 14(3): 150-63.
[http://dx.doi.org/10.1016/j.drup.2011.01.003] [PMID: 21330184]

[24]   Zhang J, Yang GY, Cheng. B Gao, Q. Qiu, JP Lu , O. Zhou. Stationary scanning x-ray source based on carbon nanotube field emitters. Appl Phys Lett 2005; 86: 184104.
[http://dx.doi.org/10.1063/1.1923750]

[25]   Jain KK. Handbook of laser neurosurgery: Charles C Thomas Pub Limited 1983.

[26]   Sacconi L, Tolić-Nørrelykke IM, Antolini R, Pavone FS. Combined intracellular three-dimensional imaging and selective nanosurgery by a nonlinear microscope. J Biomed Opt 2005; 10(1): 14002.
[http://dx.doi.org/10.1117/1.1854675] [PMID: 15847583]

[27]   Yanik MF, Cinar H, Cinar HN, Chisholm AD, Jin Y, Ben-Yakar A. Neurosurgery: functional regeneration after laser axotomy. Nature 2004; 432(7019): 822.
[http://dx.doi.org/10.1038/432822a] [PMID: 15602545]

[28]   Riviere CN, Patronik N, Zenati M, Eds. Prototype epicardial crawling device for intrapericardial intervention on the beating heart Heart Surg Forum. Citeseer 2004.

[29]   Cale TS, Lu J-Q, Gutmann RJ. Three-dimensional integration in microelectronics: Motivation, processing, and thermomechanical modeling. Chem Eng Commun 2008; 195(8): 847-88.
[http://dx.doi.org/10.1080/00986440801930302]

[30]   Adleman LM. On constructing a molecular computer. DNA based computers. 1995; 27: 1-21.

[31]   Hamdi M, Ferreira A. Multiscale design and modeling of protein-based nanomechanisms for nanorobotics. Int J Robot Res 2009; 28(4): 436-49.
[http://dx.doi.org/10.1177/0278364908099888]

[32]   Jhaveri H, Balaji P. Nanotechnology: The future of dentistry. J Indian Prosthodont Soc 2005; 5: 1.

[33]   Srivastava S, Kabra P. Nanorobotics-A novel shift towards an era of hands free dentistry. Dental Sci 2017; 6(4): 2437-40.

[34]   Ahmad MA, Kamal A, Ashraf F, Ansari AF. A review on current scenario in the field of nanorobotics. Int J Eng SCI Res Tech 2014; 3: 6.

[35]   Verma SK, Chauhan R. Nanorobotics in dentistry–A review. Indian J Dent 2014; 5: 62-70.
[http://dx.doi.org/10.1016/j.ijd.2012.12.010]

[36]   Verma SK, Prabhat KC, Goyal L, Rani M, Jain A. A critical review of the implication of nanotechnology in modern dental practice. Natl J Maxillofac Surg 2010; 1(1): 41-4.
[http://dx.doi.org/10.4103/0975-5950.69166] [PMID: 22442549]

[37]   Genov R, Stanacevic M, Naware M, Cauwenberghs G, Thakor N. 16-channel integrated potentiostat for distributed neurochemical sensing. IEEE Trans Circuits Syst I Regul Pap 2006; 53(11): 2371-6.
[http://dx.doi.org/10.1109/TCSI.2006.884425]

[38]   Cavalcanti A. Assembly automation with evolutionary nanorobots and sensor-based control applied to nanomedicine. IEEE Trans NanoTechnol 2003; 2(2): 82-7.
[http://dx.doi.org/10.1109/TNANO.2003.812590]

[39]   Hogg T. Coordinating microscopic robots in viscous fluids. Auton Agent Multi Agent Syst 2007; 14(3): 271-305.
[http://dx.doi.org/10.1007/s10458-006-9004-3]

[40]   Cavalcanti A, Freitas RA Jr. Autonomous multi-robot sensor-based cooperation for nanomedicine. Int J Nonlinear Sci Numer Simul 2002; 3(3/4): 743-6.

[41] Buchanan J Jr, Kleinstreuer C. Simulation of particle-hemodynamics in a partially occluded artery segment with implications to the initiation of microemboli and secondary stenoses 1998.
[http://dx.doi.org/10.1115/1.2798013]

[42] Casal A, Hogg T, Cavalcanti A. Nanorobots as cellular assistants in inflammatory responses. IEEE BCATS Biomedical Computation at Stanford 2003 Symposium 2003.

[43] Elder JB, Hoh DJ, Oh BC, Heller AC, Liu CY, Apuzzo ML. The future of cerebral surgery: a kaleidoscope of opportunities. Neurosurgery 2008; 62(6) (Suppl. 3): 1555-79.
[http://dx.doi.org/10.1227/01.neu.0000333820.33143.0d] [PMID: 18695575]

[44] Freitas RA Jr. What is nanomedicine? Nanomed 2005; 1(1): 2-9.
[http://dx.doi.org/10.1016/j.nano.2004.11.003] [PMID: 17292052]

[45] Fukuda S, Hashimoto N, Naritomi H, *et al.* Prevention of rat cerebral aneurysm formation by inhibition of nitric oxide synthase. Circulation 2000; 101(21): 2532-8.
[http://dx.doi.org/10.1161/01.CIR.101.21.2532] [PMID: 10831529]

[46] Fukuda T, Kawamoto A, Arai F, Matsuura H, Eds. Mechanism and swimming experiment of micro mobile robot in water. Proceedings of the 1994 IEEE International Conference on Robotics and Automation.
[http://dx.doi.org/10.1109/ROBOT.1994.351388]

[47] Mason M, Swain J, Matthews BD, Harold KL. Use of video capsule endoscopy in the setting of recurrent subacute small-bowel obstruction. J Laparoendosc Adv Surg Tech A 2008; 18(5): 713-6.
[http://dx.doi.org/10.1089/lap.2007.0156] [PMID: 18803514]

[48] Jain KK. Nanomedicine NanoBioTechnology. Springer 2008; pp. 303-27.
[http://dx.doi.org/10.1007/978-1-59745-218-2_12]

[49] Saljoughian M. Gastrointestinal Bleeding: An Alarming Sign. US Pharm 2009; 12: 17.

[50] Bawarski WE, Chidlowsky E, Bharali DJ, Mousa SA. Emerging nanopharmaceuticals. Nanomed 2008; 4(4): 273-82.
[http://dx.doi.org/10.1016/j.nano.2008.06.002] [PMID: 18640076]

[51] Marcato PD, Durán N. New aspects of nanopharmaceutical delivery systems. J Nanosci Nanotechnol 2008; 8(5): 2216-29.
[http://dx.doi.org/10.1166/jnn.2008.274] [PMID: 18572633]

[52] Carey L, Winer E, Viale G, Cameron D, Gianni L. Triple-negative breast cancer: disease entity or title of convenience? Nat Rev Clin Oncol 2010; 7(12): 683-92.
[http://dx.doi.org/10.1038/nrclinonc.2010.154] [PMID: 20877296]

[53] Folkman J, Kalluri R. Cancer without disease. Nature 2004; 427(6977): 787.
[http://dx.doi.org/10.1038/427787a] [PMID: 14985739]

[54] Ravasco P, Monteiro-Grillo I, Vidal PM, Camilo ME. Cancer: disease and nutrition are key determinants of patients' quality of life. Support Care Cancer 2004; 12(4): 246-52.
[http://dx.doi.org/10.1007/s00520-003-0568-z] [PMID: 14997369]

[55] Brown JM, Wilson WR. Exploiting tumour hypoxia in cancer treatment. Nat Rev Cancer 2004; 4(6): 437-47.
[http://dx.doi.org/10.1038/nrc1367] [PMID: 15170446]

[56] DeVita VT Jr, Chu E. A history of cancer chemotherapy. Cancer Res 2008; 68(21): 8643-53.
[http://dx.doi.org/10.1158/0008-5472.CAN-07-6611] [PMID: 18974103]

[57] Dranoff G. Cytokines in cancer pathogenesis and cancer therapy. Nat Rev Cancer 2004; 4(1): 11-22.
[http://dx.doi.org/10.1038/nrc1252] [PMID: 14708024]

[58] Fetting J, Anderson P, Ball H, Benear J, Benjamin K, Bennett C, *et al.* Outcomes of cancer treatment for technology assessment and cancer treatment guidelines. J Clin Oncol 1996; 14(2): 671-9.

[http://dx.doi.org/10.1200/JCO.1996.14.2.671] [PMID: 8636786]

[59]   Garrod LP, O'grady F. Antibiotic and chemotherapy. 1971.

[60]   Holland JF, Glidewell O, Cooper RG. Adverse effect of radiotherapy on adjuvant chemotherapy for carcinoma of the breast. Surg Gynecol Obstet 1980; 150(6): 817-21.
[PMID: 7376042]

[61]   Ladas EJ, Jacobson JS, Kennedy DD, Teel K, Fleischauer A, Kelly KM. Antioxidants and cancer therapy: a systematic review. J Clin Oncol 2004; 22(3): 517-28.
[http://dx.doi.org/10.1200/JCO.2004.03.086] [PMID: 14752075]

[62]   Relling MV, Pui C-H, Sandlund JT, *et al.* Adverse effect of anticonvulsants on efficacy of chemotherapy for acute lymphoblastic leukaemia. Lancet 2000; 356(9226): 285-90.
[http://dx.doi.org/10.1016/S0140-6736(00)02503-4] [PMID: 11071183]

[63]   Ahmad MZ, Alkahtani SA, Akhter S, *et al.* Progress in nanotechnology-based drug carrier in designing of curcumin nanomedicines for cancer therapy: current state-of-the-art. J Drug Target 2016; 24(4): 273-93.
[http://dx.doi.org/10.3109/1061186X.2015.1055570] [PMID: 26066739]

[64]   Bhattarai P, Hameed S, Dai Z. Recent advances in anti-angiogenic nanomedicines for cancer therapy. Nanoscale 2018; 10(12): 5393-423.
[http://dx.doi.org/10.1039/C7NR09612G] [PMID: 29528075]

[65]   Bor G, Mat Azmi ID, Yaghmur A. Nanomedicines for cancer therapy: current status, challenges and future prospects. Ther Deliv 2019; 10(2): 113-32.
[http://dx.doi.org/10.4155/tde-2018-0062] [PMID: 30678550]

[66]   Dawidczyk CM, Russell LM, Searson PC. Nanomedicines for cancer therapy: state-of-the-art and limitations to pre-clinical studies that hinder future developments. Front Chem 2014; 2: 69.
[http://dx.doi.org/10.3389/fchem.2014.00069] [PMID: 25202689]

[67]   Pillai G. Nanomedicines for cancer therapy: an update of FDA approved and those under various stages of development. SOJ Pharm Pharm Sci 2014; 1(2): 13.

[68]   Sebastian R. Nanomedicine-the future of cancer treatment: A review. J Cancer Prev Curr Res. 2017; 8(1): 00-265.

[69]   Schultheiss TE, Hanks GE, Hunt MA, Lee WR. Incidence of and factors related to late complications in conformal and conventional radiation treatment of cancer of the prostate. Int J Rad Oncol Biol Phy 1995; 32(3):643-9. 32(3): 643-9.
[http://dx.doi.org/10.1016/0360-3016(95)00149-S]

[70]   Alam M, Massoud Y, Eds. An accurate closed-form analytical model of single nanoshells for cancer treatment. 48th Midwest Symposium on Circuits and Systems 2005.
[http://dx.doi.org/10.1109/MWSCAS.2005.1594503]

[71]   Bardhan R, Lal S, Joshi A, Halas NJ. Theranostic nanoshells: from probe design to imaging and treatment of cancer. Acc Chem Res 2011; 44(10): 936-46.
[http://dx.doi.org/10.1021/ar200023x] [PMID: 21612199]

CHAPTER 2

Nanotechnology in Stem Cell Research

Sifeng Lucy Chen[1,*] and **Fahad Hassan Shah**[2]

[1] *Department of Life Sciences, Imperial College London, London, United Kingdom*

[2] *Department of Biological Sciences, College of Natural Sciences, Kongju National University, Gongju 32588, Republic of Korea*

Abstract: Nanotechnology encompasses the production of materials at the nanoscale level and has been applied to many fields, including medicine. Within nanoscale ranges, the physical properties of particles are dominated by quantum mechanics, thus resulting in chemical behaviours that are distinct from that of bulk substances. Nano-based therapeutics and medical devices take advantage of these specific properties in order to better image and model the underlying biochemical and biophysical changes in a system, especially in diseases that progress over time. More specifically, advances in stem cell research have been aided by the use of nanoscale materials, enabling scientists to enhance stem cell behaviours for precise gene editing, regenerative medicine, and drug delivery. The interdisciplinary application of nanotechnology has great potential in clarifying the fundamentals of stem cell biochemistry, thus accelerating the development of future regenerative therapies.

Keywords: Chemical Behaviour, Nanomaterials, Nanotechnology, Physical Properties, Regenerative Medicine, Stem Cells.

1. INTRODUCTION

Nanotechnology is an emerging field focused on the production of materials at the nanoscale level. The underlying principles of its use in various fields include the observed phenomenon that size directly affects the physiochemical properties of the substance, generating different behaviours to that of bulk structures. In recent years, the application of nanotechnology to the medical field (thus term nanomedicine has garnered substantial interest due to their flexible engineering towards therapeutics, imaging, and diagnostics. In this chapter, the prevalence of nanotechnology in stem cell research will be explored by analyzing the ways in which the physicochemical properties of specifically-engineered nanoparticles can

* **Corresponding author Sifeng Lucy Chen:** Imperial College London, United Kingdom South Kensington, London SW7 2BU, United Kingdom; E-mail: sc8118@imperial.ac.uk

Shahid Ali Khan, Saad Salman, Youssef O. Al-Ghamd (Eds.)

All rights reserved-© 2021 Bentham Science Publishers

supplement stem cell function in therapeutics. The advantages and disadvantages of these various technologies will also be discussed. Although much of the biochemistry behind stem cells has yet to be fully understood, they provide a promising outlook for many fields, including organ transplantation and the treatment of congenital disorders. However, limitations towards its clinical use remain, which could potentially be overcome by the incorporation of biomimetic nanoparticles.

1.1. What are Stem Cells?

Stem cells are unspecialized, with the ability to differentiate into a number of different cell types, and are present in both adult and embryonic tissues [1]. They are part of the repair system, providing a supply of correctly-differentiated cells in situations where these cells need to be continually replaced. Stem cells are characterised by their ability for self-renewal, enabling them to divide indefinitely under specific conditions [2]. This is in part due to the higher level of telomerase within stem cells as compared to other somatic cells, which allows them to replenish chromosomal cappings. However, attrition of these regions over time may lead to aberrations in replication; some stem cell types are susceptible to the formation of teratomas, which are non-cancerous tumours that contain diverse mixtures of semi-developed tissues such as teeth, hair and cartilage [3]. Stem cells are also potent, with the ability to specialise into various cell types, the diversity of which is limited by the stage of development from which the stem cell is obtained. The specialisation process is influenced by many different signals, both external and internal, including physical cell-cell contact and fluctuations in gene expression.

1.2. Types and Biogenesis of Stem Cells

The ability for stem cells to differentiate into various cell lineages is determined by the stage at which it is extracted; embryonic or adult. These cells, therefore, display different behaviours and are generated through distinct lineages. The therapeutic potential of both will be evaluated and compared.

1.2.1. Embryonic Stem Cells

Embryonic stem cells (ESCs) are derived from the inner cell mass of a human blastocyst, a structure that forms approximately five days after fertilization [4]. The zygote, the cell immediately resulting from fertilisation is totipotent. Totipotency is characterised by the ability to differentiate into any other cell line;

the developmental potency of a cell becomes more restricted as it progresses further down distinct pathways of specialisation [5]. A series of mitotic cell divisions results in a structure known as the morula, a sphere of 32-64 totipotent cells. This then develops into the blastocyst, the cell types of which are separated into the peripheral cells and the inner cell mass; peripheral cells later form extraembryonic membranes and the placenta, whereas the inner cell mass forms the foetus (Fig. 1). Thus, the inner cell mass is not totipotent but instead pluripotent, with the ability to differentiate into any cell type excepting those derived from the peripheral blastocyst cells [6]. Cultured ESCs are pluripotent and can be engineered to differentiate into the three germ layers: ectoderm, mesoderm, and endoderm, from which all mature cell types found in the adult organism develop [7]. This presents a number of innovative applications into further understanding of the development and disease progression, as well as therapeutic tools for the treatment of currently incurable disorders such as neurological injury, type I diabetes, and cardiovascular conditions.

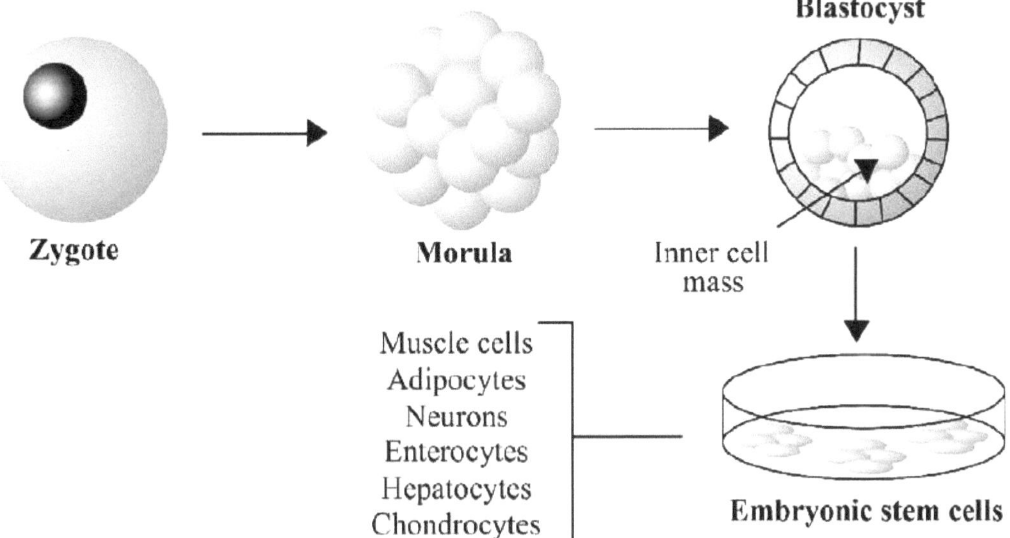

Fig. (1). Embryonic stem cell development and culture for *in vitro* differentiation into various tissues [8].

ESC lines are kept in the undifferentiated state *via* strictly controlled conditions in permanent culture containing bovine serum and feeder cells, which are inactivated to supply growth factors for the stem cells [9, 10]. However, the establishment of these stem cells has been ethically controversial as the extraction of the inner cell mass results in the destruction of the blastocyst in most cases. Whether blastocysts can be considered human lives has not yet been scientifically determined; thus, alternative methods of obtaining pluripotent cells have been developed in order to avoid the use of human embryos. One such method is the engineering of induced pluripotent stem cells (iPSCs), which are reprogrammed from adult somatic cells wherein the gene expression of mature cells is altered, reversing the differentiation state back to pluripotency (Fig. **2**) [11].

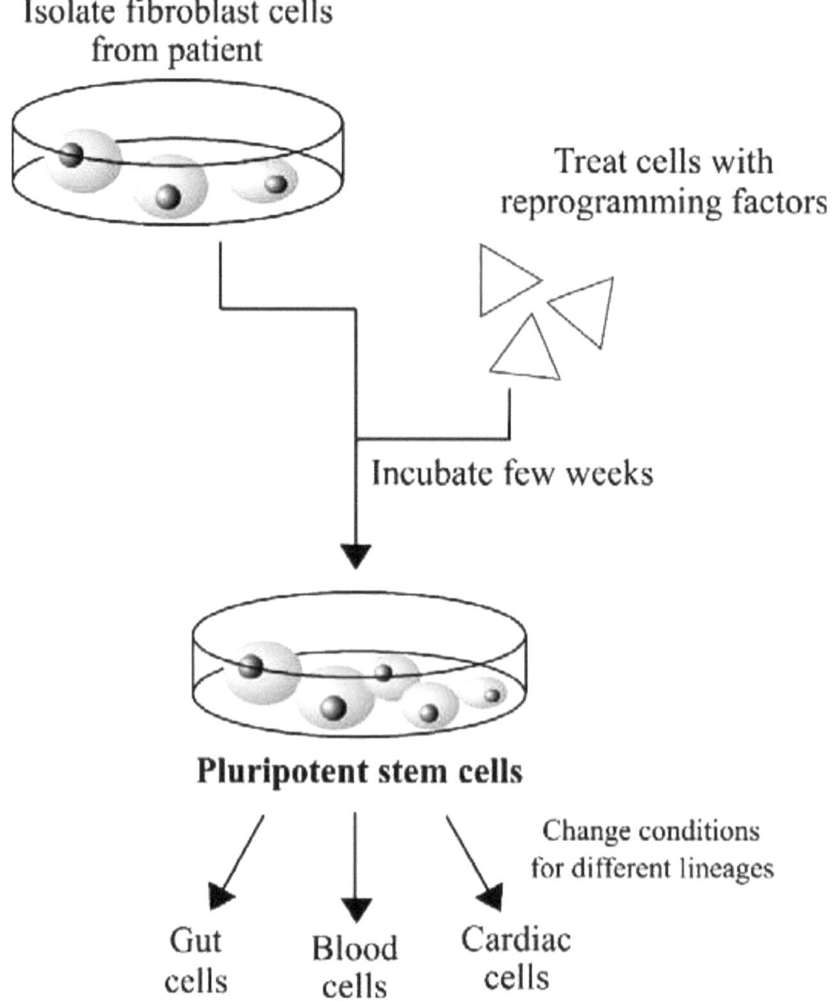

Fig. (2). Reprogramming of somatic cells to induced pluripotent stem cells *in vitro* [5].

This breakthrough reprogramming was performed in human fibroblasts by Yamanaka *et al.*, which are cells that produce the constituents of the extracellular matrix, and mediate cell-cell communication [12]. Fibroblasts are commonly used in skin repair, due to their function in maintaining the intercellular space. Genetic manipulation was conducted *via* the specific expression of four transcription factors: Oct4, Sox2, Klf4, and c-Myc, *via* retroviral transduction [13]. The latter half was shown to be upregulated in tumour cells and contributed to rapid proliferation rates, whereas the former was essential for maintaining pluripotency. Klf4 is a dual-function transcriptional factor with roles in both tumour suppression and oncogenesis, depending on its interaction with various cell cycle markers [14]. C-Myc also has dual functions, but primarily activates expression of various pro-proliferative genes, and increases the rate of translation by recruiting elongation factors and inducing RNA Pol II pause release [15]. Sox2 is characterised by a conserved DNA-binding high-mobility group box domain and binds cooperatively with Oct4; their target sites are adjacent to one another. This interaction is crucial to activate the transcription of downstream pluripotency factors [4]. Their respective genes OCT4, SOX2, and an additional gene NANOG were previously shown to participate in autoregulation as well as regulatory feedforward loops, with one regulator controlling another, and both binding a shared set of genes. This two-regulator system enables flexible changes in the activity; if both were positive, the output activity would be independent of fluctuations in input. If one was positive and the other negative, the overall loop would perform switch functions, one cancelling the effects of the other with a slight delay between nodes. This architecture is responsible for establishing pluripotency whilst also providing sensitive responses to differentiation signals; the downstream genes that are controlled by this core set are involved in numerous pathways, such as chromatin remodelling and growth factor signalling [16].

The interaction of these four essential transcription factors leads to changes in downstream targeting; c-Myc is known to associate with histone deacetylation complexes (HAT) and thus induces global acetylation to facilitate the binding of Oct4 and Sox2 to their respective targets [12]. The balance of expression between c-Myc and Klf4 is significant in that Klf4 has both positive and negative effects on the transcription of ES-cell specific genes *via* repression of the cell cycle protein p53, whereas c-Myc inhibits this antiproliferative signal [17].

iPSCs were a new development in stem cell research for accurately modelling ESC behaviours; both cell types share the same gene expression, surface markers, and chromatin methylation patterns, as well as similar observed culture kinetics and teratoma formation [18]. This has since driven hundreds of disease modelling studies and therapy strategies, as iPS cell lines can be derived from the somatic cells of any patient, thus avoiding the risk of immunogenic response. Notably, cell lines have been generated from patients with complex and rare genetic disorders, thus accelerating the path to achieving genetic therapy.

However, although theoretically it may be sufficient to assume that a specific disease state can be modelled to an equal accuracy in both ESCs and iPSCs, there are still uncontrolled differences between these cell types. In transcriptome studies, iPSCs have been shown to retain DNA methylation patterns shared with their parental somatic cells, evidence of incomplete reprogramming [19]. These epigenetic divergences may result in unpredictable phenotypic changes; the reprogramming process also involves deleterious effects on the genome itself, leading to chromosomal instability [20].

1.2.2. Adult Stem Cells

Adult stem cells (ASCs) are comparatively rare, with limited self-renewal capabilities. They are quiescent cells that exist in a reversible G0 state, and are characterised by the ability to re-enter the cell cycle upon specific stimuli. ASCs are responsible for repairing tissues by replacing senescent cells, and most have the ability to differentiate into all the cell types from their organ of origin, a phenomenon known as multipotency. Thus, they provide the therapeutic potential for tissue, organoid or whole-organ regeneration [21]. The major classifications of adult stem cells are the following: mesenchymal, which are pluripotent and present in many tissues; neural, which form nerve cells and supporting glial cells; haematopoietic, which form all blood cell types; and skin, primarily responsible for replacing the keratinocytes that form the protective epidermal layer (Fig. 3) [22]. The haematopoetic stem cells (HSCs) are the most thoroughly characterised, and have potential for regenerative medicine and transplantation, the advances in which will be later discussed (Fig. 4) [23].

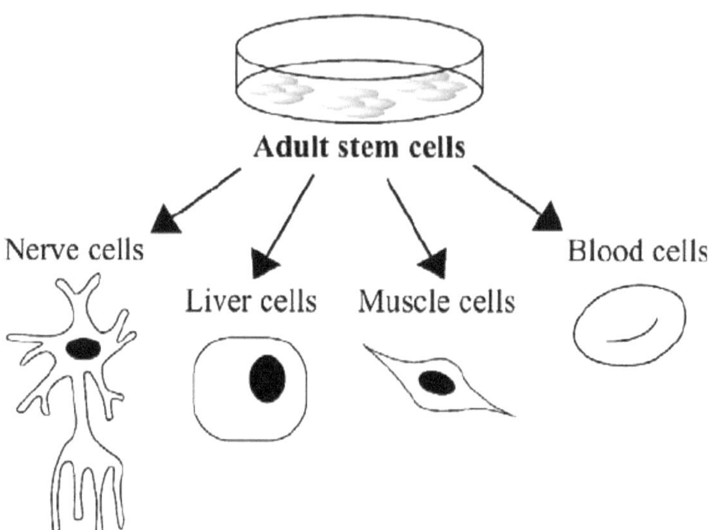

Fig. (3). Classifications of adult stem cells in various somatic tissues [24].

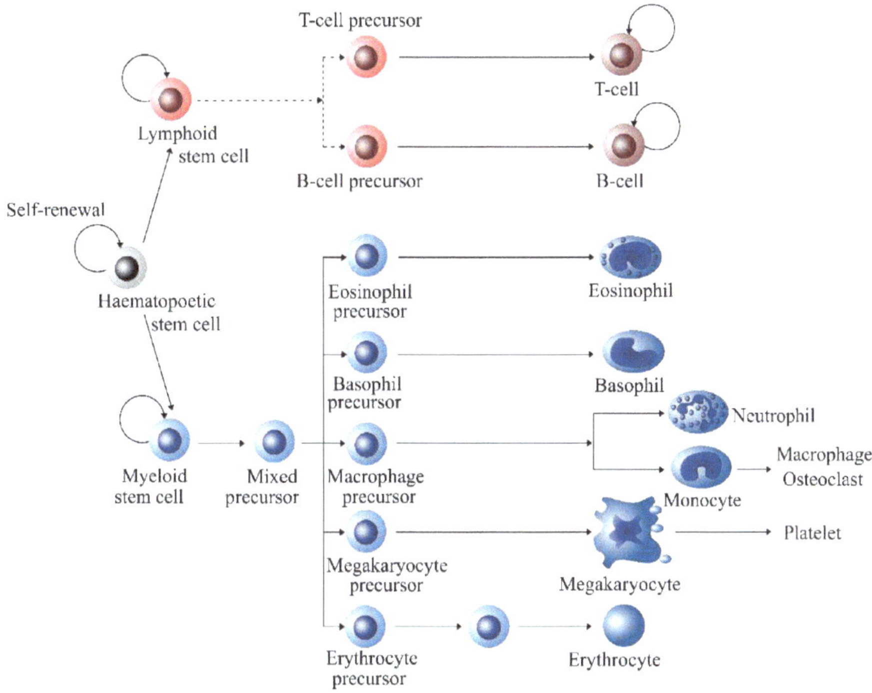

Fig. (4). Hierarchical differentiation pathways for the hematopoietic stem cell family [9].

1.2.3. Limitations in Stem Cell Therapy

Recent applications of stem cells in medicine have focused on the improper differentiation steps that lead to serious medical conditions or birth defects. Existing therapies include hematopoietic stem cell transplantation, which utilises the most characterised cell type. Target cells are derived from the bone marrow or peripheral blood; the multipotency of the stem cell type ensures that all functional haematopoetic lineages can be generated to create anemia or leukemia. However, key limitations are that there are a limited number of transplantable cells, and given that these cells are ASCs, finding an antigen-matched donor is often challenging. The transplantation process is also high-risk, and thus the use of iPSCs has become increasingly popular in this regard. Stem cell therapy has also been shown to be effective in delaying the progression of neurodegenerative disorders such as Parkinson's or Alzheimer's disease by tackling the problem at its source; neural stem cells in particular have improved cognitive function in rodent models of Alzheimer's [25]. Notably, as the neuronal degeneration in

Parkinson's disease is initially localised and specialized to the dopaminergic neurons, fully-functioning cells can be easily generated from iPSCs [26].

Due to their prevalence throughout the human body, ASCs have been proposed as promising clinical targets for the replacement of damaged tissues, especially in genetic disorders. The main advantage of ESCs over ASCs is their increased potency and subsequent clinical versatility, despite the continuing ethical concerns over ESC use and numerous studies suggesting their potential tumourigenicity. Indeed, the directed differentiation of stem cells is essential to avoid teratoma formation; thus, an in-depth understanding of the underlying signalling pathways and control over the extracellular environment are necessary. Different growth factors drive the establishment of germ layers, such as bone morphogenic proteins (BMP) or the WNT superfamily of transforming growth factors (β-TGF-β) [27]. However, due to the nature of stem cell specialisation, the exact concentrations and durations of influence these factors may have on a cell are unknown; lower concentrations of the TGF-β family proteins have been shown to trigger mesodermal differentiation, but this is still poorly understood. This has led to a major limitation in the progression of clinically-relevant ASC tools, as attempts to define the universal set of genes underlying all adult stem cells have not been successful, unlike in ESCs. The steps in differentiation for hematopoietic stem cells, for instance, are well defined and demonstrate a hierarchical organisation of growth factors and cell surface markers, but these are not seen in the regeneration of other tissues. Thus, methods for labelling and tracking are at the forefront of stem cell research, in order to gain a better understanding of the biochemical changes [5].

iPSCs have advanced further than ESCs in clinical applications due to the avoidance of ethical issues, but they have also shown genetic instability in some studies. New advances in regenerative medicine have shifted focus from iPSCs to a new protocol of generating pluripotent cells, namely, human somatic cell nuclear transfer (SCNT)-ESCs. SCNT involves the transfer of the nucleus of a somatic cell into the cytoplasm of an enucleated egg (Fig. **5**). Spindle removal and cytoplast activation are essential for patient-specific cellular reprogramming [28]. Transcriptional analysis demonstrates that SCNTs have upregulated pluripotent genes, with a greater divergence from parental somatic gene expression than that of iPSCs.

Therefore, these cells have a primary advantage in that they convey increased similarity to ESCs in terms of gene expressions and genetic alteration patterns; the differences between iPSCs and SCNT-ESCs have come under contention. Thus, a clearer definition of pluripotency would be crucial in allowing scientists to identify which cell type is more suitable for modelling specific disease states [29].

A further limitation in stem cell therapy is the ability to identify the correct dosage, especially in cardiac repair. Optimal administration is ideally determined by accurate and continuous cell imaging. Methods such as MRI scanning or optical fluorescence labelling are limited by false positives and photobleaching rates respectively; thus, techniques with higher resolution and precision must be developed in order to predict *in vivo* stem cell behaviour and visualise on a smaller scale [30, 31].

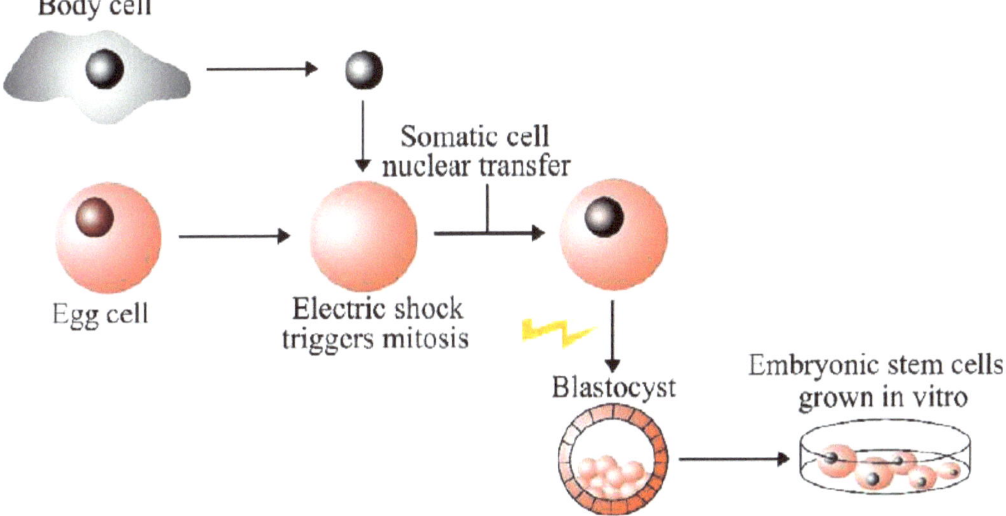

Fig. (5). Somatic Cell Nuclear Transfer reprogramming to derive human ESCs (hESCs) [28].

2. NANOTHERAPEUTIC AGENTS

Nanomedicine is a developing field with the aim to improve public health *via* the application of tools that have dimensions on a nanoscale. In nanotherapeutics, technologies are applied to the treatment of diseases, wherein nanoscale molecules are delivered to target sites with high specificity, thus reducing systemic toxicity and off-target side effects. Nanomedicine encompasses a wide variety of applications, including diagnostics, medical devices, biosensor development, and imaging [32]. Advances in genetics, proteomics, mathematical modelling, and engineering have all contributed to its development, utilising cellular biology concepts and manipulating its underlying systems on a nanoscale level. Many biologically significant molecules such as glucose, proteins, antibodies and receptors are sized within the nanoscale range, thus prompting the design of devices that can interact with or measure the concentrations of these molecules when linked to various disease pathologies.

2.1. Physical and Chemical Properties of Nanoparticles

Nanoparticles (NPs) are structures with at least one dimension being between 1 and 100 nm; this includes diameters of spherical particles and fibrous structures that are less than 100 nm in two dimensions. The properties of NPs are distinct from those of the same substance in bulk form, which provides several advantages over existing tools when applied to a medical context. First, nanoparticles have a larger area to volume ratio; thus, the volume of the surface layer becomes a more significant fraction of the total NP volume, where the surface layer constitutes all matter within a few atomic diameters of the particle's surface (Fig. **6**) [33].

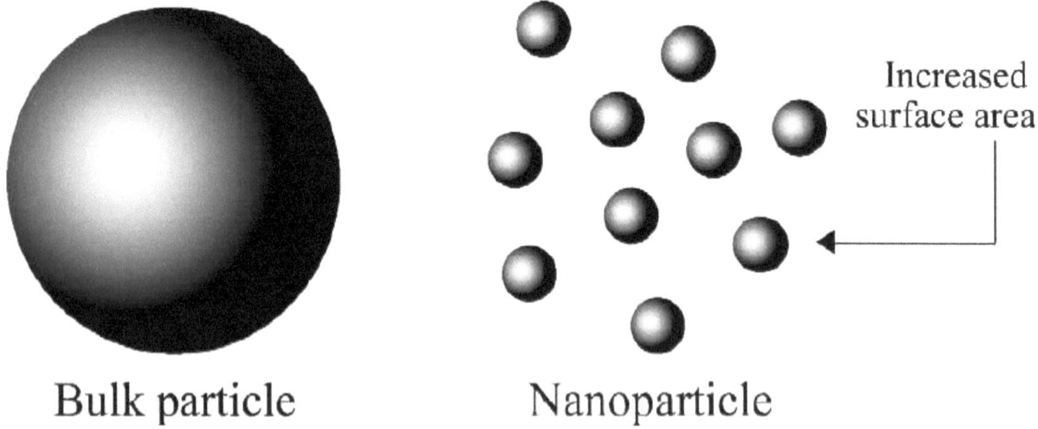

Fig. (6). The increased surface area to volume ratio effect in nanoparticles as compared to bulk [33].

This greater surface area results in an increased reactivity of approximately 1000-fold, with high rates of ion diffusion at lower temperatures and rapid equilibration of the whole material due to its small particle diameter. The change in surface layer for nanoparticles may also result in a lower melting point as a function of decreasing particle radius, due to the comparatively lower number of neighbouring molecules and subsequent lower binding energy as opposed to that of the bulk substance. This relationship is quantified by the Gibbs-Thomson formula (Fig. **7**) [34].

Thus, it is crucial to consider the surrounding environment of a nanoparticle; both the molecules present in the interfacial layer when dispersed through a distinct medium, and the possible engineered coatings of the nanoparticle itself, all of which can change the catalytic behaviour, chemical stability, and physical properties of the nanoparticle [36]. Quantum mechanics also plays a major role in observed nanoparticle properties; the physics of electrons in particles are primarily hidden in macroscopic matter but dominate at a sufficiently low threshold particle size, wherein particle properties such as chemical reactivity, fluorescence, and electrical conductivity may change as a function of particle size [37]. Quantum confinement refers to this change in electronic and optical properties as a result of the electrons being squeezed into a dimension that approaches a critical value known as the exciton Bohr radius. This leads to a quantised energy spectrum and observed magnetic moments from the unpaired electron spins of nanoparticles, an effect that is manipulated in medical applications such as tumour therapy, where different sizes of gold nanoparticles react differently with light and thus can enable specific imaging and photothermal destruction of cancerous cells whilst selectively avoiding healthy tissues [38].

NP shape and solidity can be engineered to suit loading capacity, transport, and interaction criteria (Fig. **8**). Hollow NPs in particular, such as liposomes or micelles, are highly effective drug carriers and can be easily surface conjugated to oligonucleotide or peptide structures that confer imaging contrast or tracking [40].

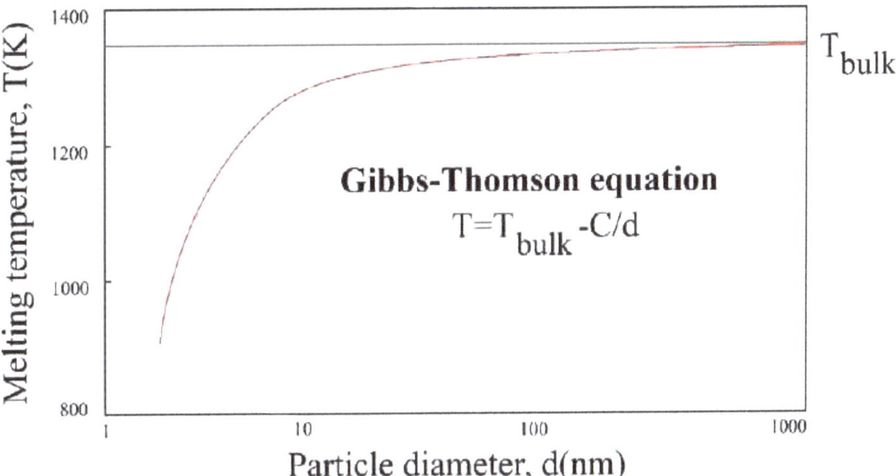

Fig. (7). Melting temperature (K) as a function of nanoparticle diameter (nm). Solid line (red) shows the generalized Gibbs-Thomson relation with asymptote at bulk melting temperature (T_{bulk}) [39].

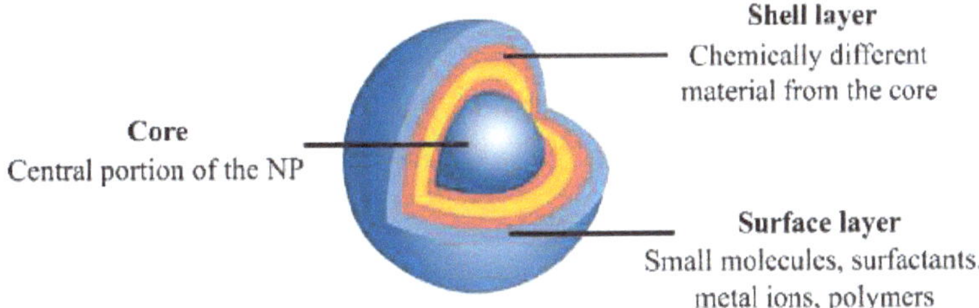

Fig. (8). Diagram representing the basic structure of a nanoparticle and the ways in which they can be modified [35].

Nanotechnology developed for medical application can be structurally classified into lipid-based and polymer-based materials, and have a wide variety of applications dependent on their artificially-determined chemical and physical behaviour *in vivo*. Lipid-based materials include nanoemulsions, solid lipid nanoparticles and nanostructured lipid carriers. For the purposes of this chapter, only polymer-based nanoparticles will be discussed, as they are more clinically relevant in stem cell research [41]. These tools must fulfil a set of criteria that allows for precise control over its interactions with biological constructs; thus, bioconjugation of both synthetic and biological systems is becoming increasingly prevalent in nanotechnology design (Fig. **9**). The composite systems must have a hierarchically organised structure to mimic that of the human body, which can only be determined by controlled design at the nano- and molecular level. Thus, understanding a system at various scales is crucial to predicting the therapeutic potential of these tools [42].

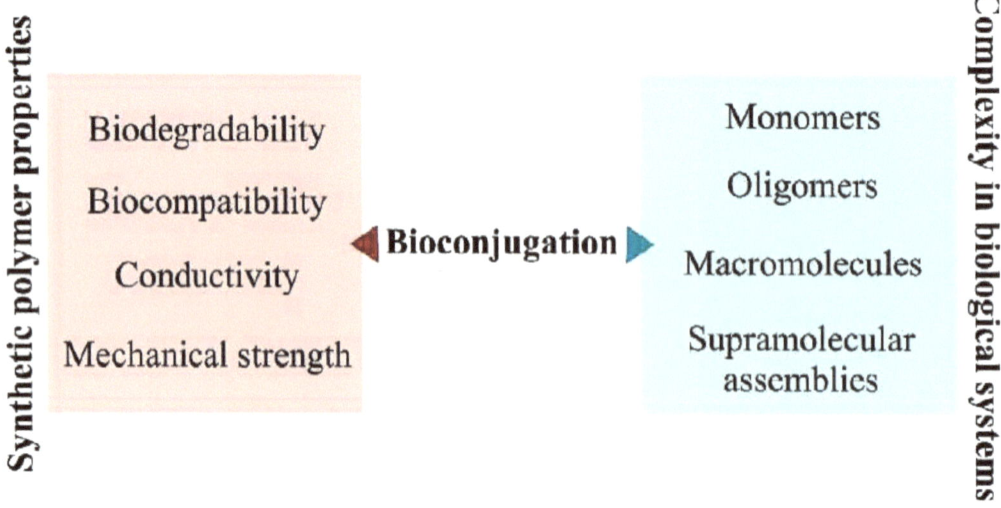

Fig. (9). Interdisciplinary combination of synthetic and biological structures at various resolutions in bioconjugation [42].

2.2. Different Types of Polymer-based Nanotechnology

2.2.1. Polymeric Nanoparticles

Polymeric nanoparticles are typically derived from synthetic polymers, as scientists can engineer specific patterns that facilitate controlled drug release behaviour at the target site. Example polymers include polylactide (PLA), which are biodegradable and aliphatic, allowing for incorporation of drugs in hydrophobic cavities as well as facilitating the passage of the NP through membranes and preventing toxicity due to the continued sequestration of the drug in the body. These improve the solubility of hydrophobic drugs by interacting at the drug surface and protecting unstable moieties from degradation [41]. The extent to which these nanopolymers are metabolised in the body can be modulated by altering their chemical composition, leading to changes in biodegradability, a property that is useful in drug delivery to avoid the need for surgical removal. The copolymer poly(lactic-co-glycolic acid) or PLGA is commonly used in drug delivery, vascular tissue grafts, and prosthetics; scientists are able to change its properties and the rate of its hydrolytic degradation in physiological conditions. The time required for degradation is negatively correlated to the content of glycolide units in its structure, a condition that can be modulated according to the relative concentrations of its constituent monomers, the cyclic dimers of glycolic and lactic acid [43].

Nanoparticles encompass both nanocapsules and nanospheres. Nanocapsules contain a liquid or solid cavity surrounded by a synthetic or natural polymer membrane, with drugs loaded into the interior to prevent the release of active moieties. Nanospheres, however, have matrix structures throughout which the drugs are dispersed uniformly either *via* adsorption to its surface or entrapment within the matrix (Fig. **10**) [44].

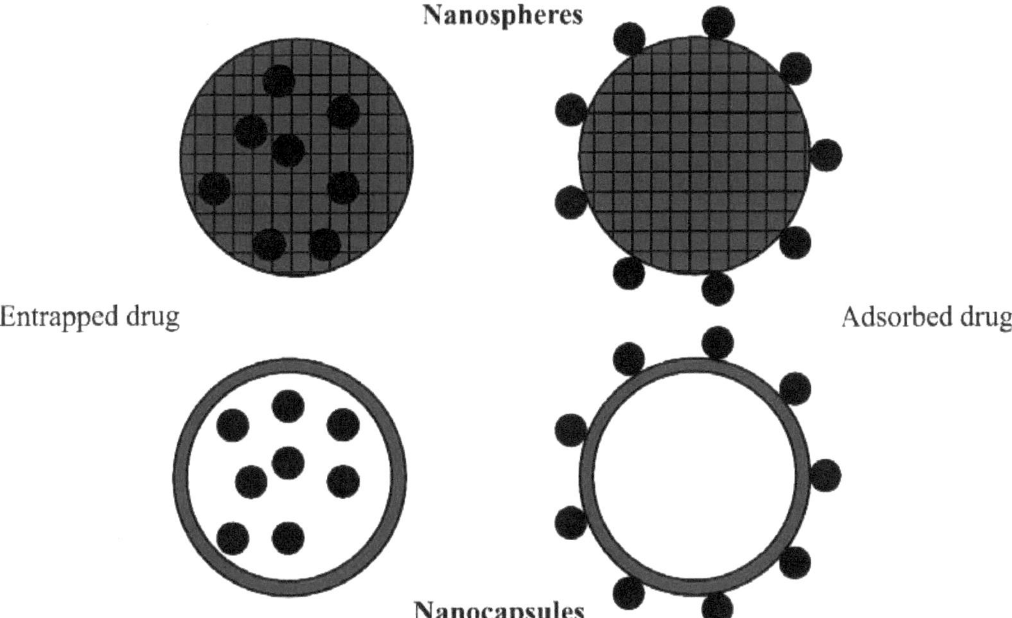

Fig. (10). Diagram showing differences in structure between nanospheres and nanocapsules [45].

2.2.2. Nanogels

Nanogels have been extensively studied as a vehicle for drug delivery, and have been demonstrated in several studies as effective due to their stability and biodegradability, which modulate circulation in the blood as well as the removal of the empty device after drug release. There are many advantageous properties, specifically their high moisture content due to the involvement of flexible hydrophilic polymers. The drug can easily be incorporated by causing the nanogel to swell in water and then adding the drug, which causes gel collapse; the decrease in solvent volume ensures tight interaction between the multivalent nanogel cavities and the drug, thus preventing premature payload release [41]. Nanogels contain crosslinked layers to ensure structural integrity and are able to carry macromolecules such as proteins and DNA without compromising the overall gel behavior (Fig. **11**). Further, the surfaces of nanogels can be bioconjugated with specific ligands that can recognize disease-specific receptors. New frontiers have been explored in generating nanohybrids, where nanogels incorporate inorganic nanomaterials for *in vivo* imaging.

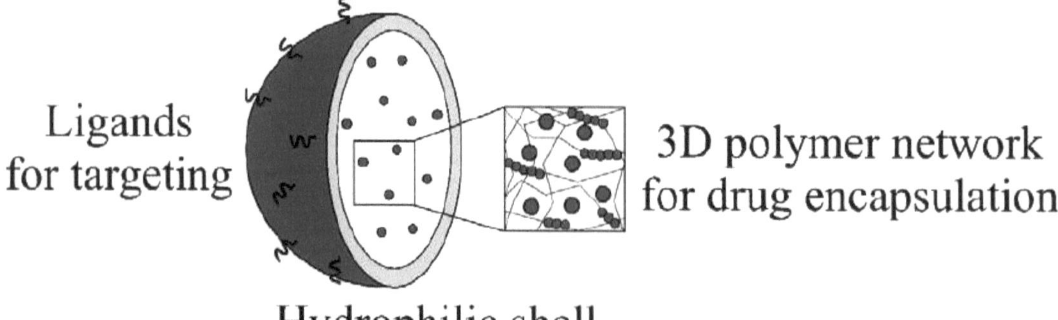

Fig. (11). Structure of a biofunctionalised nanogel with modifications for specific clinical applications [46].

A major clinical advantage over polymeric nanoparticles is that nanogels are stimuli-responsive, wherein a swelling conformational change occurs as a result of the external environment; this can be within the body such as changes in pH or temperature, or artificially applied such as magnetic field intensity [41]. This structural modification may involve the ionization of acidic and basic functional groups directly on the polymer chains, which subsequently alter the overall hydrophobicity of the nanogel and therefore change the extent to which it interacts with the surrounding water molecules. The sensitivity of this response can be altered simply by changing the number of ionisable functional groups, which may result in an increase of osmotic pressure [47]. Thus, swelling is dependent on a number of modifiable parameters that determine the physical dimensions of the nanogel, such as the chemical nature of crosslinkers, degree of crosslinking, and resulting elasticity of the polymer network [48]. In contrast, macroscale gels of similar chemical and physical composition have been shown to have limited swelling rates in response to changes in environmental conditions, making them unpredictable for applications *in vivo* [49].

In order to retain drug carriers in circulation, structures must be designed to have long half-lives, avoiding removal from the body for a sufficient amount of time such that the proportion of active drug delivered to the target site is nternali. Nanogels achieve this in a number of ways: preventing rapid clearance *via* immune cells and preventing metabolism-based breakdown of its actual structure [50]. Nanocarriers are prone to nternalizat *via* macrophages in the liver and spleen, wherein the drug vehicles are marked for phagocytosis and efficiently removed from circulation. Efforts to avoid this have been made, which primarily involve increasing its overall hydrophilicity and preventing recognition *via* steric hindrance. However, one feature unique to nanogels that enables the avoidance of an immune response is its deformability. Particles were shown to pass through pores that were roughly 10-fold smaller in diameter than that of the original particle. Changes in the polymeric composition enabled high compressibility, which resulted from rapid deswelling and reswelling as it emerged from the other side of the membrane [51]. The probability of successful pore traversing was also indicated to be a function of polymer chain connectivity; a less linear polymer provided more conformational freedom and thus increased probability of passage [52]. Studies into the elasticity of nanogels demonstrated that the Young modulus of the nanoparticle is correlated with the mechanism of nternalization *via* macrophages. Nanogels with intermediate flexibility were taken up by multiple entry mechanisms including clathrin- and caveolae-mediated endocytosis, which subsequently led to higher internal concentrations and higher clearance rate than that of nanogels with extremes in elasticity [53]. This study indicated a link between the uptake kinetics of nanoparticles and their physical structure, thus proving that control of its mechanical properties provided a new avenue for designing carriers with more successful *in vivo* delivery.

2.2.3. Dendrimers

Dendrimers have been implicated in nanoparticle-mediated drug delivery due to their globular, highly-branched architecture and high-water solubility. The number of cavities in the interior as well as the multiple functional groups at the periphery allow for versatile chemical activity towards drug targeting and conjugation (Fig. **12**). Both nanogels and dendrimers are self-assembled polymeric nanotechnologies; the most investigated dendrimer family towards drug delivery is the polyamidoamine (PAMAM) dendrimer, the initial substrate of which is the amine functional core, which is then reacted with methyl acrylate units in a series of Michael addition reactions. The overall structure generated is branched, with an ester terminal group that may be further amidated to form full-generation amine-terminated chains [41]. These amine groups can then bind various target molecules; it is crucial that the number of exposed amino groups is kept to a minimum, as primary amines are quite cytotoxic, and so are not biocompatible [54]. As the generation of dendrimers is repetitive and stepwise, the size and structure can be highly modified, making it a promising avenue for specific drug delivery behaviours *in vivo*. Recent studies have focused on engineering novel dendrimers with the ability to release drugs under specific conditions. Drug molecules may be covalently attached to the biocompatible surface chain ends, as demonstrated with methotrexate chemotherapeutic agents; this is of particular advantage due to the large number of terminal groups and thus high-density drug capacity per dendrimer [55].

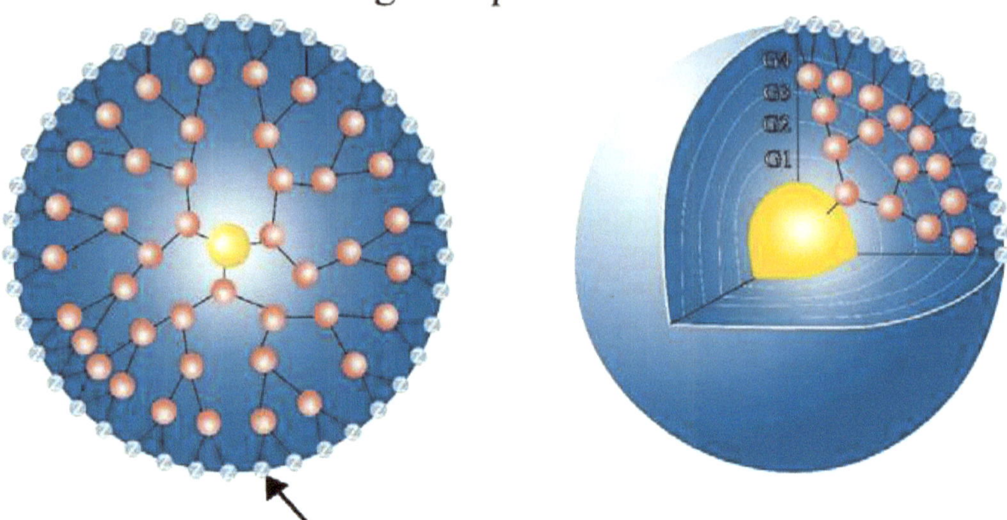

Fig. (12). Schematic of overall dendrimer structure with modifiable groups labelled [56].

Another method of drug delivery is to encapsulate the drug within the interior cavities of the dendrimer itself, which are often lined with hydrophobic tertiary amines. Thus, similar to micellar structures, dendrimers are able to solubilise hydrophobic compounds in aqueous solutions, by conjugating surface hydrophilic chain ends. Previous studies tackled the biocompatibility problem by covalently attaching Poly(ethylene glycol) or PEG polymers to PAMAM dendrimers, thus avoiding the risk of rapid clearance. PEG has been shown to improve the immunogenicity of proteins as well as other nanoscale structures such as liposomes [57]. The rate of drug release from PEG-attached PAMAM dendrimers was found to be a function of both the molecular weight of conjugated PEG and the hydrophobicity of the dendrimer itself, where PEG-attached dendrimers showed higher retention of hydrophobic drugs; this is also dependent on the chemical nature of the drug and its affinity of interaction with the interior capsule.

2.2.4. Metallic Nanoparticles

Inorganic nanoparticles have been used in the development of nanodevices in the pharmaceutical industry. Iron oxide particles are most commonly applied for this purpose. Supramagnetic iron oxide NPs have been utilised in increasing MRI contrast, cell separation, and tissue repair, which will be further discussed later [58]. Gold nanoparticles and nanorods have been used in cell imaging; absorption and scattering efficiencies of wavelengths of light are calculated using the discrete dipole approximation method.

Many metallic NPs have potential in cancer diagnosis due to the surface plasmon resonance-enhanced light absorption, which is converted into localised heat for specific laser-based photothermal destruction of tumours. Silver NPs are also being used in wound dressings due to their antimicrobial activity [59]. These NPs can be functionalised with groups to overcome specific microbial species.

2.3. Applications of Nanotherapeutic Agents in Stem Cell Research

Polymeric nanoparticles and dendrimers have been commonly used for targeted delivery and release of peptides that have significant biological activity in various metabolic, neurological, and cardiovascular disorders. Inorganic nanoparticles have supplemented existing stem cell imaging methods, providing a novel system in which therapeutics can be tracked precisely over longer periods of time. Developments in understanding both stem cell biology and nanotechnology have led to innovations in the medical field, the most notable of which will now be discussed.

2.3.1. Improving Tissue Engineering Scaffolds

Tissue engineering involves the use of cells and relevant factors to replace biological tissues that have been damaged due to disease or congenital abnormalities, and is an emerging field at the intersection between engineering, cellular biology, and biomaterials. Common targets include bone, blood vessels, and muscle tissues, all of which have characteristic mechanical properties that are conducive to healthy function. Thus, the aim of tissue engineering is to create an artificial structural framework that will mimic the properties of the tissue enough to provide a temporary compensation in function, whilst also creating a microenvironment in which newly generated cells can eventually replace the entire tissue (Fig. **13**). In order to achieve this, specific criteria must be met: (a) cells with the correct function, (b) a scaffold to provide the correct growth environment, (c) the presence of growth factors and other stimulants that induce rapid replication, and (d) the application of mechanical forces to influence growth on a macro scale [60].

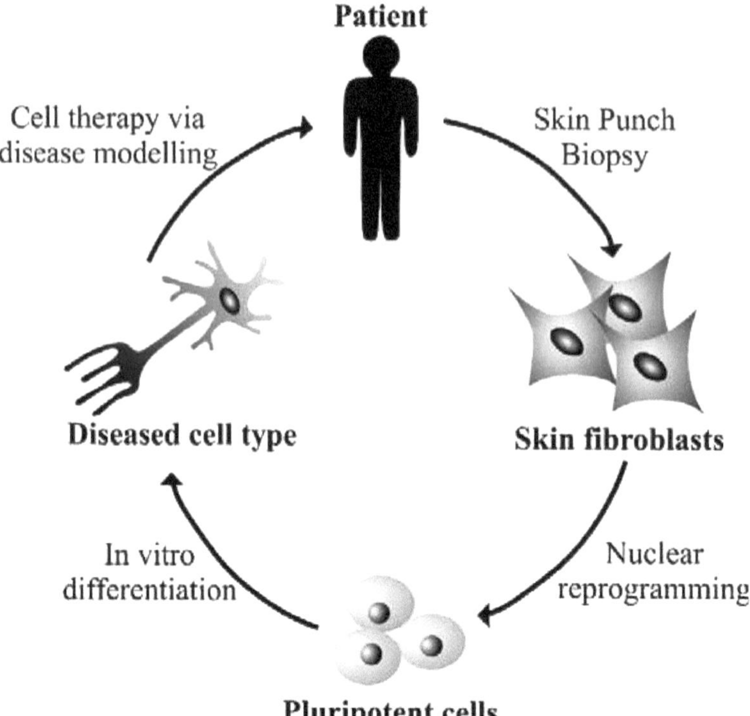

Fig. (13). Fundamental steps and applications of tissue engineering with reprogrammed pluripotent stem cells [61].

Many different cell types may be used; the tissue engineering methods which use stem or progenitor cells are classified under regenerative medicine. Progenitor cells can be viewed as a middle-ground between stem cells and fully differentiated cells in that they are oligopotent, although they cannot divide indefinitely, and include blast cells during the formation of B and T lymphocytes, satellite cells essential for muscle injury recovery, and radial glial cells found in developing regions of the brain [62, 63]. The distinction between progenitor and stem cells has been a topic of controversy for many years. Cells are generally extracted from the patient to avoid immunogenicity, although some exceptions have been made in skin tissue engineering. Scaffolds are derived from donor tissue or synthetic polymers with attachment sites for biomolecules and hormones. They function to drive the *in vitro* differentiation of stem cells into the desired lineage, and their major role is to ensure complete tissue functionality by establishing tissue volume and specific microenvironments that maintain correct cell behaviours. To achieve this, scaffolds must be able to mimic in vivo conditions as closely as possible, and scientists have developed various protocols in which the extracellular matrix (ECM) is artificially reproduced.

The ECM consists of a hierarchically organised network of fibres and macromolecules that provide structural support to cells and mediate cell-cell interactions; the exact composition of the ECM differs between tissue types, but all have shared function in cell adhesion and differentiation [64]. Modelling the extracellular environment is key to understanding the development of stem cells, in order to apply them towards tissue engineering. Scaffolds should have specific physicochemical characteristics: they must be three-dimensional and highly porous to allow for transport of nutrients and metabolic waste during cell growth, and must be biocompatible with controlled degradation and resorption rates, as well as sufficient surface chemistry to allow for cell attachment, proliferation, and differentiation.

A number of synthetic biodegradable polymers such as polylactic acid (PLA) have been used to form the overall network. Their controlled hydrolysis ensures that the scaffold is removed during a sequential transition wherein the regenerated tissue increases in function as the scaffold degrades. Similar polymers such as polycaprolactone (PCL) are more hydrophobic despite having similar structural integrity and ability to be fabricated into specific shapes, rendering them less effective [65]. In contrast, hydrogels such as PEG are highly suitable for in vivo use but are susceptible to deformation underpressurised conditions due to their absorbent polymer chain cross-linked three-dimensional structure [66]. Composite materials have been developed wherein both hydrophobic polymers and hydrogels are integrated to form fibrous matrices (Fig. **14**) [67]. Stable structures have been generated from the localised polymerisation of hydrogels on the surface of electrospun fibres, which are polymer solutions of nanoscale diameter generated from applying a high voltage to a liquid droplet. This generates electrostatic repulsion, which counteracts the surface tension of the droplet, thus stretching the liquid and drying it until the charge migrates from the droplet surface to the fibre (Fig. **15**) [68]. Having a hydrogel layer would provide novel water-absorbing properties, thus mimicking the role of hyaluronic acid and other glycosaminoglycans (GAGs) in the ECM, resisting tissue compression by counteracting with turgor.

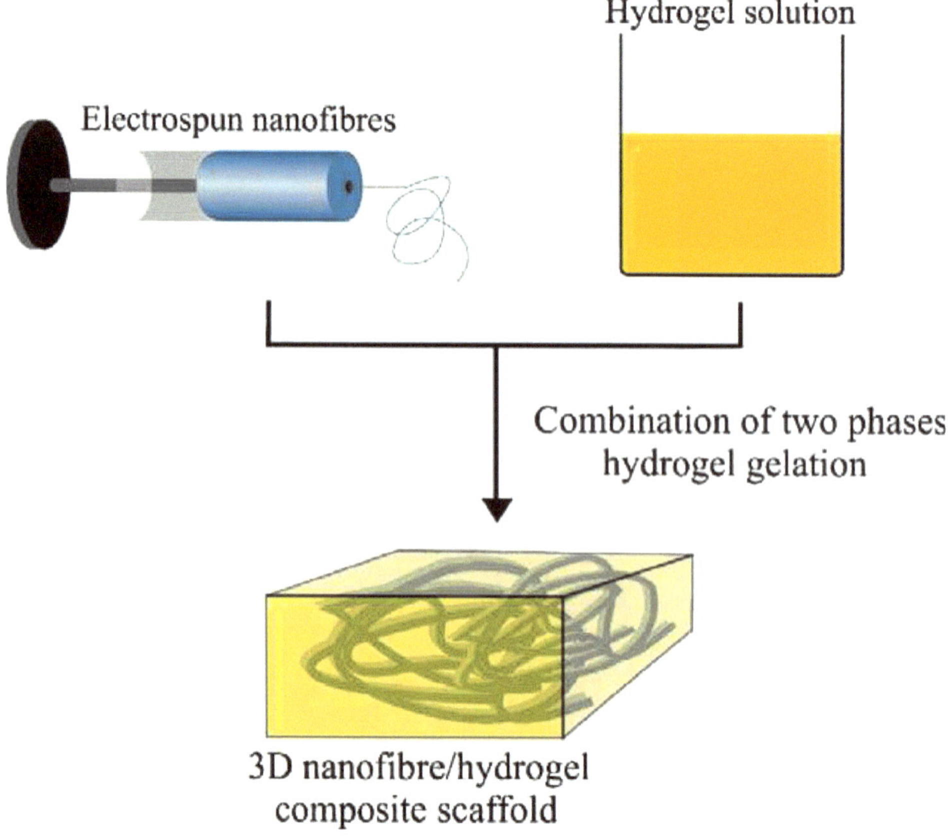

Fig. (14). Creation of nanohybrid electrospun fibres and hydrogel mixture [67]. This hybrid structure was synthesised by immobilising a trithiocarbonate-based chain transfer agent (CTA) onto the surface of electrospun PCL fibres, which subsequently facilitate the attachment of PEG layers through reversible polymerisation reactions [68].

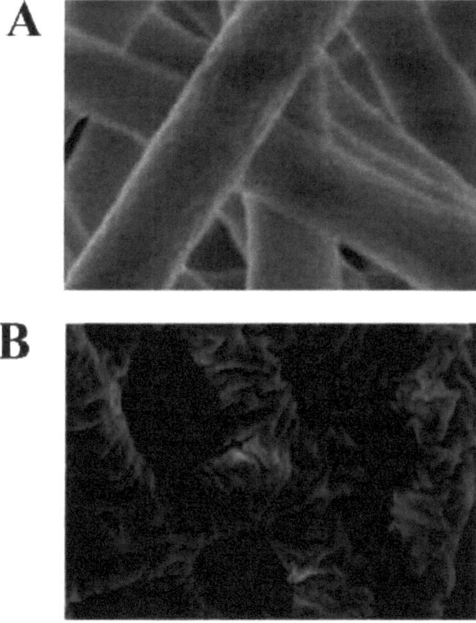

Fig. (15). Electron microscopy imaging of microfibers before and after polymerisation. Panel **A**: PCL microfiber without surface polymerisation indicates low surface area, leading to hydrophobicity. Panel **B**: Polymerisation with PEG layers generates hydrogel-microfibre hybrid with increased capacity for water absorption [68].

This confers a number of advantages: the hydrogel coatings have a nanoscale width, preserving the pores in the PCL fibres to allow transport of seeded cells and blood vessels throughout the scaffold. This also ensured that the layers could expand without causing changes in total macro volume or affecting any bulk mechanical properties. Thus, the flexibility of the hydrogels was maintained whilst also ensuring the overall support framework was kept intact. Previous studies had involved the crosslinking of hydrogels within nanofibers, but this study improved upon the stability of this interaction by direct covalent linkages at the surface instead of within the framework.

Natural polymers such as collagen and chitosan have also been used to replicate the fibrous phase of the ECM, but their use is limited in comparison to synthetic polymers, which are reacted in a reproducible manner to generate the same polymeric composition in bulk and retain precise control over physical, chemical, and mechanical properties. Adhesion proteins such as laminins and fibronectins have been replaced by specific RGD peptide motifs and IKVAV laminin sequences which can be conjugated to the matrix backbone; the highly-charged nature of the side chain residues renders highly-sensitive control of cell adhesion in the surrounding environment [69]. Other chemical modifications that functionalise the backbone include sulfation with perlecan to control growth factor concentration gradients; percelan is a heparin sulfate proteoglycan found in basement membranes, and contain five domains that are essential for cell proliferation and ECM formation [70]. The heparin sulfate chains act as stabilised stores of growth factors, preventing them from proteolytic degradation [71]. Thus, tissues are highly sensitive to local and systemic changes, with the ability to spatially sequester growth factors and generate gradients of proteins needed to change cell fate.

Although some tissue engineering methods are widely applied, such as the regeneration of artificial skin to treat surface burns, the field currently faces limited implementation in human patients due to the inconsistent maintenance of scaffolds over time. Specifically, the original purpose of a scaffold merely guiding the differentiation process has been proven insufficient for effective tissue engineering. Whether or not the target niche is closely replicated in a scaffold has always been an uncertainty; the surrounding environment changes during the process of stem cell specialisation, expressing different ECM components over time [60]. Current collagen-based scaffolds cannot change in the same way to accommodate for the cell niche as the tissue develops; therefore, alternative methods have been proposed. A promising example is the use of multiple nanotopographies; like scaffolds, these structures also drive specific differentiation lineages, but they can be more easily combined to generate implanted devices that are multifunctional, with each function demarcated into different zones [72].

2.3.2. Nanotopographies in Directing Stem Cell Differentiation

The natural extracellular environment differs from that of *in vitro* surfaces in the various topographies that cells may be subjected to; that is, the arrangement of the physical features of the surrounding area. Macroscale topographies include surface topologies of bones or ligaments; microscale topographies include the morphology and projections of surrounding cells; nanoscale topographies include protein conformations, ligand presentation, and collagen banding [73]. Thus, topography is crucial when considering the three-dimensional environment of a stem cell, as it can be represented on multiple different levels and provides biomechanical cues for cell development. One of the most promising innovations in the field of tissue engineering is the nanotopographic patterning of implanted surfaces to generate nanodot arrays, which are fabricated using precision techniques such as electron beam lithography, polymer phase separation, and colloidal lithography. In the body, cells are dependent on information detected from their surroundings to determine their relative orientation, a phenomenon that drives many biological processes such as wound healing [74]. Therefore, adhesion is a major parameter that affects cell behaviour, and mediates interactions between cells and substrates in the ECM. Integrins are transmembrane proteins that form αβ heterodimers, creating focal contacts by binding to ECM proteins *via* the RGD peptide sequence in their extracellular domains. This leads to changes in cytoskeletal tension, applying force across cell-matrix interfaces, and triggers downstream intracellular signalling to regulate the formation of stress fibres that ultimately change cell shape [75]. The effect of cell shape on its function has been well documented in various studies, where reduced cell spreading within a confined space leads to apoptosis, and the reverse leads to increased proliferation [76]. This has also been seen in MSC lineages, where the commitment of fat or bone tissue is dependent on cytoskeletal tension [77]. Therefore, substrate topography induces changes to cell shape, which then affect gene expression and mediates differentiation of stem cells. Nanotopography affects the relative alignment of cells, guiding them along micron-sized grooves which causes them to elongate, whereas many cell types do not adhere to pillared structures; these behaviours can be exploited to drive specific cell-cell clustering and fabricate differentiated cells. Groove depth affects the degree of cellular alignment, with the threshold being roughly 2μm; nearly all cell types respond to grooves of width above this value (Fig. **16**) [78].

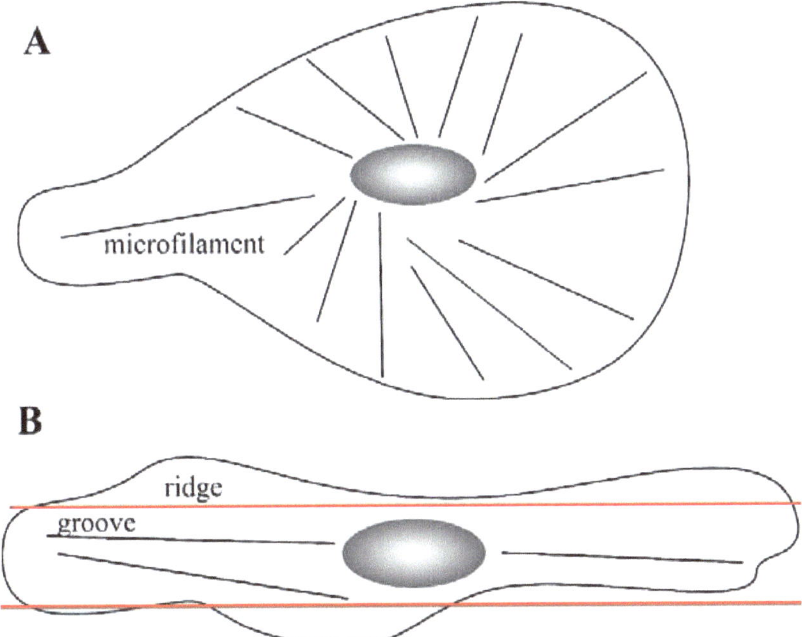

Fig. (16). Diagram of changes in the cytoskeleton in response to encountering a groove. **(A)** The cytoskeleton of a cell on a flat surface is arranged stretching from the nucleus to the periphery. **(B)** The cytoskeleton of a cell on a grooved surface is reorganised laterally along the direction of the groove [78].

Lithographic patterning has enabled precise control over topography, wherein a nanoscale surface can be patterned with both adhesive and non-adhesive areas, thus resulting in regions of different function (Fig. **17**). The extent of adhesion is determined by the number of surface-associated protein molecules (SAMs) that are immobilised onto the surface. These molecules bind with high specificity to integrins and thus can mimic ECM interactions [78]. A similar phenomenon is shown in conventional scaffolds, such as the stacking of paper saturated with cell culture, which generates three-dimensional oxygen and nutrient gradients to control cell localisation; however, the nanotopographic patterning is a far more accurate method [79]. The ability to modulate cell adhesion is highly advantageous; when observing tendon cells on a polystyrene substrate with 60 nm pillars spaced at 300 nm intervals, the number of cells in the patterned area decreased over time. The underlying cause has been hypothesised to involve a lower number of focal contacts or a change in surface energy as a result of pillared structures [73]. This lack of adhesion can be applied to many medical contexts, such as the removal of implants or tubing in vascular repair [80].

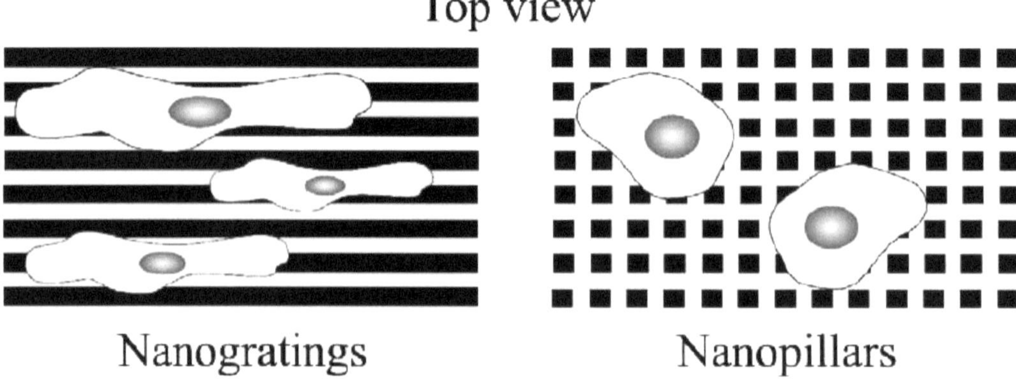

Fig. (17). Various cell behaviours on different nanotopographies. Nanopillars disrupt the development of focal adhesions, whereas continuous contact is maintained with nanogratings, causing elongated cell shape [81].

Scaffolds are distinct from nanodot arrays in that they provide porous regions for cells to travel through and are usually on the micrometre scale as opposed to the nanometre, whereas nanodot arrays drive cell differentiation primarily *via* cell adhesion, although both are modelled after specific chemical or mechanical properties of the natural ECM. However, new frontiers in scaffold formation are utilising nanometre scales for improved control of cell adhesion.

The application of nanotechnology to scaffold fabrication has been a fairly recent development, and is of particular interest due to having properties of a similar chemistry and physical scale as that of components within the existing ECM.

Towards this, molecular self-assembly methods have been generated, which involves the scaffold generating its own extracellular matrix by using the remaining components at the site of damage. Further applications include the incorporation of metallic, polymeric, or carbon-based NPs within crosslinked nanoscale hydrogels to tailor the scaffold functionality, as well as carbon and titanium dioxide nanotubes for replacement bone therapies due to their high tensile and mechanical strength. Graphene and its oxide (GO) are specifically used in tissue engineering due to their enhanced surface area and electrical properties. The overall aim is to generate biomimetic scaffolds that are closer models to the natural ECM, which will be achieved on the advent of improved photolithography and other design technologies.

Tissue engineering may also be applied in a more indirect context, as biosensors or chips to detect chemical toxicity when developing novel therapies. NPs can be used to improve or provide function where polymeric structures cannot; carbon nanotubes are commonly used to improve matrix tensile strength and conductivity. Nanospheres have also been engineered to facilitate controlled release of biomolecules and magnetic NPs that control cell morphology. Titanium and gold nanowires have been shown to improve cell adhesion and allow precise localization control within the entire scaffold [41].

3. NANOTECHNOLOGY FOR STEM CELL TRANSPLANTATION

Stem cell transplantation differs from tissue engineering in that the main focus of transplantation is to replace damaged stem cells with healthy stem cells, which can be done through a number of procedures and is usually designed to treat rare congenital disorders. Stem cell transplantation is most commonly used with MSCs in leukaemia patients, to replenish cells that have been destroyed immediately following chemotherapy. The stem cells are transfused directly into a vein, where they settle in the bone marrow and differentiate into new healthy blood cells, a process known as engraftment. Transplantation is a high-risk treatment, and challenges persist in finding appropriate donors and managing graft-vs-host disease, which is inflammation of the tissue site as a result of an immunologic reaction to tissue that is not genetically identical to that of the patient [82]. The aim of stem cell transplantation is to provide a novel cure for diseases, whereas tissue engineering may involve a number of different applications.

Nanogels have been applied to cardiac repair following myocardial infarctions by encapsulating the stem cells and delivering them into the damaged tissues; previous experiments used synthetic P(NIPAM-AA) gels which were used in mouse models of myocardial infarction-mediated damage (Fig. **18**). The nanogels were thermosensitive with multiple carboxylate groups for improved cell proliferation and engraftment after transplantation [83]. The increased retention may have been due to the scaffolding of the polymer itself acting as a steric hindrance to prevent the entry of T cells that may have triggered an immune response. Further, the porous structure of the nanogel resulted in more rapid delivery of factors secreted cardiac stem cells such as VEGF and IGF-1, which would lead to recruitment of endogenous stem cells into the site of injury [84].

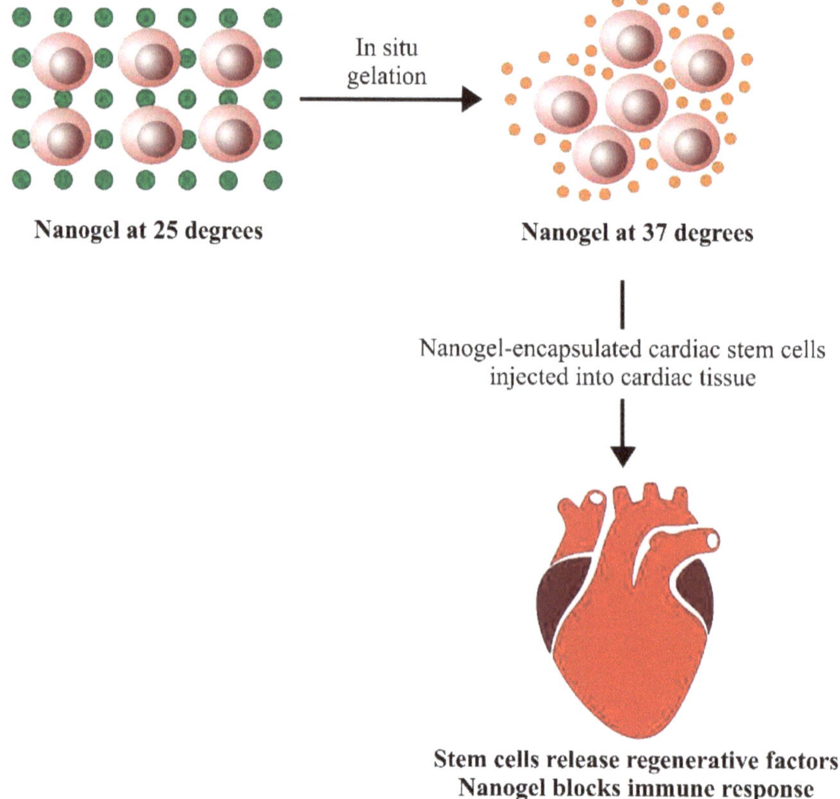

Fig. (18). Nanogel-coated CSCs for cardiac tissue repair [85].

3.1. Labelling Stem Cells for NP Drug Delivery

Targeted nanoparticle drug delivery has commonly exploited the enhanced permeation and retention effect in which nanosized molecules passively accumulate in tumour tissue to a greater degree than in normal tissues. This is most likely due to the changes in aggregate structure of solid tumours, which involves stimulating angiogenesis through growth factors; the production of blood vessels from existing ones provides a constant nutrient and oxygen supply to facilitate rapid proliferation. However, these new tumour-associated vessels are abnormally formed, lacking a smooth muscle layer with defective endothelial cells and large fenestrations between cells, which all lead to altered fluid transport dynamics. The lack of lymphatic drainage around the solid tumours leads to an accumulation of particles which would have otherwise been filtered out under healthy conditions. However, although this in theory would facilitate highly selective delivery of nanoparticle-conjugated drugs, only around 0.7% of the total dosage reaches the tumour site [86]. Thus, the EPR effect may not be a phenomenon present in all tumours. There is a clear need for delivery methods that can target tumours that are not reliant solely on the EPR effect, and exploit molecules that are actively and selectively trafficked to tumour sites.

Mesenchymal adult stem cells (MSCs) travel to tumours in response to chemokine signals secreted by neutrophils and macrophages invading the area. MSCs can be modified to express antitumour peptides such as interleukin (IL)-12, and have shown promising inhibition of melanoma and breast tumours. In this way, stem cells themselves have become active therapeutics, but their roles in delivering cytotoxic drugs have been limited by the overexpression of efflux transporters such as P-glycoprotein, which leads to rapid clearance and poor retention of the stem cell internal drug concentration. Therefore, alternative methods have emerged where the drug is not sequestered directly inside the stem cell, but instead contained within a nanocarrier that is then stably conjugated to the cell surface. Previous studies have involved similar methodologies with different cells, such as platelets and erthyrocytes, but stem cells provide an advantage in their high level of molecular recognition moieties, which can be precisely engineered to modulate interaction and therefore affinity towards tumour sites [87].

Nanogels have presented potential in NP-MSC-mediated drug delivery to tumour sites. A novel carrier (SCMGs) designed by Gao *et al.* generated stem cell membranes by reassembling the vesicles from lysed MSCs [88]. The vesicles were then cloaked in gelatin nanogels *via* co-extrusion through a porous polycarbonate membrane; the nanogels were loaded with doxorubicin (DOX), a fluorescent anticancer drug. This process demonstrated only 3.5% drug loss during extrusion, thus demonstrating high loading capacity. *In vivo* experiments showed that the SCMGs accumulated selectively at tumour tissues *via* intravenous injection, which led to enhanced antitumour efficiency as compared to gelatin-DOX. This is most likely due to the fact that particles sized above 200nm are susceptible to spleen and liver-mediated clearance, as well as activation of the complement system; the SCMGs, however, were sized at 146nm, allowing them to retain antitumour function.

The drug release mechanism for these engineered SCMGs was pH-based, as the isoelectric point of DOX is 9.06 and thus will be released in the acidic conditions surrounding tumour tissue due to hypoxia and the accumulation of lactic acid. A future development may improve the specificity of drug release by combining the pH-based mechanism with a thermal-based sensitivity as well, as nanogels with specific polymer compositions may undergo hydrophobic to hydrophilic transitions at various threshold temperatures; the lower critical solution temperature (LCST). This is due to a change in interaction forces; when the temperature is below the LCST, the amide groups on the surface of the nanogel form hydrogen bonds with surrounding water molecules, but these are replaced with intermolecular forces when the temperature is above the LCST, resulting in a change of swelling state and facilitating drug release.

Other possible vehicles include dendrimers, which have been used to deliver specific genes to stem cells with minimised cytotoxicity, enabled *via* the removal of amine groups from the dendrimer surface to decrease its cationic character [89]. As cell surface integrins are overexpressed in many MSCs, RGD peptide ligands were conjugated to the dendrimer in order to recognise target cells and facilitate specific interactions. The entrapment of gold nanoparticles in the dendrimer cavity also served to maintain the structural integrity of the interior, which ensured more efficient DNA molecule compaction (Fig. **19**) [90]. MSCs were transfected with hBMP-2 genes, which enabled the stem cells to differentiate into osteoblastic lineages, thus demonstrating that selective nanoparticle structures can facilitate the determination of cell fate. Further experiments have yet to be conducted on whether these novel nanohybrids can also perform dual function in photothermal destruction of tumour tissues.

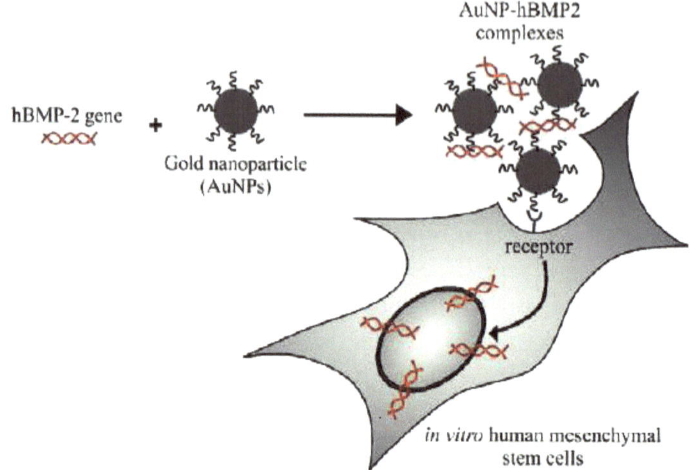

Fig. (19). Dendrimer-mediated gene delivery into MSCs [90].

3.2. Nanotechnology for Stem Cell Tracking

Although stem cells have high medical potential, many therapies are not successfully translated to the clinic, the reasons for which are not fully understood. In order to avoid this, a better understanding of the long-term behavior of transplanted stem cells is necessary. This would enable the monitoring of grafting efficiency, and possibly prevent immunogenic responses. In tissue engineering, the monitoring of stem cells could be a method of ensuring correct tissue function as the scaffold is removed or degraded over time. A number of methods have been developed, including MRI scanning and radiolabeled nanoparticles to provide higher contrast. Additionally, a recent technique known as multispectral optoacoustic tomography (MSOT) has become increasingly prevalent due to its high optical imaging sensitivity and high ultrasound resolution. The underlying process involves the generation of ultrasound after light of a specific wavelength is absorbed; the scattering in this procedure is roughly three orders of magnitude lower than that of conventional photon scattering for other optical techniques, which allows for visualization at 5 cm deep into tissues [91, 92].

MSOT works to identify areas of contrast in tissues, a phenomenon that is observed as a result of specific labelling with exogenous contrast agents that have sharp absorption bands in the near-infrared region. The most notable of these agents is the gold nanorod (GNR) (Fig. **20**) [93]. A key limitation to this is the plasmon coupling effect, which occurs when the distance between GNRs is a few nanometers in length, leading to a loss of intensity in the absorbance band and therefore a decrease in the overall optical signal. To compensate for this, silica coatings have been developed for GNRs to provide steric hindrance in interactions; it is transparent in the visible and near-infrared spectra, and therefore will not affect the absorption properties of the nanorods. To assess the effectiveness of this new nanostructure, MSCs were labelled with silica-coated GNRs and incubated for 24 hours using varying GNR concentrations.

The resulting spectra showed that absorbance increased with concentration, but the width of the band was maintained at 100pM, which was the highest nanorod concentration, showing that even under compact conditions, the optical signature could still be recognized *via* MSOT. The labelled MSCs exhibited a high signal-to-noise ratio, which allowed for monitoring of cells for up to 15 days, providing a method by which the proliferation rate of cell clusters could be observed (Fig. **21**) [95]. Thus, the major advantage of gold nanorods is the modified surface plasmon band (SPR), which allows for near-infrared (NIR) absorption, providing deeper penetration into living tissues. Through this, cancerous and non-cancerous cells can be distinguished for highly-specific drug targeting [94]. As can be seen in Fig. (**20**), gold nanorods can be easily functionalized with conjugated groups, enabling different surface chemistries.

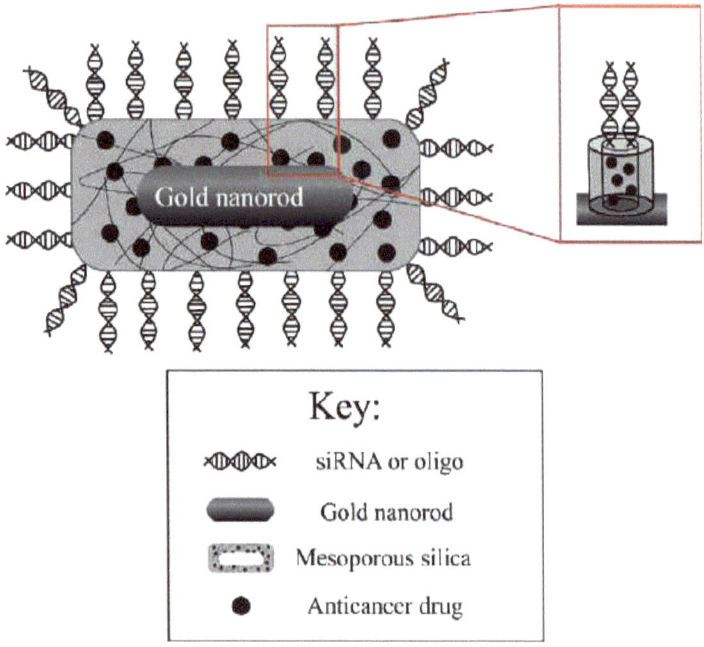

Fig. (20). Silica-coated gold nanorods and various functionalities [94].

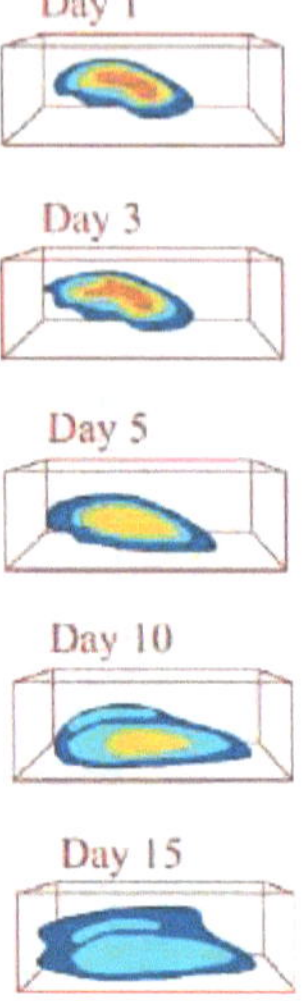

Fig. (21). Monitoring MSC growth in cell clusters; the dimensions of all boxes are in mm [91].

Other inorganic nanoparticles involved in cell imaging include iron oxide NPs, which are limited by their low uptake into target stem cells, and are rapidly diluted with increased cell proliferation and migration *in vivo* leading to a lower detection signal.

Quantum dots are also highly promising nanoscale alternatives for imaging, and are semiconductor particles. Upon excitation *via* UV light, electrons in quantum dots transition from the valence to the conductance band, and its return to ground state involves the emission of light at a given wavelength determined by the energy difference between the two bands. In previous experiments, semi-conducting quantum dots were taken up into mesenchymal stem cells for cardiac repair and observed *in vivo* for 8 weeks. These cells continued to proliferate for more than 6 weeks *in vitro* and the quantum dots were specifically internalised by stem cells without being transported to adjacent cells. This was highly significant, as previous attempts of tracking stem cells in cardiac tissue were limited by the autofluorescence of the host tissue. Further, the precise three-dimensional locations of all injected stem cells were maintained and identified accurately, indicating a possible loading approach in which cardiac tissue can then be reconstructed in a controlled manner (Fig. **22**) [96]. One of the major advantages of this particular study was that a passive loading approach was utilised instead of more commonly used methods such as lipofection or receptor-mediated endocytosis, which resulted in uniform cytoplasmic distribution of labels instead of aggregation at the nucleus; an observation closely linked to loss of cell function [97].

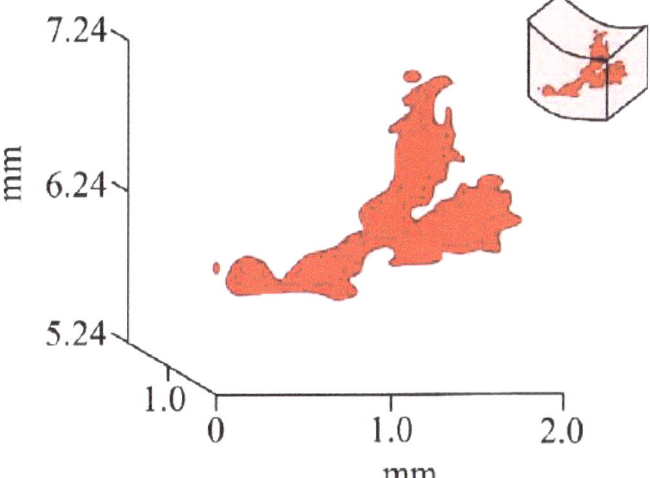

Fig. (22). Schematic of QD-hMSC reconstruction of tissue in an animal that was terminated 1 hour after injection based on nanoparticle imaging coordinates [96].

CONCLUSION AND FUTURE DEVELOPMENTS

In this chapter, the applications of various nanotechnologies in stem cell research have been summarized. Labelling and tracking devices supplemented with magnetic and iron oxide nanoparticles have led to breakthroughs in the *in vivo* visualization of stem cell behaviour. This not only helps in ensuring the safety of stem cell therapies, but also allows scientists to better understand the underlying processes of differentiation, especially in adult stem cells. However, advances still need to be made in understanding the fate of inorganic nanoparticles, including the mechanisms through which they are cleared from the body [98].

Driving stem cell differentiation for tissue engineering and developmental studies has been a key focus for many years, and the use of patterned nanosurfaces has provided an alternative method through which cell behaviour can be manipulated. These topographies may provide more flexibility than conventional polymeric scaffolds, but limitations remain in their ability to fine-tune cell fate; as cells grow, they secrete biochemical cues into the surrounding environment, thus overriding the specific delineation of the surface topography [78]. The possibility of nanotopographies that are sensitive to these cellular changes is still being explored, and may represent a new innovation in the biomimetic reproduction of the extracellular matrix. Towards this, promising avenues include a polydimethylsiloxane substrate that is sensitive to strain and forms dynamic buckling patterns to exert spatial control over MSCs. This patterning is reversible, as demonstrated using a biaxial stretching system to reorient the grooved intervals [99].

Nanogels and dendrimers are two polymer-based nanotechnologies that have shown great promise in the labelling of stem cells, as well as drug and gene delivery applications, respectively. Dendrimers, in particular, may entrap gold nanoparticles to ensure correct uptake of novel genes into MSCs, providing a platform for specific cell targeting and DNA compaction. Nanogels affixed to stem cell surfaces have also generated potential delivery systems for anticancer drugs that will reduce off-target effects. However, limitations remain in the understanding of the long-term behaviour of these devices in vivo, as well as the mechanism of clearance from the body [100].

Nanomedicine is an emerging field at the intersection between engineering and biology, utilising materials with nanoscale dimensions in a therapeutic context. The unique size of these materials enables specific characteristics that are not observed in bulk, which have been manipulated to suit a variety of applications including imaging, disease treatment, and diagnostics. In this chapter, the various applications of nanotechnology to stem cells have been summarised, including relevant protocols and models of possible *in vivo* behavior. Scientists now aim to engineer nanoparticles that can supplement stem cell function and overcome their natural limitations in medicine. The advantages and possible limitations of these technologies have been evaluated, along with a discussion of the outlook of nanoparticle use in stem cells. Stem cells provide the potential to revolutionise many fields, including organ transplantation and the treatment of congenital disorders. Further developments in this interdisciplinary field indicate a promising horizon for therapeutics.

CONSENT FOR PUBLICATION

Not applicable.

CONFLICT OF INTEREST

The author declares no conflict of interest, financial or otherwise.

ACKNOWLEDGEMENTS

Throughout the writing of this chapter I have received much support and assistance. I would first like to thank Dr. F. H. Shah, whose patient guidance and expertise were invaluable in the formulation of the research topic and the formatting of the chapter itself. In addition, I would like to thank my parents for their continual support. Finally, I would like to thank my friends, who have always been a source of inspiration for me and are some of the most hardworking people I know.

REFERENCES

[1]   Alberts B, Johnson A, Lewis J, Raff M, Roberts K, Walter P. Molecular Biology of the Cell. New York: Garland Science 2014; pp. 1217-63.

[2]   Chen Y, Podlevsky JD, Logeswaran D, Chen JJ. A single nucleotide incorporation step limits human telomerase repeat addition activity. EMBO J 2018; 37(6): e97953.
[http://dx.doi.org/10.15252/embj.201797953] [PMID: 29440226]

[3]   Nelakanti RV, Kooreman NG, Wu JC. Teratoma formation: A tool for monitoring pluripotency in stem cell research. Curr. Protoc. Stem Cell Biol 2015; 32(1): 4A.8.1-4A.8.17.
[http://dx.doi.org/10.1002/9780470151808.sc04a08s32]

[4]   Chambers I, Tomlinson SR. The transcriptional foundation of pluripotency. Development 2009; 136(14): 2311-22.
[http://dx.doi.org/10.1242/dev.024398] [PMID: 19542351]

[5]   Zakrzewski W, Dobrzyński M, Szymonowicz M, Rybak Z. Stem cells: past, present, and future. Stem Cell Res Ther 2019; 10(1): 68.
[http://dx.doi.org/10.1186/s13287-019-1165-5] [PMID: 30808416]

[6]   Lanza R, Gearhart J, Hogan B, Melton D, Pedersen R, Thomas ED, *et al.* Essentials of Stem Cell Biology. 3rd ed. Amsterdam: Elsevier Publishing. 2014; pp. 387-98.

[7]   Vazin T, Freed WJ. Human embryonic stem cells: derivation, culture, and differentiation: a review.

Restor Neurol Neurosci 2010; 28(4): 589-603.
[http://dx.doi.org/10.3233/RNN-2010-0543] [PMID: 20714081]

[8]   Chagastelles PC, Nardi NB. Biology of stem cells: an overview. Kidney Int Suppl 2011; 1(3): 63-7.
[http://dx.doi.org/10.1038/kisup.2011.15] [PMID: 25028627]

[9]   Stem Cells and the Future of Regenerative Medicine. Washington, DC: National Academies Press 2002.

[10]   Mountford JC. Human embryonic stem cells: origins, characteristics and potential for regenerative therapy. Transfus Med 2008; 18(1): 1-12.
[http://dx.doi.org/10.1111/j.1365-3148.2007.00807.x] [PMID: 18279188]

[11]   Rippon HJ, Bishop AE. Embryonic stem cells. Cell Prolif 2004; 37(1): 23-34.
[http://dx.doi.org/10.1111/j.1365-2184.2004.00298.x] [PMID: 14871235]

[12]   Takahashi K, Tanabe K, Ohnuki M, *et al.* Induction of pluripotent stem cells from adult human fibroblasts by defined factors. Cell 2007; 131(5): 861-72.
[http://dx.doi.org/10.1016/j.cell.2007.11.019] [PMID: 18035408]

[13]   Morita S, Kojima T, Kitamura T. Plat-E: an efficient and stable system for transient packaging of retroviruses. Gene Ther 2000; 7(12): 1063-6.
[http://dx.doi.org/10.1038/sj.gt.3301206] [PMID: 10871756]

[14]   Tapia N, Schöler HR. P53 connects tumorigenesis and reprogramming to pluripotency. J Exp Med 2010; 207(10): 2045-8.
[http://dx.doi.org/10.1084/jem.20101866] [PMID: 20876313]

[15]   Marks H, Kalkan T, Menafra R, *et al.* The transcriptional and epigenomic foundations of ground state pluripotency. Cell 2012; 149(3): 590-604.
[http://dx.doi.org/10.1016/j.cell.2012.03.026] [PMID: 22541430]

[16]   Shin M, Alev C, Wu Y, Nagai H, Sheng G. Activin/TGF-beta signaling regulates Nanog expression in the epiblast during gastrulation. Mech Dev 2011; 128(5-6): 268-78.
[http://dx.doi.org/10.1016/j.mod.2011.03.001] [PMID: 21402155]

[17]   Rowland BD, Bernards R, Peeper DS. The KLF4 tumour suppressor is a transcriptional repressor of P53 that acts as a context-dependent oncogene. Nat Cell Biol 2005; 7(11): 1074-82.
[http://dx.doi.org/10.1038/ncb1314] [PMID: 16244670]

[18]   Halevy T, Urbach A. Comparing ESC and iPSC-Based models for human genetic disorders. J Clin Med 2014; 3(4): 1146-62.
[http://dx.doi.org/10.3390/jcm3041146] [PMID: 26237596]

[19]   Ma H, Morey R, O'Neil RC, *et al.* Abnormalities in human pluripotent cells due to reprogramming mechanisms. Nature 2014; 511(7508): 177-83.
[http://dx.doi.org/10.1038/nature13551] [PMID: 25008523]

[20]   Yung SK, Tilgner K, Ledran MH, *et al.* Brief report: human pluripotent stem cell models of fanconi anemia deficiency reveal an important role for fanconi anemia proteins in cellular reprogramming and survival of hematopoietic progenitors. Stem Cells 2013; 31(5): 1022-9.
[http://dx.doi.org/10.1002/stem.1308] [PMID: 23280624]

[21]   Mahla RS. Stem cells applications in regenerative medicine and disease therapeutics. Int J Cell Biol 2016; 2016(1): 6940283.
[http://dx.doi.org/10.1155/2016/6940283] [PMID: 27516776]

[22]   Wagers AJ, Weissman IL. Plasticity of adult stem cells. Cell 2004; 116(5): 639-48.
[http://dx.doi.org/10.1016/S0092-8674(04)00208-9] [PMID: 15006347]

[23]   Prentice DA. Adult stem cells: Successful standard for regenerative medicine. Circ Res 2019; 124(6): 837-9.
[http://dx.doi.org/10.1161/CIRCRESAHA.118.313664] [PMID: 30870122]

[24]   Kørbling M, Estrov Z. Adult stem cells for tissue repair - a new therapeutic concept? N Engl J Med 2003; 349(6): 570-82.
[http://dx.doi.org/10.1056/NEJMra022361] [PMID: 12904523]

[25]   Wang Q, Matsumoto Y, Shindo T, *et al.* Neural stem cells transplantation in cortex in a mouse model of Alzheimer's disease. J Med Invest 2006; 53(1-2): 61-9.
[http://dx.doi.org/10.2152/jmi.53.61] [PMID: 16537997]

[26]   Mahajani S, Raina A, Fokken C, Kügler S, Bähr M. Homogenous generation of dopaminergic neurons from multiple hiPSC lines by transient expression of transcription factors. Cell Death Dis 2019; 10(12): 898.
[http://dx.doi.org/10.1038/s41419-019-2133-9] [PMID: 31776327]

[27]   Ring A, Kim YM, Kahn M. Wnt/catenin signaling in adult stem cell physiology and disease. Stem Cell Rev Rep 2014; 10(4): 512-25.
[http://dx.doi.org/10.1007/s12015-014-9515-2] [PMID: 24825509]

[28]   Tachibana M, Amato P, Sparman M, *et al.* Human embryonic stem cells derived by somatic cell nuclear transfer. Cell 2013; 153(6): 1228-38.
[http://dx.doi.org/10.1016/j.cell.2013.05.006] [PMID: 23683578]

[29]   Ohnuki M, Takahashi K. Present and Future Challenges of Induced Pluripotent Stem Cells. Philos Trans R Soc Lond B Biol Sci 1680; 370(1680): 20140367.

[30]   von der Haar K, Lavrentieva A, Stahl F, Scheper T, Blume C. Lost signature: progress and failures in *in vivo* tracking of implanted stem cells. Appl Microbiol Biotechnol 2015; 99(23): 9907-22.
[http://dx.doi.org/10.1007/s00253-015-6965-7] [PMID: 26373727]

[31]   Xu C, Miranda-Nieves D, Ankrum JA, *et al.* Tracking mesenchymal stem cells with iron oxide nanoparticle loaded poly(lactide-co-glycolide) microparticles. Nano Lett 2012; 12(8): 4131-9.
[http://dx.doi.org/10.1021/nl301658q] [PMID: 22769232]

[32]   Ventola CL. The nanomedicine revolution: part 2: current and future clinical applications. P&T 2012; 37(10): 582-91.
[PMID: 23115468]

[33]   Naito M, Yokoyama T, Hosokawa K, Nogi K. Nanoparticle Technology Handbook. Amsterdam: Elsevier Publishing 2018; pp. 3-47.

[34]   Roduner E. Size matters: why nanomaterials are different. Chem Soc Rev 2006; 35(7): 583-92.
[http://dx.doi.org/10.1039/b502142c] [PMID: 16791330]

[35]   Mohamad AT, Kaur J, Sidik NA, Rahman S. Nanoparticles: A review on their synthesis, characterization and physicochemical properties for energy technology industry. J Adv Res Fluid Mech Therm Sci 2018; 46(1): 1-10.

[36]   Batista CA, Larson RG, Kotov NA. Nonadditivity of nanoparticle interactions. Sci 2015; 350(6257): 1242477.
[http://dx.doi.org/10.1126/science.1242477] [PMID: 26450215]

[37]   Son Y, Park M, Son Y, *et al.* Quantum confinement and its related effects on the critical size of GeO2 nanoparticles anodes for lithium batteries. Nano Lett 2014; 14(2): 1005-10.
[http://dx.doi.org/10.1021/nl404466v] [PMID: 24392754]

[38]   Goodrich GP, Bao L, Gill-Sharp K, Sang KL, Wang J, Payne JD. Photothermal therapy in a murine colon cancer model using near-infrared absorbing gold nanorods. J Biomed Opt 2010; 15(1): 018001.
[http://dx.doi.org/10.1117/1.3290817] [PMID: 20210487]

[39]   Buzea C, Pacheco II, Robbie K. Nanomaterials and nanoparticles: sources and toxicity. Biointerphases 2007; 2(4): MR17-71.
[http://dx.doi.org/10.1116/1.2815690] [PMID: 20419892]

[40]   Farokhzad OC, Cheng J, Teply BA, *et al.* Targeted nanoparticle-aptamer bioconjugates for cancer

chemotherapy *in vivo*. Proc Natl Acad Sci USA 2006; 103(16): 6315-20.
[http://dx.doi.org/10.1073/pnas.0601755103] [PMID: 16606824]

[41]   Prasad M, Lambe UP, Brar B, *et al*. Nanotherapeutics: An insight into healthcare and multi-dimensional applications in medical sector of the modern world. Biomed Pharmacother 2018; 97: 1521-37.
[http://dx.doi.org/10.1016/j.biopha.2017.11.026] [PMID: 29793315]

[42]   Neamtu I, Rusu AG, Diaconu A, Nita LE, Chiriac AP. Basic concepts and recent advances in nanogels as carriers for medical applications. Drug Deliv 2017; 24(1): 539-57.
[http://dx.doi.org/10.1080/10717544.2016.1276232] [PMID: 28181831]

[43]   Samadi N, Abbadessa A, Di Stefano A, *et al*. The effect of lauryl capping group on protein release and degradation of poly(D,L-lactic-co-glycolic acid) particles. J Cont Rel 2013; 172(2): 436-43.
[http://dx.doi.org/10.1016/j.jconrel.2013.05.034] [PMID: 23751568]

[44]   Mohapatra S, Ranjan S, Dasgupta N, Kumar R, Thomas S. Characterization and biology of nanomaterials for drug delivery: nanoscience and nanotechnology in drug delivery. Amsterdam: Elsevier Publishing 2018.

[45]   Jawahar N, Meyyanathan SN. Polymeric nanoparticles for drug delivery and targeting: A comprehensive review. Int J Health Allied Sci 2012; 1(4): 217-23.
[http://dx.doi.org/10.4103/2278-344X.107832]

[46]   Raemdonck K, Demeester J, de Smedt S. Advanced nanogel engineering for drug delivery. Soft Matter 2009; 5(4): 707-15.
[http://dx.doi.org/10.1039/B811923F]

[47]   Tamura G, Shinohara Y, Tamura A, Sanada Y, Oishi M, Akiba I, *et al*. Dependence of the Swelling Behavior of a PH-Responsive PEG-Modified Nanogel on the Cross-Link Density. Polym J 2012; 44(3): 240-4.
[http://dx.doi.org/10.1038/pj.2011.123]

[48]   Pikabea A, Aguirre G, Miranda JI, Ramos J, Forcada J. Understanding of nanogels swelling behavior through a deep insight into their morphology. J Polym Sci A Polym Chem 2015; 53(17): 2017-25.
[http://dx.doi.org/10.1002/pola.27653]

[49]   Eichenbaum GM, Kiser PF, Simon SA, Needham D. pH and Ion-triggered volume response of anionic hydrogel microspheres. Macromolecules 1998; 31(15): 5084-93.
[http://dx.doi.org/10.1021/ma970897t] [PMID: 9680449]

[50]   Soni KS, Desale SS, Bronich TK. Nanogels: An overview of properties, biomedical applications and obstacles to clinical translation. J Control Release 2016; 240: 109-26.
[http://dx.doi.org/10.1016/j.jconrel.2015.11.009] [PMID: 26571000]

[51]   Hendrickson GR, Lyon LA. Microgel translocation through pores under confinement. Angew Chem Int Ed Engl 2010; 49(12): 2193-7.
[http://dx.doi.org/10.1002/anie.200906606] [PMID: 20183836]

[52]   Fox ME, Szoka FC, Fréchet JM. Soluble polymer carriers for the treatment of cancer: the importance of molecular architecture. Acc Chem Res 2009; 42(8): 1141-51.
[http://dx.doi.org/10.1021/ar900035f] [PMID: 19555070]

[53]   Banquy X, Suarez F, Argaw A, *et al*. Effect of mechanical properties of hydrogel nanoparticles on macrophage cell pptake. Soft matter 2009; 5(20): 3984-91.
[http://dx.doi.org/10.1039/b821583a]

[54]   Abbasi E, Aval SF, Akbarzadeh A, *et al*. Dendrimers: synthesis, applications, and properties. Nanoscale Res Lett 2014; 9(1): 247.
[http://dx.doi.org/10.1186/1556-276X-9-247] [PMID: 24994950]

[55]   Kono K, Liu M, Fréchet JM. Design of dendritic macromolecules containing folate or methotrexate residues. Bioconjug Chem 1999; 10(6): 1115-21.

[http://dx.doi.org/10.1021/bc990082k] [PMID: 10563782]

[56]   Fréchet JM, Tomalia DA. Dendrimers and other dendritic polymers. New York: Wiley & Sons 2001.
[http://dx.doi.org/10.1002/0470845821]

[57]   Basu A, Yang K, Wang M, *et al.* Structure-function engineering of interferon-β-1b for improving stability, solubility, potency, immunogenicity, and pharmacokinetic properties by site-selective mono-PEGylation. Bioconjug Chem 2006; 17(3): 618-30.
[http://dx.doi.org/10.1021/bc050322y] [PMID: 16704199]

[58]   Laurent S, Forge D, Port M, *et al.* Magnetic iron oxide nanoparticles: synthesis, stabilization, vectorization, physicochemical characterizations, and biological applications. Chem Rev 2008; 108(6): 2064-110.
[http://dx.doi.org/10.1021/cr068445e] [PMID: 18543879]

[59]   AshaRani PV, Low Kah Mun G, Hande MP, Valiyaveettil S. Cytotoxicity and genotoxicity of silver nanoparticles in human cells. ACS Nano 2009; 3(2): 279-90.
[http://dx.doi.org/10.1021/nn800596w] [PMID: 19236062]

[60]   Williams DF. Challenges with the development of biomaterials for sustainable tissue engineering. Front Bioeng Biotechnol 2019; 7: 127.
[http://dx.doi.org/10.3389/fbioe.2019.00127] [PMID: 31214584]

[61]   Arai F, Suda T. Quiescent Stem Cells in the Niche StemBook. Harvard Stem Cell Institute 2008.

[62]   Morgan JE, Partridge TA. Muscle satellite cells. Int J Biochem Cell Biol 2003; 35(8): 1151-6.
[http://dx.doi.org/10.1016/S1357-2725(03)00042-6] [PMID: 12757751]

[63]   Mason JO, Price DJ. Building brains in a dish: Prospects for growing cerebral organoids from stem cells. Neuroscience 2016; 334: 105-18.
[http://dx.doi.org/10.1016/j.neuroscience.2016.07.048] [PMID: 27506142]

[64]   Frantz C, Stewart KM, Weaver VM. The extracellular matrix at a glance. J Cell Sci 2010; 123(Pt 24): 4195-200.
[http://dx.doi.org/10.1242/jcs.023820] [PMID: 21123617]

[65]   Hutmacher DW. Scaffolds in tissue engineering bone and cartilage. Biomat 2000; 21(24): 2529-43.
[http://dx.doi.org/10.1016/S0142-9612(00)00121-6] [PMID: 11071603]

[66]   Pasut G, Veronese FM. State of the art in PEGylation: the great versatility achieved after forty years of research. J Control Release 2012; 161(2): 461-72.
[http://dx.doi.org/10.1016/j.jconrel.2011.10.037] [PMID: 22094104]

[67]   Bosworth LA, Turner LA, Cartmell SH. State of the art composites comprising electrospun fibres coupled with hydrogels: a review. Nanomedicine 2013; 9(3): 322-35.
[http://dx.doi.org/10.1016/j.nano.2012.10.008] [PMID: 23178282]

[68]   Wang JY, Wang K, Gu X, Luo Y. Polymerization of hydrogel network on microfiber surface: synthesis of hybrid water-absorbing matrices for biomedical applications. ACS Biomater Sci Eng 2016; 2(6): 887-92.
[http://dx.doi.org/10.1021/acsbiomaterials.6b00143] [PMID: 33429497]

[69]   Re'em T, Tsur-Gang O, Cohen S. The effect of immobilized RGD peptide in macroporous alginate scaffolds on TGFbeta1-induced chondrogenesis of human mesenchymal stem cells. Biomat 2010; 31(26): 6746-55.
[http://dx.doi.org/10.1016/j.biomaterials.2010.05.025] [PMID: 20542332]

[70]   Casper CL, Yang W, Farach-Carson MC, Rabolt JF. Coating electrospun collagen and gelatin fibers with perlecan domain I for increased growth factor binding. Biomacromol 2007; 8(4): 1116-23.
[http://dx.doi.org/10.1021/bm061003s] [PMID: 17326680]

[71]   Newman DR, Li CM, Simmons R, Khosla J, Sannes PL. Heparin affects signaling pathways stimulated by fibroblast growth factor-1 and -2 in type II cells. Am J Physiol Lung Cell Mol Physiol

2004; 287(1): L191-200.
[http://dx.doi.org/10.1152/ajplung.00284.2003] [PMID: 14966081]

[72]   McNamara LE, McMurray RJ, Biggs MJ, Kantawong F, Oreffo RO, Dalby MJ. Nanotopographical control of stem cell differentiation. J Tissue Eng 2010; 2010: 120623.
[http://dx.doi.org/10.4061/2010/120623] [PMID: 21350640]

[73]   Kulangara K, Leong KW. Substrate topography shapes cell function. Soft Matter 2009; 5(21): 4072-6.
[http://dx.doi.org/10.1039/b910132m]

[74]   Li L, He Y, Zhao M, Jiang J. Collective cell migration: Implications for wound healing and cancer invasion. Burns Trauma 2013; 1(1): 21-6.
[http://dx.doi.org/10.4103/2321-3868.113331] [PMID: 27574618]

[75]   Discher DE, Janmey P, Wang YL. Tissue cells feel and respond to the stiffness of their substrate. Science 2005; 310(5751): 1139-43.
[http://dx.doi.org/10.1126/science.1116995] [PMID: 16293750]

[76]   Kwon HK, Lee JH, Shin HJ, Kim JH, Choi S. Structural and functional analysis of cell adhesion and nuclear envelope nano-topography in cell death. Sci Rep 2015; 5(1): 15623.
[http://dx.doi.org/10.1038/srep15623] [PMID: 26490051]

[77]   McBeath R, Pirone DM, Nelson CM, Bhadriraju K, Chen CS. Cell shape, cytoskeletal tension, and RhoA regulate stem cell lineage commitment. Dev Cell 2004; 6(4): 483-95.
[http://dx.doi.org/10.1016/S1534-5807(04)00075-9] [PMID: 15068789]

[78]   Wilkinson CD, Riehle M, Wood M, Gallagher J, Curtis AS. The use of materials patterned on a nano- and micro-metric scale in cellular engineering. Mater Sci Eng C 2002; 19(1): 263-9.
[http://dx.doi.org/10.1016/S0928-4931(01)00396-4]

[79]   Derda R, Laromaine A, Mammoto A, *et al.* Paper-supported 3D cell culture for tissue-based bioassays. Proc Natl Acad Sci USA 2009; 106(44): 18457-62.
[http://dx.doi.org/10.1073/pnas.0910666106] [PMID: 19846768]

[80]   Casey BG, Monaghan W, Wilkinson CD. Embossing of Nanoscale Features and Environments. Microelectron Eng 1997; 35(1): 393-6.
[http://dx.doi.org/10.1016/S0167-9317(96)00208-0]

[81]   Shi L, Wang K, Yang Y. Adhesion-based tumor cell capture using nanotopography. Colloids Surf B Biointerfaces 2016; 147: 291-9.
[http://dx.doi.org/10.1016/j.colsurfb.2016.08.008] [PMID: 27526289]

[82]   The evolving role of stem cell transplantation. Lancet Haematol 2020; 7(4): e271.
[http://dx.doi.org/10.1016/S2352-3026(20)30075-2] [PMID: 32220336]

[83]   Cui X, Dini S, Dai S, Bi J, Binder BJ, Green JEF, *et al.* A mechanistic study on tumour spheroid formation in thermosensitive hydrogels: experiments and mathematical modelling. RSC Advances 2016; 6(77): 73282-91.
[http://dx.doi.org/10.1039/C6RA11699J]

[84]   Li TS, Cheng K, Malliaras K, *et al.* Direct comparison of different stem cell types and subpopulations reveals superior paracrine potency and myocardial repair efficacy with cardiosphere-derived cells. J Am Coll Cardiol 2012; 59(10): 942-53.
[http://dx.doi.org/10.1016/j.jacc.2011.11.029] [PMID: 22381431]

[85]   Tang J, Cui X, Caranasos TG, *et al.* Heart repair using nanogel-encapsulated human cardiac stem cells in mice and pigs with myocardial infarction. ACS Nano 2017; 11(10): 9738-49.
[http://dx.doi.org/10.1021/acsnano.7b01008] [PMID: 28929735]

[86]   Wilhelm S, Tavares AJ, Dai Q, Ohta S, Audet J, Dvorak HF, *et al.* Analysis of nanoparticle delivery to tumours. Nat Rev Mater 2016; 1(5): 16014.
[http://dx.doi.org/10.1038/natrevmats.2016.14]

[87]   Uccelli A, Moretta L, Pistoia V. Mesenchymal stem cells in health and disease. Nat Rev Immunol 2008; 8(9): 726-36.
[http://dx.doi.org/10.1038/nri2395] [PMID: 19172693]

[88]   Gao C, Lin Z, Jurado-Sánchez B, Lin X, Wu Z, He Q. Stem cell membrane-coated nanogels for highly efficient *in vivo* tumor targeted drug delivery. Small 2016; 12(30): 4056-62.
[http://dx.doi.org/10.1002/smll.201600624] [PMID: 27337109]

[89]   Munro N, Srinageshwar B, Shalabi F, *et al.* A novel approach to label bone marrow-derived mesenchymal stem cells with mixed-surface PAMAM dendrimers. Stem Cell Res Ther 2019; 10(1): 71.
[http://dx.doi.org/10.1186/s13287-019-1171-7] [PMID: 30819246]

[90]   Shan Y, Luo T, Peng C, *et al.* Gene delivery using dendrimer-entrapped gold nanoparticles as nonviral vectors. Biomaterials 2012; 33(10): 3025-35.
[http://dx.doi.org/10.1016/j.biomaterials.2011.12.045] [PMID: 22248990]

[91]   Ntziachristos V, Razansky D. Molecular imaging by means of multispectral optoacoustic tomography (MSOT). Chem Rev 2010; 110(5): 2783-94.
[http://dx.doi.org/10.1021/cr9002566] [PMID: 20387910]

[92]   Wang LV, Hu S. Photoacoustic tomography: *in vivo* imaging from organelles to organs. Science 2012; 335(6075): 1458-62.
[http://dx.doi.org/10.1126/science.1216210] [PMID: 22442475]

[93]   Taruttis A, Lozano N, Nunes A, *et al.* siRNA liposome-gold nanorod vectors for multispectral optoacoustic tomography theranostics. Nanoscale 2014; 6(22): 13451-6.
[http://dx.doi.org/10.1039/C4NR04164J] [PMID: 25301102]

[94]   Song Y, Li Y, Xu Q, Liu Z. Mesoporous silica nanoparticles for stimuli-responsive controlled drug delivery: advances, challenges, and outlook. Int J Nanomedicine 2016; 12: 87-110.
[http://dx.doi.org/10.2147/IJN.S117495] [PMID: 28053526]

[95]   Comenge J, Fragueiro O, Sharkey J, *et al.* Preventing plasmon coupling between gold nanorods improves the sensitivity of photoacoustic detection of labeled stem cells *in vivo.* ACS Nano 2016; 10(7): 7106-16.
[http://dx.doi.org/10.1021/acsnano.6b03246] [PMID: 27308890]

[96]   Rosen AB, Kelly DJ, Schuldt AJ, *et al.* Finding fluorescent needles in the cardiac haystack: tracking human mesenchymal stem cells labeled with quantum dots for quantitative *in vivo* three-dimensional fluorescence analysis. Stem Cells 2007; 25(8): 2128-38.
[http://dx.doi.org/10.1634/stemcells.2006-0722] [PMID: 17495112]

[97]   Hsieh SC, Wang FF, Hung SC, Chen YJ, Wang YJ. The internalized CdSe/ZnS quantum dots impair the chondrogenesis of bone marrow mesenchymal stem cells. J Biomed Mater Res B Appl Biomater 2006; 79(1): 95-101.
[http://dx.doi.org/10.1002/jbm.b.30517] [PMID: 16470833]

[98]   Feliu N, Docter D, Heine M, *et al. In vivo* degeneration and the fate of inorganic nanoparticles. Chem Soc Rev 2016; 45(9): 2440-57.
[http://dx.doi.org/10.1039/C5CS00699F] [PMID: 26862602]

[99]   Guvendiren M, Burdick JA. Stem cell response to spatially and temporally displayed and reversible surface topography. Adv Healthc Mater 2013; 2(1): 155-64.
[http://dx.doi.org/10.1002/adhm.201200105] [PMID: 23184470]

[100]   Kong L, Alves CS, Hou W, *et al.* RGD peptide-modified dendrimer-entrapped gold nanoparticles enable highly efficient and specific gene delivery to stem cells. ACS Appl Mater Interfaces 2015; 7(8): 4833-43.
[http://dx.doi.org/10.1021/am508760w] [PMID: 25658033]

CHAPTER 3

The Role of Nanotherapeutic Agents in Hematology and Related Diseases

Veena Ganti[1,*]

[1] *William Mason High School, 6100 Mason Montgomery Rd, Mason, OH 45040, United States*

Abstract: Hematological anomalies are becoming more prevalent in the world and are comprised of blood-related diseases. They either disrupt normal blood circulation or reduce the blood volume and, consequently, death. Therapies are available to treat and alleviate these diseases, but they adversely interact with other organs/tissues to provoke them. To avoid such adverse scenarios, NT graced medicine to deliver therapeutic agents in nanocarriers that are engineered to transport them to their target site, averting untoward effects and functioning for a long time. In this chapter, we will be highlighting the role of NT in the treatment of hematological and other related diseases.

Keywords: Blood Related disease, Hematology, Nanotechnology, Targeted delivery, Treatment.

1. INTRODUCTION

Biomedical applications and pharmacology rely on nanotherapeutic agents. These applications rely on nanotherapeutic agents (NT) which is an example of a microscale form of disease treatment. A growing number of people are embracing NT in today's world, due to the transition to focused treatment [1], where medication retention capacities can be improved. As part of the treatment, healthy cells are often destroyed. However, targeted treatment only addresses the aberrant cells, which prevents any injury to the surrounding healthy cells [2]. While previous medical discoveries have made use of similar technologies, it is possible that in the future, as nanomedicine (NM) and technology come together, more solutions will be found. Due to these considerations, NM has been (and continues to be) exposed to new domains in medicine [3]. Particularly, NM has impacted the field of Hematology. In its essence, Hematology is the branch of medicine that focuses on blood, its formation, and blood-related diseases. Hematologists are physicians who look for patterns in the behavior of blood cells and interpret those

* **Corresponding author Veena Ganti:** William Mason High School, 6100 Mason Montgomery Rd, Mason, OH 45040, United States; E-mail: veenamganti@gmail.com

Shahid Ali Khan, Saad Salman, Youssef O. Al-Ghamd (Eds.)

patterns to find correlations in the Cardiovascular and Lymphatic systems [4]. Hematologists can diagnose diseases from Anemia all the way to leukemia (LA) and lymphoma. Within this chapter, you will find common diseases that hematologists diagnose and how NT has impacted treatment methods and overall results for these diseases.

2. TYPES OF BLOOD DISORDERS AND ROLE OF NANOPARTICLES

In addition, you will find a correlation between lipid-based nanoparticles and these diseases. The diseases that we will explore are Sickle Cell Anemia, High Cholesterol, Hemophilia, and LA.

2.1. Sickle Cell Anemia

Sickle cell anemia occurs when there is a deformation of the red blood cell. A mutation in the HBB gene is what causes this deformation. The HBB gene regulates the production of Hemoglobin, which binds to the oxygen molecule. Hemoglobin has four subunits: two alpha-globin subunits and two Beta-globin subunits [5]. An individual will develop Sickle cell Anemia when there is a mutation in at least one of the beta-globin subunits. The beta-globin subunit switches with hemoglobin S. This disease is an alteration in the hemoglobin, which is slightly different from B. Thalassemia. As a result, RBC will take the shape of a crescent instead of a circle, as shown in Fig. (**1**).

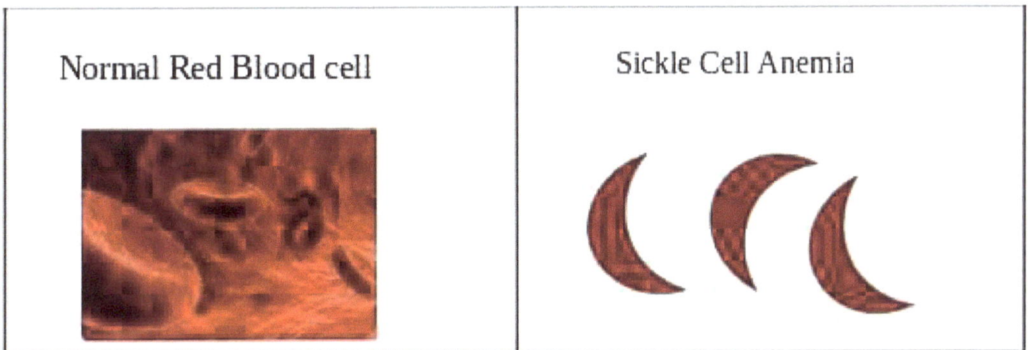

Fig. (1). Structural comparison of Normal Blood and Sickle Cell.

For individuals with sickle cell anemia, their cells cannot take adequate amounts of oxygen and transport it to the rest of the body [6]. This is why one of the most common symptoms is shortness of breath. In addition, sickle cells can also block the flow of other RBC in the blood vessels [7]. If enough sickle cells build up to block blood flow in the blood vessels, individuals can be at risk for a stroke due to oxygen deprivation in the brain 6. Circular RBCs are shaped in such a way that they can fold and move easily throughout the cardiovascular system, unlike sickle cells. Unfortunately, there is no cure for Sickle Cell Anemia. Treatment is used to alleviate symptoms and pain and prevent further complications for patients. Some treatment methods include blood transfusions [8], stem cell transplants [9], increased vitamin intake [10], and Hydroxyurea (a chemotherapy drug) [11].

Hydroxyurea is effective in Sickle-cell Anemia because it introduces fetal hemoglobin to RBC. Due to the increase in fetal hemoglobin, the risk of organ damage is reduced [12]. However, the side effects of Hydroxyurea make this option less appealing. Common side effects include nausea, loss of appetite, diarrhea, reduction of hemolysis, and mouth sores [13, 14]. In addition, this drug can elevate hepatic enzymes, which can cause inflammation in the liver. Hemolysis is the destruction of RBC. Essentially this is the apoptosis process for RBC.

If Hydroxyurea has been shown to decrease sickle cells in the blood, then why are other treatment possibilities considered? Just because Hydroxyurea eliminates sickle cells in the blood, it does not mean that it's the most effective way without placing a toll on the body. What specifically does Hydroxyurea do to the bloodstream? Hydroxyurea can reduce the number of platelets (Thrombocytes), RBC (Erythrocytes), and white blood cells (Leukocytes) produced from the bone marrow. As a result, patients can be susceptible to infection as there are fewer white blood cells to fight bacteria. Bruising and bleeding are also common due to fewer platelets to clot the blood. Hydroxyurea can also cause Anemia - a condition where there is less healthy (RBC) in the blood. This is dangerous because individuals with Sickle Cell disease develop an Anemia, but with even lower healthy RBC, patients can be at risk for various other conditions. This is why Sickle cell patients will take Vitamin C, Iron, and even Zinc supplements to combat red blood cell loss.

With new advancements in technology, NM continues to prove promising results. NM treatment continues to be researched because it can provide patients a happier and healthier outcome with minimal side effects [15]. There are other drugs like Hydroxyurea that are similar. For the purpose of this section, we studied Hydroxyurea because it was one of the most common drugs for treatments. Other drugs used for Sickle cell Anemia include Endari, Oxybryta, and Adaveko. Endari increases the amount of glutamine (amino acid) in the blood [16]. Oxybryta strengthens the binding of hemoglobin to oxygen molecules. Adaveko, which contains an antibody, is used to mitigate pain for Sickle cell Anemia patients. For these drugs, there are unintended side effects as well. Endari can enlarge the spleen, which can potentially, if left untreated, lead to a ruptured spleen and severe bleeding. Oxybryta can lead to abdominal pain, headaches, dizziness, and Nausea. With Adaveko, joint pain, diarrhea, and chest pain can occur. Even though these drugs might mitigate sickle cell disease to a certain level, there will always be side effects.

CRISPR allows scientists and researchers to edit the genome. Currently, CRISPR-Cas9 is used on somatic cells. This new gene-editing tool has been tested with individuals who have Sickle Cell disease facilitated by NT to allow targeted gene editing [17]. There have been clinical trials proving fewer adverse side effects for patients, but more prospective and research studies are necessary to obtain a thorough understanding of NT in Sickle cell Anemia [18]. Overall, NM and CRISPR prove to be promising treatment options compared to Chemotherapy drugs.

In addition to CRISPR, lentiviral vectors have also been tested with individuals who have sickle cell anemia. These vectors work very similarly to retroviruses. As a result, viral DNA gets transcribed and translated, and eventually inserted into a host's genome.

2.2. High Cholesterol (Ch)

High Ch is becoming more common around the world. Ch is found in the food you eat, but too much can cause complications to your cardiovascular system. Your body needs adequate amounts of Ch to build cells. Ch is also made from the liver. Ch circulates through the blood on lipoproteins, however, too much can obstruct blood flow throughout the arteries. There are two types of Ch that determine the risk of plaque buildup: HDL (good Ch) and LDL (bad Ch). When Ch and Triglycerides, a type of fat, build up in the arteries, blood flow to the brain and heart can be impaired, as depicted in Fig. (**2**). This is known as Atherosclerosis. As a result, this can cause heart disease, heart attack, and stroke.

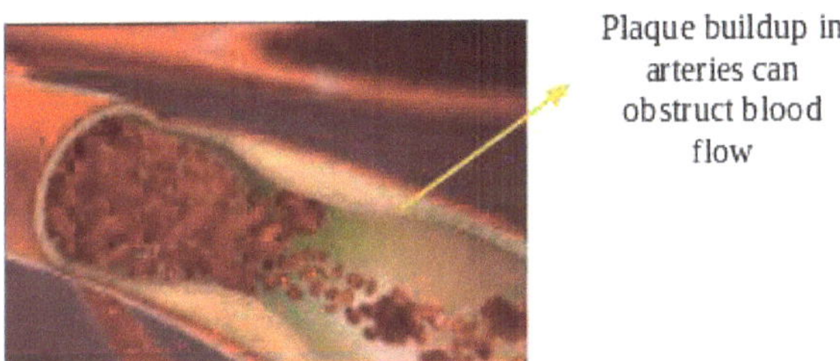

Fig. (2). Illustration of Plaque buildup in the blood vessel impeding blood flow in the arteries.

High levels of Ch can have negative implications for the bloodstream and cardiovascular health. In order to mitigate further complications from arising, medications are taken. Normal levels of HDL are below 100 mg/dL and 50 mg/dL or higher for HDL [19]. One common form of treatment includes Statins, which are drugs to block the liver from overproducing Ch and also help to increase HDL levels. There are many different types of statins: atorvastatin, fluvastatin, simvastatin, pravastatin, pitavastatin, rosuvastatin, and lovastatin [20]. These statins differ based on the amount of HDL increase and LDL decrease. These drugs also have different side effects. For example, lovastatin does not cause many muscle problems compared to other drugs. In general, statins can cause muscle pain and weakness. Muscle pain and weakness experienced from statins are not as life-threatening as Rhabdomyolysis [20]. In addition, patients using statins will have to take a liver enzyme test to see if there is any inflammation in the liver. In any case, these drugs will have side effects to a certain degree.

The PCSK9 inhibitor is more recent than statins. PCSK9 inhibitors are synthetically made proteins. These inhibitors prevent the PCSK9 protein from performing its function. In the liver, there are receptors to remove excess Ch, but the PCSK9 protein destroys these receptors. The PCSK9 inhibitor attaches itself to the proteins to prevent them from blocking the liver receptors. In some cases, PCSK9 inhibitors can be taken with statins to increase the overall effect on Ch [21]. This method of treatment can cause increased muscle and joint pain along with nausea and back pain.

Fibrates are used to lower triglyceride levels. Fibrates can increase HDL levels, but they are not effective in decreasing LDL levels [22]. If Fibrates are used for many years, then the gallbladder can develop stones inside. These are known as gallstones. In fact, individuals with Sickle cell Anemia are more likely to have gallstones.

There have been technological advancements in reducing the buildup of Ch and triglycerides in arteries. One common method of treatment for an enlarged artery is balloon Angioplasty. This is when a balloon from a catheter, surrounded by a metal stent, is inserted at the site of thrombosis. The balloon will pop out the excess Ch in the artery and the stent will support the artery. Stents are typically used to support narrowed arteries.

How exactly has NT impacted patients with Hyperlipidemia?

Nanoparticles have been used in vascular testing. In this case, vascular imaging has been developed to obtain various organ structures [23]. Nanoparticles can attach to proteins, antibodies, or other molecules to target certain cells or receptors. These nanoparticles can then be present in new vessels or along the walls of existing vessels. In addition, nanoparticles can also transmit glucocorticoids, which is a hormone used for the reduction of inflammation. In order for nanoparticles to be effective, they need to extravasate from the blood through the phagocyte system. Despite current experimentation, researchers are developing lipid-based nanoparticles that will have a stronger performance in combating plaque and atherosclerosis [24, 25]. Ch is a rising issue for many people around the world. One of the most therapeutic ways to decrease Ch levels is eating foods with a high level of HDL. Oils, in particular, have higher triglycerides and HDL levels. By minimizing the number of oils consumed, bad Ch levels can also decrease.

2.3. Hemophilia

Hemophilia is relatively rare compared to high Ch levels. Hemophilia is a condition that affects the body's ability to clot blood due to the lack of platelets. For patients who have Hemophilia, internal bleeding in organs is a major concern. Like Sickle Cell Anemia, Hemophilia is a genetic disorder that can only be inherited. Based on an Individual's clotting factors, various symptoms can occur. Common symptoms include frequent nosebleeds, bruises, and excessive bleeding from cuts. For individuals with severe Hemophilia, bleeding in the brain from a bump can cause critical injuries. There are two main types of Hemophilia [26]: Hemophilia A and Hemophilia B. Hemophilia A is more common with patients. Hemophilia A occurs when there is a mutation in the F8 genes, which codes for the factor VIII protein. Hemophilia B is a mutation on gene 9, which codes for the factor IX protein. Both these chromosomes belong to the X chromosome of women. In either case, men have a higher chance of inheriting the disease.

There are misconceptions that people with Hemophilia can die from excessive bleeding from a wound. This is not necessarily true. When a person has Hemophilia, their blood vessel narrows, just like in a person without Hemophilia. However, those with the disease, they are not able to make a Fibrin clot. Fig. (3) depicts blood flow due to the lack of a Fibrin clot. Due to the lack of certain clotting factors, a fibrin clot becomes so thin or is not able to be made that the bleeding continues to occur for the individual. Typically, people with hemophilia will bleed longer, but not necessarily faster. There can be situations where there is a spontaneous bleed. Most spontaneous internal bleeding situations occur in the knee, ankles, or elbows. This is more common with bruises. Bruises occur when there is damage to the capillaries, which are microvessels that connect arteries and veins together. In the body, blood can go into spaces between organs or joints. If untreated, this can damage organs and tissues. Most trials with Hemophilia have mainly incorporated testing on mice. This includes inserting the gene for the human factor-VIII protein into the mice's genome and observing whether transcription and translation of the gene are successful.

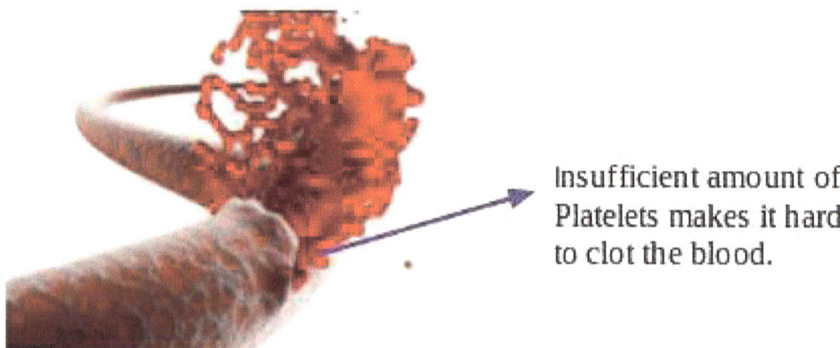

Fig. (3). Graphical illustration of Hemophilia.

Another form of treatment is Capsule therapy. This is when a small capsule that is inserted into the stomach reaches the small intestines. The high pH levels of the stomach will degrade the outer layer of the capsule, releasing a drug that promotes protein synthesis. This can help patients to synthesize the necessary clotting factor proteins that are lacking in individuals who have Hemophilia.

2.4. Leukemia

LA is a cancer that affects the bone marrow. Individuals with LA have a high white blood cell count. These LA white blood cells do not fight infection as they should, and eventually, they will start to damage organs. A mutation in the CEBPA gene will impact the CCAAT protein [27]. This protein is involved in the specialization of blood cells. The gene also regulates the division of abnormal cells. This gene is found on chromosome 19. There are two types of LA: Acute and Chronic. Acute LA progresses more quickly than Chronic LA. In Acute LA there are more abnormal cells that can't perform the right function compared to Chronic LA. Of the different types of LA, Acute Myeloid LA is the most common.

Types of LA:

- Acute Myeloid LA
- Chronic Myeloid LA
- Acute Lymphocytic LA

- Chronic Lymphocytic LA
- Hairy Cell LA

Current treatment options for LA include chemotherapy, radiation therapy, stem cell transplant, immunotherapy, and target therapy using inflammation drugs. As discussed in the Sickle Cell Anemia section, the effects of chemotherapy can be less appealing for patients. Radiation therapy uses radiation to kill LA cells. This form of treatment is much more targeted compared to chemotherapy. Stem cell transplant replaces the bone marrow with healthy bone marrow. Immunotherapy allows your body to kill and recognize cancerous cells. Target treatment includes inflammatory drugs like Imatinib that help to suppress tumor growth. Nanotherapeutic agents also fall under this category.

One example of a Nanotherapeutic agent in LA is a Dendrimer [28]. Dendrimers are artificial macromolecules that help to detect agents in diseases by using a dye. Dendrimers are nano-sized and have both an inner and outer shell. In addition, gold nanoparticles have been explored for radiation therapy. Eventually, Nanoparticles will be able to detect immature white blood cells at early stages and have attraction-like abilities to cancerous cells.

One form of treatment to eradicate LA and even lymphoma cells is through Gold Quantum Dots inorganic nanoparticles [29, 30]. These nanoparticles target the antigens present in these cells. In this way, nanoparticles serve as a detection mechanism for cancer cells.

It is essential to note that plasmonic nonlinear optical reaction is a versatile method for determining specific properties in biological media. The activity of dynamical reaction with physical characteristics of biofluids in conjunction with Gold Nanoparticles (AuNPs) has significantly changed. When moving in unsafe fluids, a fast response from AuNPs was observed. This experiment indicates that the mechanical properties of unhealthy fluids (cell intensity or elasticity module) are poor, which could explain AuNPs' rapid movement. The mechanical properties of stable and unhealthy cells in biofluids may be interesting for a more accurate description of the parameters corresponding to these circumstances.

For the analysis of biofluid samples, shape, size and surface functioning correlated with AuNPs are important factors in the biodistribution and toxicity impact. The sensitivity of the two-wave combination to classify the plasmonic response decreases through the usage of larger AuNPs but increases with the smaller AuNPs. For the experimental settings, the scale of the nanoparticles appears to be a significant effect on the signature of a sample. This is due to the increased surface-to-volume ratio of studied NPs that the development of mechanical and non-linear optical properties shown by AuNPs seems to be exacerbated [31].

A polypeptide, a protein, a nucleotide, or a tiny molecule medication could be the active ingredient. It indicates that NM can circumvent the body's defence mechanisms, lower clearance rates, prevent tissue injury through controlled drug release and improve the pharmacokinetics and biodistribution of a drug compared to traditional medicine. Liposomes, Polymer NPs, carbon nanotubes, metal NPs, and molecularly targeted NPs are some of the nanoscale components needed to make an NM. Typical polymer nanoparticles, *e.g.*, are made of a hydrophobic core and a hydrophilic shell, both of which have been coated. Polyamidoamine dendrimer was used to transport methotrexate, folic acid, and fluorescein. NPs were used as an adjuvant therapy to traditional intravenous and oral drugs to treat lung infection illness. With the help of contrast agents and high-density lipoprotein mimicking NPs.

CONCLUSION

Nanoparticles continue to be explored in various hematological diseases. Nanoparticles are able to enhance pre-diagnosis capabilities while improving treatment outcomes. In this chapter, we focused on how nanoparticles are used in Sickle Cell Anemia, High Ch, Hemophilia, and LA. Nanotherapeutic agents will continue to be the future for targeted treatment.

CONSENT FOR PUBLICATION

Not applicable.

CONFLICT OF INTEREST

The author declares no conflict of interest, financial or otherwise.

ACKNOWLEDGEMENTS

Declared none.

REFERENCES

[1]   Goorani S, Koohi MK, Morovvati H, Hassan J, Ahmeda A, Zangeneh MM. Application of natural compounds–based gold nanoparticles for the treatment of hemolytic anemia in an anemic mouse model: Formulation of a novel drug from relationship between the nanotechnology and hematology sciences. Appl Organomet Chem 2020; 34(4): e5475.
[http://dx.doi.org/10.1002/aoc.5475]

[2]   Zhang Y, Li M, Gao X, Chen Y, Liu T. Nanotechnology in cancer diagnosis: progress, challenges and opportunities. J Hematol Oncol 2019; 12(1): 137.

[http://dx.doi.org/10.1186/s13045-019-0833-3] [PMID: 31847897]

[3]   Kabiri M, Tafaghodi M, Sankian M, Sadri K, Oldenburg J. Nanomedicine and Pharmaceutical Nanotechnology. NanoMed 2017.

[4]   Ciesla B. Hematology in practice. Fa Davis 2018.

[5]   Eaton WA, Bunn HF. Treating sickle cell disease by targeting HbS polymerization. Blood 2017; 129(20): 2719-26.
[http://dx.doi.org/10.1182/blood-2017-02-765891] [PMID: 28385699]

[6]   Wood JC. Brain O_2 reserve in sickle cell disease. Blood 2019; 133(22): 2356-8.
[http://dx.doi.org/10.1182/blood-2019-04-901124] [PMID: 31147375]

[7]   Porter M. Rapid fire: Sickle cell disease. Emerg Med Clin 2018; 36(3): 567-76.
[http://dx.doi.org/10.1016/j.emc.2018.04.002] [PMID: 30037443]

[8]   Howard J. Sickle cell disease: when and how to transfuse. Hematology (Am Soc Hematol Educ Program) 2016; 2016(1): 625-31.
[http://dx.doi.org/10.1182/asheducation-2016.1.625] [PMID: 27913538]

[9]   Fitzhugh CD, Walters MC. The case for HLA-identical sibling hematopoietic stem cell transplantation in children with symptomatic sickle cell anemia. Blood Adv 2017; 1(26): 2563-7.
[http://dx.doi.org/10.1182/bloodadvances.2017007708] [PMID: 29296908]

[10]   Boadu I, Ohemeng A, Renner LA. Dietary intakes and nutritional status of children with sickle cell disease at the Princess Marie Louise Hospital, Accra - a survey. BMC Nutr 2018; 4(1): 33.
[http://dx.doi.org/10.1186/s40795-018-0241-z] [PMID: 32153894]

[11]   McGann PT, Niss O, Dong M, *et al.* Robust clinical and laboratory response to hydroxyurea using pharmacokinetically guided dosing for young children with sickle cell anemia. Am J Hematol 2019; 94(8): 871-9.
[http://dx.doi.org/10.1002/ajh.25510] [PMID: 31106898]

[12]   Lemonne N, Möckesch B, Charlot K, *et al.* Effects of hydroxyurea on blood rheology in sickle cell anemia: A two-years follow-up study. Clin Hemorheol Microcirc 2017; 67(2): 141-8.
[http://dx.doi.org/10.3233/CH-170280] [PMID: 28759962]

[13]   Singh A, Xu YJ. The cell killing mechanisms of hydroxyurea. Genes (Basel) 2016; 7(11): 99.
[http://dx.doi.org/10.3390/genes7110099] [PMID: 27869662]

[14]   Keikhaei B, Yousefi H, Bahadoram M. Hydroxyurea: clinical and hematological effects in patients with sickle cell anemia. Glob J Health Sci 2015; 8(3): 252-6.
[http://dx.doi.org/10.5539/gjhs.v8n3p252] [PMID: 26493428]

[15]   Zhang N, Wei M-Y, Ma Q. Nanomedicines: A potential treatment for blood disorder diseases. Front Bioeng Biotechnol 2019; 7: 369.
[http://dx.doi.org/10.3389/fbioe.2019.00369] [PMID: 31850329]

[16]   Telen MJ. Beyond hydroxyurea: new and old drugs in the pipeline for sickle cell disease. Blood 2016; 127(7): 810-9.
[http://dx.doi.org/10.1182/blood-2015-09-618553] [PMID: 26758919]

[17]   Deng H, Huang W, Zhang Z. Nanotechnology based CRISPR/Cas9 system delivery for genome editing: progress and prospect. Nano Res 2019; 12(10): 2437-50.
[http://dx.doi.org/10.1007/s12274-019-2465-x]

[18]   Demirci S, Leonard A, Haro-Mora JJ, Uchida N, Tisdale JF. CRISPR/Cas9 for sickle cell disease: applications, future possibilities, and challenges. Adv Exp Med Biol 2019; 1144: 37-52.
[http://dx.doi.org/10.1007/5584_2018_331] [PMID: 30715679]

[19]   Fernández-Friera L, Fuster V, López-Melgar B, *et al.* Normal LDL-cholesterol levels are associated with subclinical atherosclerosis in the absence of risk factors. J Am Coll Cardiol 2017; 70(24): 2979-91.

[http://dx.doi.org/10.1016/j.jacc.2017.10.024] [PMID: 29241485]

[20]   Pinal-Fernandez I, Casal-Dominguez M, Mammen AL. Statins: pros and cons. Med Clin (Barc) 2018; 150(10): 398-402. [English Edition].
[http://dx.doi.org/10.1016/j.medcli.2017.11.030] [PMID: 29292104]

[21]   Page MM, Watts GF. PCSK9 inhibitors - mechanisms of action. Aust Prescr 2016; 39(5): 164-7.
[http://dx.doi.org/10.18773/austprescr.2016.060] [PMID: 27789927]

[22]   Sahebkar A, Serban MC, Mikhailidis DP, *et al.* Head-to-head comparison of statins *versus* fibrates in reducing plasma fibrinogen concentrations: A systematic review and meta-analysis. Pharmacol Res 2016; 103: 236-52.
[http://dx.doi.org/10.1016/j.phrs.2015.12.001] [PMID: 26657419]

[23]   Liu J, Cai X, Pan HC, *et al.* Molecular engineering of photoacoustic performance by chalcogenide variation in conjugated polymer nanoparticles for brain vascular imaging. Small 2018; 14(13): e1703732.
[http://dx.doi.org/10.1002/smll.201703732] [PMID: 29411945]

[24]   Szebeni J, Simberg D, González-Fernández Á, Barenholz Y, Dobrovolskaia MA. Roadmap and strategy for overcoming infusion reactions to nanomedicines. Nat Nanotechnol 2018; 13(12): 1100-8.
[http://dx.doi.org/10.1038/s41565-018-0273-1] [PMID: 30348955]

[25]   Vigne J, Cabella C, Dézsi L, *et al.* Nanostructured lipid carriers accumulate in atherosclerotic plaques of ApoE$^{-/-}$ mice. Nanomedicine 2020; 25: 102157.
[http://dx.doi.org/10.1016/j.nano.2020.102157] [PMID: 31982616]

[26]   Zaree M, Sabzevari MS, Ahmadi A, Ramezanzadeh M, Bereshneh AH. Hemophilia Gene Therapy; Clinical and Molecular Aspects. J Hum Genet Genomics 2018; 2(1) ; e80764.
[http://dx.doi.org/10.5812/jhgg.80764]

[27]   Mustafa MI, Mohammed ZO, Murshed NS, Elfadol NM, Abdelmoneim AH, Hassan MA. *In Silico* Genetics revealing 5 mutations in *CEBPA* gene associated with acute myeloid leukemia. Cancer Inform 2019; 18: 1176935119870817.
[http://dx.doi.org/10.1177/1176935119870817] [PMID: 31621694]

[28]   Michlewska S, Ionov M, Szwed A, *et al.* Ruthenium dendrimers against human lymphoblastic leukemia 1301 cells. Int J Mol Sci 2020; 21(11): 4119.
[http://dx.doi.org/10.3390/ijms21114119] [PMID: 32526993]

[29]   Houshmand M, Garello F, Circosta P, *et al.* Nanocarriers as magic bullets in the treatment of leukemia. Nanomaterials (Basel) 2020; 10(2): 276.
[http://dx.doi.org/10.3390/nano10020276] [PMID: 32041219]

[30]   Peer D, Karp JM, Hong S, Farokhzad OC, Margalit R, Langer R. Nanocarriers as an emerging platform for cancer therapy. Nano-Enabled Medical Applications 2020; 61-91.
[http://dx.doi.org/10.1201/9780429399039-2]

[31]   Morales-Bonilla S, Martines-Arano H, Torres-Torres D, *et al.* Dynamic and plasmonic response exhibited by Au nanoparticles suspended in blood plasma and cerebrospinal fluids. J Mol Liq 2019; 281: 1-8.
[http://dx.doi.org/10.1016/j.molliq.2019.02.073]

[31]   Nan Z, Wei M-Y, Qiang M. Nanomedicines: A potential treatment for blood disorder diseases. Front Bioeng Biotechnol 2019; 369(7): 1-16.

CHAPTER 4

Properties and Biomedical Applications of Graphene-based Nanotechnologies

Fabeha Shafaat[1,*], Roberto Parisi[2], Arpan Dey[3], Nipun Gorantla[4] and Fahad Hassan Shah[5]

[1] *Bolton School, Chorley New Rd, Bolton BL1 4PA, United Kingdom*

[2] *Department of Medicine, Surgery and Dentistry, University of Salerno, Baronissi, Salerno*

[3] *Delhi Public School, West Bengal, India*

[4] *Marvin Ridge High School, North Carolina, United States*

[5] *Department of Biological Sciences, College of Natural Sciences, Kongju National University, Gongju 32588, Republic of Korea*

Abstract: Graphene is a 2-dimensional allotropic structure and crystalline form of carbon in which atoms of carbons are supported by sigma bonds and arranged in a hexagonal-shaped lattice. These carbon allotropes contain unpaired electrons providing them with unique physiochemical properties and are further exploited in the formation of graphene derivatives. *i.e.*, Graphene oxide and reduced graphene oxide. These graphene derivatives caused a huge revolution in nanotechnological research. The nanocomposites of graphene derivatives are employed in drug delivery, nucleic acid delivery, tissue engineering, imaging, and biosensing. This chapter is focused on discussing the physiochemical properties of graphene nanoparticles and their biomedical applications.

Keywords: Diagnostics, Drug Delivery, Graphene, Nanoparticles, Nucleic Acid Delivery, Physiochemical Properties, Tissue Engineering.

1. INTRODUCTION

Modern branches of science, like solid-state physics, organic chemistry and molecular biology, are ultimately based on the principles of quantum mechanics. While some people have pondered on the limits of the universe, others have strived to answer the fundamental question: What is everything made of? What is the smallest possible unit? All these led to the discovery of the atom and paved the way for a new science called quantum mechanics, the science of the subatomic

---

* **Corresponding author Fabeha Shafaat.**: Bolton School, Chorley New Rd, Bolton BL1 4PA, United Kingdom; E-mail: g20114@boltonschool.org.uk

world. Humans discovered the strange behavior of subatomic particles. Nothing acts like a point particle at such scales – but exhibit a wave-like behavior as well, with an intrinsic uncertainty that never allows us to simultaneously know, with certainty, its momentum and position. All these have given rise to philosophical debates and the theory of the parallel universe. But on the other hand, it has also given rise to more practical technologies as well. A question that inevitably arises at this point is whether we could manipulate the particles at that scale to create drastic results in the output. The answer is yes. This is where nanotechnology comes into play.

Nanotechnology refers to the technology dealing with the manipulation of atoms at the atomic, molecular, or supramolecular scale [1, 2]. According to the National Nanotechnology Initiative, nanotechnology is the manipulation of matter with at least one dimension sized from 1 to 100 nanometres [3, 4]. Quantum-mechanical effect becomes significant at such scales, and thus, this science is very different from the macroscopic sciences. It is one of the most promising sciences that have sprung up from researches in the physical sciences. Nanotechnology holds the promise of developing new materials, which may have an unimaginable significance in the fields of engineering, medicine, and more [5, 6].

As we move from larger to smaller scales, things become more and more complex. Modern synthetic chemistry is capable of preparing small molecules for any structure. A wide variety of useful substances, like Graphene, can be prepared this way, thus making this technology a highly important one in pharmaceuticals.

Nanomedicine refers to the field which deals with the medical applications of nanotechnology. Nanotechnology makes it possible to transport drugs to specific target cells in the body, a process known as drug delivery. This way, it can be ensured that the drug is consumed, in the right amounts, only by the target cells. This helps to minimize side effects and has great potential in medicine. Currently, complex drug delivery systems are under development.

Tissue engineering is another field where nanotechnology is applied. Tissue engineering refers to the replacement or modification of existing tissue using a combination of cells, nanoparticles, and other methods. Further research is going on to develop nanoparticles for a wide range of applications.

2. APPROACHES IN NANOTECHNOLOGY RESEARCH

There are many approaches that are used in nanotechnology research. Two major approaches are the top-down approach and the bottom-up approach [7, 8].

Simply put, top-down refers to the approach of synthesizing smaller nanoparticles/devices while using larger particles to do so. This approach seeks to miniaturize current technologies and is an easy and convenient method since the parts are patterned and built-in place. On the other hand, the bottom-up approach does the opposite. The bottom-up method seeks to arrange smaller units in more complex patterns. It is, thus, basically a self-assembly process. The ultimate achievement of the bottom-up way would be to recreate life itself; since the Urey-Miller experiment justifies, life on earth was formed due to simple units clustering together to form complex molecules [9, 10].

Both the above approaches are important and successful enough in their respective applications. Top-down approaches are good for producing structures with long-range order and for making macroscopic connections, while bottom-up approaches are suitable for assembly and establishing short-range order at nanoscale dimensions. The integration of top-down and bottom-up techniques is expected to provide the best combination of tools for nanofabrication eventually.

Researchers are optimistic enough to believe that, one day, autonomous nanobots could be inserted into the body for sensitive medical operations without having to develop any cut in the body. It is beyond doubt that nanotechnology holds the key to a better understanding of the complex biochemical processes that give rise to life. At the same time, nanoparticles may have certain unintended effects. As research in nanotoxicology suggests, the manufacture and use of nanoparticles on an industrial scale can ultimately be harmful to the environment. Thus, like all new technology, the debate whether the use of nanotechnology should be regulated or not goes on.

2.1. Graphene

Graphene is a single layer of graphite, as it is the first material that is 2D, which means that it is one layer of atoms thick. This material is an allotrope (2 or more different physical forms in which an element can exist) of carbon, and these carbon atoms are bonded in a very special way. Graphene is a layer of interlocking hexagonal rings of carbon atoms. Each carbon atom is covalently bonded to 3 others in its giant 2D structure. In 2004 at Manchester University, the scientists Andre Geim and Konstantin Novoselov obtained the crystals of Graphene by sticking sticky tape onto a graphite rock and pulled it off [11]. They viewed the piece of sticky tape under a powerful electron microscope. They were awarded the Nobel Prize in Physics 2010 "for groundbreaking experiments regarding the two-dimensional material Graphene."

2.1.1. Properties

This giant covalent structure has a formula of C, and its melting and boiling points are very high because they need to break the strong covalent bonds. Graphene is an excellent conductor of electricity and thermal energy because it has delocalised electrons that can carry the charge throughout the structure, and it's very strong due to having strong covalent bonds [12, 13]. An amazing property that Graphene has is being only one atom thick, which means that it is the lightest and the thinnest object, it's also bendable and flexible, and it's transparent. Furthermore, Graphene can take any form, which means it will have a lot of future uses [14 - 16]. The fact that it has a low density means that it can be used to make lightweight sports equipment, for example, a tennis racket. Even though the sports equipment will be light, this does not mean that it won't be strong because pieces of Graphene are incredibly strong for their mass, and Graphene is actually the most reactive form of carbon.

2.1.2. Applications

Graphene has properties that make it useful in electronics and composites. Flexible electronic displays are likely to be Graphene's first application on a huge scale. This means that it will help create new advancements in the future for the electronics industry. Moreover, Graphene could be used to make more powerful and rapid computer chips, which will aid the electronics industry, especially in making popular devices like mobile phones and tablets. Graphene's amazing only one atom thick property will allow this to be possible. Other industries that Graphene could be used in are aerospace, automotive, cookery, oil, biomedical, communication, energy stores, coatings and paint, and solar.

Due to all of Graphene's properties, it will have many useful applications in the future. Some examples include biofunctionalization with proteins, gene delivery, small molecular drug delivery, biosensing and bioimaging, cancer treatment, antibacterial effects, differentiation of stem cells and scaffolds for mammalian cell culture, bone and teeth implantation [17], absorbing radioactive compounds, which would be really useful in medical equipment, and due to many of the above, improved medical treatments.

3. MATHEMATICAL ANALYSIS OF GRAPHENE'S STRUCTURE AND APPLICATIONS IN NANOTECHNOLOGY

For one to truly understand the potential applications of Graphene in the nanotechnological aspect, there must be a close examination of the structure of

Graphene, including the mathematical framework which the structure of Graphene is composed of. Graphene itself is composed of a thick atom sheet of graphite and has been regularly praised for its intrinsic structure, which provides the potential to essentially reform the age of nanotechnology and further advancement and modernization of the field. Indeed, this two-dimensional (2D) material's properties fundamentally depend on its shape and the characterizations of this shape which allows us to utilize it in such advanced nanotechnology [18]. To understand the shape of Graphene and to derive a basic understanding of the molecular web, this material forms that allow us to make generalizations about its functions in order to apply it to function in the nanotechnology field, a mathematical framework known as discrete differential geometry is being used [19, 20]. Using this mathematical model, an individual will be able to fully grasp the functionalities of Graphene's morphology and electronic properties, which ultimately results in successful functionalization in the nanotechnology perspective.

Graphene's fundamental properties consist of elastic membranes which are atom-thin, a tendency to conform to hard surfaces, and the ability to be deconstructed into regimes that can then be utilized in order to operationalize an electric response [13, 19]. This electric response is the most sought-after property needed in the utilization of nanotechnology. Throughout the remainder of this section, the properties of Graphene will be observed, explained, and modeled through a primarily mathematical perspective.

3.1. Electrical Properties

For the passage of electrical properties in Graphene, one critical functionality and property of Graphene must be considered: gate dependence in single layer Graphene. Gate dependency in single layer Graphene can be defined as the electrical resistance of a single layer of Graphene in conflict with the gate voltage seen in this single layer of Graphene. This gate dependence effect can be seen as a result of the thinnest Graphene samples. The samples from numerous other layers portray the weak gate dependence due to the isolation of this electric field by other layers in the Graphene. Indeed, the resistivity proves the high rate of conductivity in the Graphene element and the astounding mobility of Graphene under low temperatures and high magnetic fields, as the Graphene quantum hall effect is seen under these conditions [15, 21 - 23]. The Quantum Hall effect can be primarily defined as the movement of charge carriers through conductors towards a magnetic attraction [24, 25]. However, in the case of Graphene, the quantum hall effect in the element shows a difference from the conventional and disciplined effects that are exhibited in the elements. This primary difference is that the plateaus in the Hall effect occur at half integers of $4e^2/h$ rather than the same typical variables. This is due to the unique band structure of Graphene. In nanotechnology, this electrical property is utilized through a rather resourceful method: the carving of Graphene into narrow ribbons that allows the momentum of the charge carriers in the oblique current to become discrete, which allows for the opening of a gap between the bands. These gap bands are primarily proportional to the width of a ribbon, which is similarly seen in the effect of carbon nanotubes, in which the nanotube has a proportional gap to the diameter of the tube.

3.2. Mechanical Properties

Graphene is an especially unique substance to utilize for nanotechnology because the elastic constants in perpendicular current are very divergent from the elastic constants along the elementary plane. A set of six equations can be utilized to functionalize the strain of a hexagonal lattice shape, such as in graphite, where the axes are parallel to the basal plane, e is strain, T is stress and S is compliance [26].

$$e_{xx} = S_{11}T_{XX} + S_{12}T_{XY} + S_{13}T_{ZZ}$$

$$e_{YY} = S_{12}T_{XX} + S_{11}T_{XY} + S_{13}T_{ZZ}$$

$$e_{ZZ} = S_{13}T_{XX} + S_{13}T_{YY} + S_{13}T_{ZZ}$$

$$e_{zz} = S_{44} + T_{zx}$$
$$e_{zy} = S_{44}T_{zy}$$
$$e_{xy} = \frac{1}{2}(S_{11} - S_{12})T_{xy}$$

The inverses can be found below, where C is the elastic modulus:

$$T_{xx} = C_{11}e_{xx} + C_{12}e_{xy} + C_{13}e_{zz}$$
$$T_{YY} = C_{12}e_{xx} + C_{11}e_{yy} + C_{13}e_{zz}$$
$$T_{zz} = C_{13}e_{xx} + C_{13}e_{yy} + C_{33}e_{zz}$$
$$T_{zx} = C_{44}e_{xx} + e_{zx}$$
$$T_{zy} = C_{44}e_{zy}$$
$$T_{xy} = \frac{1}{2}(C_{11} - C_{12})e_{xy}$$

The experimental procedures for measuring the value of C and S are acoustic wave propagation and flexural vibrations, respectively.

Through solving these equations, the relations between S and C can be derived as follows:

$$C_{44} = (S_{44})^{-1}$$

$$(C_{11} - C_{12}) = (S_{11} - S_{12})^{-1}$$

$$\frac{C_{13}}{X} = -S_{13}$$

$$\frac{C_{33}}{X} = S_{11} + S_{12}$$

$$\frac{C_{11} + C_{12}}{X} = S_{33}$$

where $X = C_{33} (C_{11}+C_{12}) - 2 (C_{13})^2 = [S_{33}(S_{11}+S_{12}) - 2 (S_{13})^2]^{-1}$

The Young's Modulus is a mechanical property that works to measure the stiffness of a certain material. In this case, the stiffness of the material Graphene can be functionalized to the basal plane both parallelly and perpendicularly. The Young's modulus to the basal plane parallelly is $1/S_{11}$ and to the basal plane perpendicularly is $1/S_{33}$. To determine the elastic properties of a certain material, we can utilize the Shear Modulus, which is the numerical constant that describes the elastic properties of a solid under the application of internal forces. The Shear Modulus for Graphene parallel to basal planes can be denoted as $G = \frac{1}{S_{44}} = C_{44}$. Furthermore, the Poisson's Ratio along the basal plane of graphite can be used in order to calculate the ratio of transverse contraction strain to longitudinal extension strain in the direction of the stretching force. The Poisson's Ratio along the basal plane of graphite is denoted as $v = -S_{12}/S_{11}$.

3.3. Fabrication and Measuring of Quasi 2-D Graphite Quantum Dots

By conducting resistivity measurements and extraction of carrier densities of 2-6 x 10^{11} holes per sheet in open dots devices, Bunch and colleagues observed the existence of Coulomb charging and blockade phenomena, which can be defined as the decreased electrical conductance at small bias voltages in small electronic devices. In this phenomenon, the device no longer functions in the currents of Ohm's Law, and instead, the relation between current and voltage in the blockade looks more like a staircase. An Atomic-Force Microscopy image of the device was fabricated using electrode methodology. White rectangular outlines represented the electrodes' size and position and proved the existence of Coulomb blockade oscillations seen in electrical activity [27].

4. BIOMEDICAL APPLICATIONS OF GRAPHENE AND ITS DERIVATIVES

4.1. Anticancer and Biological Activity

There is strong evidence in the literature of some cytotoxic effects caused by Graphene and its derivates. In human skin keratinocytes [28], long-term exposure to low doses (0.1 µg/L) of GO or FLG (Few Layers Graphene) may cause the onset of mild mitochondrial and plasma membrane damages, although there is no evidence of a reduction in cell proliferation. The process of mitochondrial damaging, after determining the inefficacy of cyclosporin-A, seems not to be dependent on the formation of the transition pore but the synthesis of ROS [29], consequently to the activation of NADH dehydrogenase and xanthine oxidase. Weakly oxidized GO may be cytotoxic for erythrocytes because of the sorption on their membranes, but it has been demonstrated that at low doses (~70 µg/L), the increase in the blood microviscosity is statistically insignificant [30].

4.2. Drug Administration

Today researchers are trying to develop biocompatible and non-toxic Graphene-based carriers in order to release specific drugs only in some predetermined regions in the human body. A typical artificial modification on Graphene oxide is PEGylation, which adds branches of polyethylene glycol (PEG), also called PEG stars. The interactions of PEG with GO are stabilized due to the reaction between carboxylic groups on Graphene and the alcohol group present on the glycol [31]. It has been demonstrated that nGO-PEG (PEGylated – nanometric Graphene oxide) tends not to be destroyed by the human reticuloendothelial system and, consequently, its time of action in the body is longer than similar nanotechnological carriers [32]. An actual application of nanometric GO is the synthesis of carriers capable of releasing insoluble aromatic anticancer drugs [33], although there is evidence that its relatively strong rigidity may represent an obstacle for the release of the desired substances into the cells [34].

A variation on the theme is nGO-SS-mPEG, a nanometric Graphene oxide that owns disulfide bridges that interact with PEG molecules. This carrier has been used to vehiculate doxorubicin, a chemotherapeutic drug, into cancer cells [35]. When DXR-nGO-SS-mPEG enters cancerous cells, the intracellular glutathione, whose levels vary depending on the specific type of tumor [36], eliminates the interactions between PEG and the Graphene-based carrier, leading to the fast release of doxorubicin in the cell. A similar process was used to create Pt-DX--nGO-PEG carriers [37], characterized by the presence of cisplatin and doxorubicin with a ratio DXR:Pt:nGO equal to 0.376:0.376:1. PEGylation was conducted with 4-arm PEG amines and cisplatin was made reactive thanks to its modification with hydrogen peroxide and succinic anhydride. In the last step, DXR has been added thanks to the π-π stacking between the structure of Graphene oxide and the quinone part of the anticancer drug. The results showed faster and more effective cell apoptosis and necrosis (18.6%), two times higher than Pt-NGO and DXR-nGO.

Chitosan (CS), a cationic linear polysaccharide, is also used to increase the biocompatibility and solubility of GO-based nanocarriers. The synthesis of CS-GO relies on the production of amide linkage during an intermediate chemical state stabilized by the adding of EDC and NHS [38]. Bao *et al.* described the creation of a GO-CS-CPT, that is a nanocarrier transporting camptothecin, a strong topoisomerase inhibitor with anticancer properties. This complex showed a good therapeutic action in HeLa cells compared to free CPT (at 29 μM, the growth inhibition was 50% vs. 20%). The same research group reported the stabilization of plasmid DNA, a useful tool to conduct gene therapy. The same chemical compound, EDC, has been used to attach Fe_3O_4 nanoparticles through amide bonds. The carrier, described by Fan *et al.* (2013), was used to transport 5-fluorouracil (FU), and it showed a strong pH dependence in HepG2 cells [39].

4.3. Gene Delivery

Usually, to increase the ability to link and then deliver genes, Graphene-based nanotechnologies should own cationic elements in their structures because they can interact with the anionic backbone of nucleic acids.

A GO-based carrier was developed to efficiently deliver genes thanks to the modification induced by adding branched polyethylenimine (BPEI), already used as a non-viral gene vector [40]. The conjugation was conducted with a covalent interaction with the carboxylic groups on the GO. The ratio BPEI:GO in the synthetized carrier was about 22. It was also noticed that GO derivates enriched with negative structure have more colloidal stability thanks to intramolecular repulsions. The research investigated the adding of double-strand pDNA to the carrier event that occurred thanks to the interaction between the negatively-charged DNA backbone and the positively-charged GO surface because of the presence of BPEI. The ability to deliver genes was studied in HeLa and PC-3 cultures with the luciferase gene expression assay and it showed the strong gene transfection ability of BPEI-GO22.

Another study described the synthesis of R8-GO (octaarginine Graphene oxide), whose ability to transfect genes was studied by investigating the expression of the green fluorescent protein in HEK293 cells, coded in the pDNA carried by the novel nanotechnological vector [41]. After an amidation process, the R8 peptide was linked to the GO support and the electrophoretic assays showed that the highest DNA loading happens at R8:GO ratios of 0.5 and 1 μmol/mg. An excessive quantity of R8 peptide may determine the onset of inter-particle crosslinking with a consequent molecular instability of the nanocarrier. The cytotoxic assay, conducted on L929 fibroblast cells, showed that the reduction in cell viability after the addition of the carrier was not statistically significant compared to the non-treated control group.

Pramod *et al.* (2019) reported the synthesis of a novel C-dot-PEG-pDNA--NF-α-CS-CGO, obtained through several chemical processes [42]. The pDNA-TNF-α complex was implemented on CS-CGO, that is chitosan-carboxylated Graphene oxide; then, in order to protect nanocarriers from the attack of the immune system and, consequently, increasing its circulation half-life, the molecular surface was engineered with the adding of 4,7,10-trioxa-1,-3-tridecanediamine, a diamine PEG, followed by the insertion of folic acid derived C-dots, fundamentally because of their interaction with folate receptors often overexpressed by tumor cells. The effective bond with pDNA happened when the CS:CGO ratio was about 5:1 or 10:1. In fact, using a 1:1 ratio, the electrophoretic assays showed migration of free DNA. An artificial tumor cell apparatus was used to evaluate the efficacy of the developed nanocarrier, showing a strong ability to target cancer cells and transfecting them with the carried nucleic acids.

In a study conducted by Li *et al.* (2017), HDAC1 and K-Ras were chosen as targets for a siRNA-mediated knockdown to treat pancreatic cancer [43]. Because of siRNA instability after injection in vivo, the nucleic acid was complexed with a GO support as a delivery system to target the pancreas. GO nanosheets were conjugated with folic acid, PEG and PAH (poly-allylamine hydrochloride) and then HDAC1 and K-Ras siRNAs were installed in the final structure. *in vitro* MIA PaCa-2 cell cultures were treated with the novel carrier and a reduction in cell proliferation greater than 80% was observed. Also, similar results were described in vivo thanks to the synergy between gene therapy and phototermal activity after the application of external NIR rays. The best mass ratio between FA-GO and siRNa was 1 µg:1 µg. In the cancer context, it is indispensable to underline the possibility of using GO nanoparticles to enhance photodynamic therapies. It has been demonstrated that PEG-GO, enriched with chlorine e6 may be used to improve cancer cell photodynamic destruction [44].

It is important to underline the efficacy of Graphene-mediated gene therapy in tissue engineering. A paradigmatic example is research completed by Khademhosseini *et al.* (2014), who developed a Graphene-based hydrogel in order to vehiculate VEGF-165 gene for myocardial regeneration [45]. A methacrylated gelatin was enriched with PEI-GO, charged with the VEGF gene. Results *in vitro* showed an increase in the proliferation of cardiac endothelial cells. Another important result of the research was the non-statistical significance of an increase in cytokine levels, showing that the new carrier did not boost inflammatory responses directed towards the carrier in the heart. Thanks to its properties, a PEI-GO enriched gelatin may be used as a gene delivery system to partially recover ischemic hearts.

4.4. Tissue Engineering

Bone tissue is prone to be damaged in conditions of cancer surgery, infections, and fractures, and it briefly consists of an initial cartilaginous coagulum followed by a temporary callous made by osteoblasts. Then the activation of osteoclasts starts the tissue re-modelling.

Classical protocols to induce the regeneration of the bone tissue include the application of collagen to create a molecular platform where new cells can grow and differentiate, regenerating the damaged bone tissue. Even with its potential, it has been demonstrated that this polymer may be responsible for the onset of an immune response in the human body [46].

Graphene oxide, combined with Ti atoms, has been tested [47] in rodents to address morphogenetic bone cells and substance P factors. The results showed that it could represent a material with optimal structural characteristics to induce and ameliorate the cellular differentiation of the osteogenic stem cells.

Graphene-based scaffolds may be implemented in liver tissue engineering to generate 3D structure mimicking the hepatic vascular architecture, a potential platform where cultured cells may proliferate. It has also been demonstrated that a co-culture with human fibroblasts may avoid the de-differentiation of hepatocytes, keeping fundamental anatomical structures like the canalicular system, and boost their ability to produce albumin [49]. Although its potential, there is still little research in hepatic tissue regeneration because there are some concerns about its biocompatibility, cytotoxicity, and clearance [48].

Graphene sheets have been used to stimulate the differentiation of induced cardiomyocytic stem cells (hiPSC-CMs) [50]. Its conductive and biomimetic structure led to cellular differentiation, increasing the myofibrillar 3D organization and the conduction velocity, a parameter correlated with the expression of connexin-43 on the Graphene layer. Also, scaffolds made of 0.01% Graphene and 15% poly-caprolactone have been designed *via* electrospinning, avoiding the conductive nanoparticles' agglomeration to create a conductive material used for cardiac tissue engineering with an external electrical stimulation [51]. The use of a low dose of Graphene correlated with its biocompatibility in the research and a point stimulation mimicked the activation of the cardiac impulse generated by the sinoatrial node.

Although purified Graphene can induce synaptogenesis in human brain cells, G-sheets are incapable of mimicking the neural environment because of the inert properties of pristine Graphene. It has been demonstrated that the use of ginseng-reduced GO, obtained by the attachment of flavanones and ginsenosides to the sheet surface, is fundamental to neuronal growth and differentiation *in vitro* [52]. Using poly-caprolactone with different doses of Graphene, several nanofibers have been developed to stimulate the differentiation of oligodendrocytes thanks to the cross-talking between neural stem cells and conductive Graphene-based nanomaterials [53].

To heal poorly regenerative skin wounds, tissue engineers usually use cell-derived ECMs that have less regenerative properties than tissue-derived ECM scaffolds. For this reason, Chuang *et al.* (2018) have generated a new ECM derived from adipose tissue and enriched it with Graphene oxide and genipin [54]. Thanks to a murine experimental model, fabricated ECMs with a medium amount of GO can be correctly excreted from the body, showing good biodegradability, and can induce lower inflammatory responses. It can be potentially used as a skin substitute and for the healing of the anterior cruciate ligament.

4.5. Imaging and Biosensing

In the last decades, much effort was made to implement Graphene derivates in the bioimaging field. The creation of novel contrast agents (CAs) and MRI seems to be the most important application for this material.

Gadolinium has been used to enrich planar GO nanosheets (GONSs) with DTPA(diethylenetriaminepentaacetic acid), which functioned as a chelator [55]. Graphene was firstly converted in GO and then reduced to r-GO-. Therefore, the resulting molecules were functionalized thanks to the adding of DTPA. Finally, chelation occurs between DTPA and gadolinium ions Gd^{3+}. The novel contrast agent was reported not to be toxic, and the Gd-rGONSs showed an increase in the effective surface area. The relaxivity r1 for Gd-rGONSs is about 16.85 mM-1s-1.

Usually, pure gadolinium is used as ions Gd^{3+} in the bioimaging field, and it can be useful for T1 imaging in MRI. Anyway, the chronic use of this lanthanide may increase the risk of the onset of systemic nephrogenic fibrosis [56, 57].

Other GO materials are harmless for the human body in bioimaging, like the studied combination of GO, manganese ions and dextran with a Graphene concentration between 10^{-1} and 10^{-2} mg/mL [58]. This substance has the same osmolarity and viscosity as human blood, and it can easily be used as a contrast agent with an intravenous injection.

Thanks to their large surface, good conductive properties, and a propension to link other molecules through chemical and physical interactions, many Graphene-based substances can be used [59] in the biosensing field to perceive several biomolecules like ATP, oligonucleotides, dopamine, and numerous amino acids. Electrochemical sensors based on Graphene have been developed in order to determine the presence, in a longer DNA sequence, of specific bases or mutations and similar structures improved the amperometric signals coming from the glucose detection. The application of Graphene for glucose biosensing may be fundamental in the future to develop new strategies to continuously control the glycemic levels in patients suffering from conditions like diabetes. Some sensors were reported to detect dopamine [60], a catecholamine deriving from the amino acid tyrosine. According to the perceived levels, serious pathologies like Parkinson's disease and schizophrenia may be diagnosed because the first disease is strongly correlated to the destruction of neural circuits releasing dopamine, while the second condition is linked to an excessive release of dopamine.

CONCLUSION

Graphene-based nanoparticles have shown promising results in different areas of nanotechnological research. It is now gradually being exploited in biomedical sciences, and its role is being thoroughly assessed in drug and gene delivery, fluorescence-based biosensing and imaging, along with tissue regeneration. To our current knowledge, almost every nanoparticle has been exploited in stem and regenerative medicine, gene therapy, antimicrobials delivery to minimize drug resistance, cell culturing scaffolds and molecular biology. However, these Graphene-based nanotechnologies are lacking behind in these leading fields. This is because of their toxicity profile; different studies have shown that Graphene-based nanoparticles show high toxicity and inflict adverse immunological effects, which might be one of the hindrances why they are not openly utilized [17]. Therefore, further studies are of imminent necessity to address the toxicity of these Graphene nanocomposites without jeopardising their physiochemical properties. Nanoparticles of Graphene have shown great promise in semiconductors and biomedical research. Still, their role needs to be further assessed in other fields of science to ameliorate technological and economic development.

CONSENT FOR PUBLICATION

Not applicable.

CONFLICT OF INTEREST

The author declares no conflict of interest, financial or otherwise.

ACKNOWLEDGEMENTS

Ms. Saritha, and Mr. Ramana for their expertise and undying support throughout writing this book chapter.

REFERENCES

[1]   Vance ME, Kuiken T, Vejerano EP, *et al.* Nanotechnology in the real world: Redeveloping the nanomaterial consumer products inventory. Beilstein J Nanotechnol 2015; 6(1): 1769-80.
        [http://dx.doi.org/10.3762/bjnano.6.181] [PMID: 26425429]

[2]   Grzybowski BA, Huck WTS. The nanotechnology of life-inspired systems. Nat Nanotechnol 2016; 11(7): 585-92.
        [http://dx.doi.org/10.1038/nnano.2016.116] [PMID: 27380745]

[3]   Dong H, Gao Y, Sinko PJ, Wu Z, Xu J, Jia L. The nanotechnology race between China and the United States. Nano Today 2016; 11(1): 7-12.
        [http://dx.doi.org/10.1016/j.nantod.2016.02.001]

[4]   Bhardwaj V, Kaushik A. Biomedical applications of nanotechnology and nanomaterials. Micromachines (Basel) 2017; 8(10): E298.
        [http://dx.doi.org/10.3390/mi8100298] [PMID: 30400488]

[5]   Heath JR. Nanotechnologies for biomedical science and translational medicine. Proc Natl Acad Sci 2015; 112(47): 14436-43.
        [http://dx.doi.org/10.1073/pnas.1515202112]

[6]   Porter AL, Garner J, Newman NC, Carley SF, Youtie J, Kwon S, *et al.* National nanotechnology research prominence. Technol Anal Strateg Manage 2019; 31(1): 25-39.

[http://dx.doi.org/10.1080/09537325.2018.1480013]

[7]   Zhou J, Shen L, Costa MD, *et al.* 2DMatPedia, an open computational database of two-dimensional materials from top-down and bottom-up approaches. Sci Data 2019; 6(1): 86.
[http://dx.doi.org/10.1038/s41597-019-0097-3] [PMID: 31189922]

[8]   Connon CJ. Approaches to corneal tissue engineering: top-down or bottom-up? Procedia Eng 2015; 110: 15-20.
[http://dx.doi.org/10.1016/j.proeng.2015.07.004]

[9]   Dick SJ. The biological universe revisited BT - space, time, and aliens: collected works on cosmos and culture. In: Dick SJ. Cham: Springer International Publishing 2020; pp. 59-69.

[10]   Neupane C. Urey-Miller Experiment: Route to the Origin of Life; an Astrobiologist Prospective.

[11]   Ball P. When graphene goes strange. Nat Mater 2020; 19(4): 368.
[http://dx.doi.org/10.1038/s41563-020-0653-4] [PMID: 32210399]

[12]   Akinwande D, Brennan CJ, Bunch JS, *et al.* A review on mechanics and mechanical properties of 2D materials-Graphene and beyond. Extreme Mech Lett 2017; 13: 42-77.
[http://dx.doi.org/10.1016/j.eml.2017.01.008]

[13]   Atif R, Shyha I, Inam F. Mechanical, Thermal, and Electrical Properties of Graphene-Epoxy Nanocomposites-A Review. Vol. 8. Polymers (Basel) 2016.
[http://dx.doi.org/10.3390/polym8080281]

[14]   Fang Q, Shen Y, Chen B. Synthesis, decoration and properties of three-dimensional graphene-based macrostructures: A review. Chem Eng J 2015; 264: 753-71.
[http://dx.doi.org/10.1016/j.cej.2014.12.001]

[15]   Liu L, Qing M, Wang Y, Chen S. Defects in graphene: generation, healing, and their effects on the properties of graphene: A review. J Mater Sci Technol 2015; 31(6): 599-606.
[http://dx.doi.org/10.1016/j.jmst.2014.11.019]

[16]   Ji X, Xu Y, Zhang W, Cui L, Liu J. Review of functionalization, structure and properties of graphene/polymer composite fibers. Compos, Part A Appl Sci Manuf 2016; 87: 29-45.
[http://dx.doi.org/10.1016/j.compositesa.2016.04.011]

[17]   Priyadarsini S, Mohanty S, Mukherjee S, Basu S, Mishra M. Graphene and graphene oxide as nanomaterials for medicine and biology application. J Nanostructure Chem 2018; 8(2): 123-37.
[http://dx.doi.org/10.1007/s40097-018-0265-6]

[18]   Naumis GG, Barraza-Lopez S, Oliva-Leyva M, Terrones H. Electronic and optical properties of strained graphene and other strained 2D materials: a review. Rep Prog Phys 2017; 80(9): 096501.
[http://dx.doi.org/10.1088/1361-6633/aa74ef] [PMID: 28540862]

[19]   Sanjuan AAP, Wang Z, Imani HP, Vanević M, Barraza-Lopez S. Graphene's morphology and electronic properties from discrete differential geometry. Phys Rev B Condens Matter Mater Phys 2014; 89(12): 121403.
[http://dx.doi.org/10.1103/PhysRevB.89.121403]

[20]   Barraza-Lopez S. Discrete differential geometry and the properties of conformal two-dimensional materials. Synth Met 2015; 210: 32-41.
[http://dx.doi.org/10.1016/j.synthmet.2015.06.025]

[21]   Ghuge AD, Shirode AR, Kadam VJ. Graphene: A Comprehensive Review. Curr Drug Targets 2017; 18(6): 724-33.
[http://dx.doi.org/10.2174/1389450117666160709023425] [PMID: 27397067]

[22]   Ke Q, Wang J. Graphene-based materials for supercapacitor electrodes – A review. J Mater 2016; 2(1): 37-54.

[23]   Meng F, Lu W, Li Q, Byun J-H, Oh Y, Chou T-W. Graphene-based fibers: A review. Adv Mater 2015; 27(35): 5113-31.

[http://dx.doi.org/10.1002/adma.201501126] [PMID: 26248041]

[24] McIver JW, Schulte B, Stein F-U, *et al.* Light-induced anomalous Hall effect in graphene. Nat Phys 2020; 16(1): 38-41.
[http://dx.doi.org/10.1038/s41567-019-0698-y] [PMID: 31915458]

[25] Wang L, Gao Y, Wen B, Han Z, Taniguchi T, Watanabe K, *et al.* Evidence for a fractional fractal quantum Hall effect in graphene superlattices. Science (80-) 2015; 350(6265): 1231-4.
[http://dx.doi.org/10.1126/science.aad2102]

[26] Kelly BT. Outstanding problems in the bonding of the graphite lattice and the theory of the thermal properties of graphite. High Temp High Press 1981; 13(3): 245-50.

[27] Bunch JS, Yaish Y, Brink M, Bolotin K, McEuen PL. Coulomb oscillations and Hall effect in quasi-2D graphite quantum dots. Nano Lett 2005; 5(2): 287-90.
[http://dx.doi.org/10.1021/nl048111+] [PMID: 15794612]

[28] Pelin M, Fusco L, León V, *et al.* Differential cytotoxic effects of graphene and graphene oxide on skin keratinocytes. Sci Rep 2017; 7(1): 40572.
[http://dx.doi.org/10.1038/srep40572] [PMID: 28079192]

[29] Pelin M, Fusco L, Martín C, *et al.* Graphene and graphene oxide induce ROS production in human HaCaT skin keratinocytes: the role of xanthine oxidase and NADH dehydrogenase. Nanoscale 2018; 10(25): 11820-30.
[http://dx.doi.org/10.1039/C8NR02933D] [PMID: 29920573]

[30] Karachevtsev VA, Kartel NT, Ivanov LV, *et al.* Change in the microviscosity of erythrocyte membranes and proteins in blood plasma after graphene oxide addition: The ESR spectroscopy study. J Spectrosc. 2019; 2019: pp. (3)1-8.

[31] Liu J, Cui L, Losic D. Graphene and graphene oxide as new nanocarriers for drug delivery applications. Acta Biomater 2013; 9(12): 9243-57.
[http://dx.doi.org/10.1016/j.actbio.2013.08.016] [PMID: 23958782]

[32] Liao C, Li Y, Tjong SC. Graphene nanomaterials: synthesis, biocompatibility, and cytotoxicity. Vol. 19. Int J Mol Sci 2018.
[http://dx.doi.org/10.3390/ijms19113564]

[33] Liu Z, Robinson JT, Sun X, Dai H. PEGylated nanographene oxide for delivery of water-insoluble cancer drugs. J Am Chem Soc 2008; 130(33): 10876-7.
[http://dx.doi.org/10.1021/ja803688x] [PMID: 18661992]

[34] Wu S-Y, An SSA, Hulme J. Current applications of graphene oxide in nanomedicine. Int J Nanomedicine 2015; 9-24.

[35] Theodosopoulos GV, Bilalis P, Sakellariou G. Polymer functionalized graphene oxide: A versatile nanoplatform for drug/gene delivery. Curr Org Chem 2015; 19: 1828-37.
[http://dx.doi.org/10.2174/1385272819666150526005714]

[36] Gamcsik MP, Kasibhatla MS, Teeter SD, Colvin OM. Glutathione levels in human tumors. Biomarkers 2012; 17(8): 671-91.
[http://dx.doi.org/10.3109/1354750X.2012.715672] [PMID: 22900535]

[37] Pei X, Zhu Z, Gan Z, *et al.* PEGylated nano-graphene oxide as a nanocarrier for delivering mixed anticancer drugs to improve anticancer activity. Sci Rep 2020; 10(1): 2717.
[http://dx.doi.org/10.1038/s41598-020-59624-w] [PMID: 32066812]

[38] Bao H, Pan Y, Ping Y, *et al.* Chitosan-functionalized graphene oxide as a nanocarrier for drug and gene delivery. Small 2011; 7(11): 1569-78.
[http://dx.doi.org/10.1002/smll.201100191] [PMID: 21538871]

[39] Fan X, Jiao G, Zhao W, Jin P, Li X. Magnetic Fe3O4-graphene composites as targeted drug nanocarriers for pH-activated release. Nanoscale 2013; 5(3): 1143-52.

[http://dx.doi.org/10.1039/c2nr33158f] [PMID: 23288110]

[40]   Kim H, Namgung R, Singha K, Oh I-K, Kim WJ. Graphene oxide-polyethylenimine nanoconstruct as a gene delivery vector and bioimaging tool. Bioconjug Chem 2011; 22(12): 2558-67.
[http://dx.doi.org/10.1021/bc200397j] [PMID: 22034966]

[41]   Imani R, Emami SH, Faghihi S. Synthesis and characterization of an octaarginine functionalized graphene oxide nano-carrier for gene delivery applications. Phys Chem Chem Phys 2015; 17(9): 6328-39.
[http://dx.doi.org/10.1039/C4CP04301D] [PMID: 25650242]

[42]   Jaleel JA, Ashraf SM, Rathinasamy K, Pramod K. Carbon dot festooned and surface passivated graphene-reinforced chitosan construct for tumor-targeted delivery of TNF-α gene. Int J Biol Macromol 2019; 127: 628-36.
[http://dx.doi.org/10.1016/j.ijbiomac.2019.01.174] [PMID: 30708020]

[43]   Yin F, Hu K, Chen Y, *et al.* SiRNA delivery with PEGylated graphene oxide nanosheets for combined photothermal and genetherapy for pancreatic cancer. Theranostics 2017; 7(5): 1133-48.
[http://dx.doi.org/10.7150/thno.17841] [PMID: 28435453]

[44]   Tian B, Wang C, Zhang S, Feng L, Liu Z. Photothermally enhanced photodynamic therapy delivered by nano-graphene oxide. ACS Nano 2011; 5(9): 7000-9.
[http://dx.doi.org/10.1021/nn201560b] [PMID: 21815655]

[45]   Paul A, Hasan A, Kindi HA, *et al.* Injectable graphene oxide/hydrogel-based angiogenic gene delivery system for vasculogenesis and cardiac repair. ACS Nano 2014; 8(8): 8050-62.
[http://dx.doi.org/10.1021/nn5020787] [PMID: 24988275]

[46]   El-Fiqi A, Lee JH, Lee E-J, Kim H-W. Collagen hydrogels incorporated with surface-aminated mesoporous nanobioactive glass: Improvement of physicochemical stability and mechanical properties is effective for hard tissue engineering. Acta Biomater 2013; 9(12): 9508-21.
[http://dx.doi.org/10.1016/j.actbio.2013.07.036] [PMID: 23928332]

[47]   Feng L, Liu Z. Graphene in biomedicine: opportunities and challenges. Nanomedicine (Lond) 2011; 6(2): 317-24.
[http://dx.doi.org/10.2217/nnm.10.158] [PMID: 21385134]

[48]   Geetha Bai R, Muthoosamy K, Manickam S, Hilal-Alnaqbi A. Graphene-based 3D scaffolds in tissue engineering: fabrication, applications, and future scope in liver tissue engineering. Int J Nanomedicine 2019; 14: 5753-83.
[http://dx.doi.org/10.2147/IJN.S192779] [PMID: 31413573]

[49]   Bhandari RNB, Riccalton LA, Lewis AL, *et al.* Liver tissue engineering: a role for co-culture systems in modifying hepatocyte function and viability. Tissue Eng 2001; 7(3): 345-57.
[http://dx.doi.org/10.1089/10763270152044206] [PMID: 11429154]

[50]   Wang J, Cui C, Nan H, *et al.* Graphene sheet-induced global maturation of cardiomyocytes derived from human induced pluripotent stem cells. ACS Appl Mater Interfaces 2017; 9(31): 25929-40.
[http://dx.doi.org/10.1021/acsami.7b08777] [PMID: 28718622]

[51]   Hitscherich P, Aphale A, Gordan R, *et al.* Electroactive graphene composite scaffolds for cardiac tissue engineering. J Biomed Mater Res A 2018; 106(11): 2923-33.
[http://dx.doi.org/10.1002/jbm.a.36481] [PMID: 30325093]

[52]   Akhavan O, Ghaderi E, Abouei E, Hatamie S, Ghasemi E. Accelerated differentiation of neural stem cells into neurons on ginseng-reduced graphene oxide sheets. Carbon N Y 2014; 66: 395-406.
[http://dx.doi.org/10.1016/j.carbon.2013.09.015]

[53]   Jakus AE, Secor EB, Rutz AL, Jordan SW, Hersam MC, Shah RN. Three-dimensional printing of high-content graphene scaffolds for electronic and biomedical applications. ACS Nano 2015; 9(4): 4636-48.
[http://dx.doi.org/10.1021/acsnano.5b01179] [PMID: 25858670]

[54]   Nyambat B, Chen C-H, Wong P-C, Chiang C-W, Satapathy MK, Chuang E-Y. Genipin-crosslinked adipose stem cell derived extracellular matrix-nano graphene oxide composite sponge for skin tissue engineering. J Mater Chem B Mater Biol Med 2018; 6(6): 979-90.
[http://dx.doi.org/10.1039/C7TB02480K] [PMID: 32254378]

[55]   Chawda N, Basu M, Majumdar D, Poddar R, Mahapatra SK, Banerjee I. Engineering of gadolinium-decorated graphene oxide nanosheets for multimodal bioimaging and drug delivery. ACS Omega 2019; 4(7): 12470-9.
[http://dx.doi.org/10.1021/acsomega.9b00883] [PMID: 31460366]

[56]   Sánchez JT. Fibrosis sistémica nefrogénica y gadolinio. Piel 2008; 23(7): 333-4.
[http://dx.doi.org/10.1016/S0213-9251(08)72299-8]

[57]   Moschella SL, Kay J, Mackool BT, Liu V. Case records of the Massachusetts General Hospital. Weekly clinicopathological exercises. Case 35-2004. A 68-year-old man with end-stage renal disease and thickening of the skin. N Engl J Med 2004; 351(21): 2219-27.
[http://dx.doi.org/10.1056/NEJMcpc049026] [PMID: 15548783]

[58]   Kanakia S, Toussaint JD, Chowdhury SM, *et al.* Physicochemical characterization of a novel graphene-based magnetic resonance imaging contrast agent. Int J Nanomedicine 2013; 8: 2821-33.
[PMID: 23946653]

[59]   Wang Y, Li Z, Wang J, Li J, Lin Y. Graphene and graphene oxide: biofunctionalization and applications in biotechnology. Trends Biotechnol 2011; 29(5): 205-12.
[http://dx.doi.org/10.1016/j.tibtech.2011.01.008] [PMID: 21397350]

[60]   Wang Y, Li Y, Tang L, Lu J, Li J. Application of graphene-modified electrode for selective detection of dopamine. Electrochem Commun 2009; 11(4): 889-92.
[http://dx.doi.org/10.1016/j.elecom.2009.02.013]

CHAPTER 5

Nanotherapeutics in Cancer Treatment

Niyati H. Patel[1,*] and **Fahad Hassan Shah**[2]

[1] *Middlesex County Academy of Allied Health and Biomedical Sciences, New Jersey, United States*

[2] *Department of Biological Sciences, College of Natural Sciences, Kongju National University, Gongju, Republic of Korea*

Abstract: Nanotherapeutics is an advancing technology and promising industry of the 21st century; with further development, it may hold secrets for the medical community and society as a whole. The development of nanotherapeutics into medicine is one of the newest developments in medical science that the scientific community has taken. The conventional approach of delivering anticancer drugs towards the targeted site is remained controversial and has numerous problems such as non-specific effects to the surrounding organs other than cancer affected, anticancer drug resistance, and chronic adverse effects. Recently, biomedical scientists have turned their attention towards nanocarriers possessing incredible activity to deliver anticancer drugs towards cancer-affected areas without being disrupted by endogenous barriers, rendering lesser toxicity and promoting anticancer response. In this chapter, the overview of nanotherapeutic agents is thoroughly assessed in the treatment of cancers.

Keywords: Anticancer Drugs, Cancer, Nanotherapeutics, Resistance, Toxicity, Targeted Delivery.

1. INTRODUCTION

Nanotherapeutic agents are emerging technologies that consist of various types of nanomaterials that have a vital role in the health care sector. These agents are atomically restructured materials used to deliver medications or other substances to ameliorate the therapeutic effect or diagnose any anomaly in the body. This can remain in the form of targeted drug therapy or even the early detection of some diseases in the human body. The body lies in a state of equilibrium, and within this state, all chemical processes can be carried out. A common example, the bicarbonate buffer system, is pivotal in the regulation of blood pH levels in humans. The bicarbonate buffer system will either donate or reserve H^+ ions depending on the pH: this being too acidic or basic for the body.

[*] **Corresponding author Niyati H. Patel:** Middlesex County Academy of Allied Health and Biomedical Sciences, New Jersey, United States; E-mail: niyup2@gmail.com

Nanotherapeutics is encompassed under a term called nanomedicine, which specifically uses nanoparticles for medical applications [1]. The alteration of said matter under the microscopic level can help form unnatural recurring properties that can benefit the use of the particles. Nanotherapeutics development requires nanoscale materials often found in the environment of the laboratory settings. This may include the biocompatible nanoparticles and nanorobots used for diagnoses, delivery of materials, sensing, and actuated purposes in a living organism [2, 3].

The most important trait of these particles is biocompatibility; they must be able to survive in the human body without the worry of the attack from the immune system as detected by a foreign agent. Rejection from the body can cause issues that can span from disease to even death for the organism. The nanorobots help with the advancement of the particles and the training into completing the multitude of tasks synchronously.

Nanomedicine has its drawbacks, comparable to any therapy that is in the modern market; these risks with nanodrugs can be unpredictable due to the variance of effects in clientele population. Repeatedly in the medical community, we have seen that the rejection of agents in the body will cause surrounding tissues within the whole system. The body functions like a factory chain. When one screw is taken out, the entire system suffers. That is mirrored in the effect of the nanoparticle rejection due to lack of biocompatibility.

We have seen nanotherapeutics in the body in many ways through the medical changes we see in the body. The interventions that help treat so many conditions that affect us in the 21st century are due to the development of nanotherapeutic medicine in the pharmaceutical development of drugs.

2. HISTORY OF NANOTHERAPEUTICS

Nanotherapeutics, regardless of the advanced nature and the new technology of the 21st century, have been around forever. Since the emergence of humans from our ape ancestors' humans remained inquisitive species, and with that comes imagination. Imagination, a new idea in the first humans that stepped foot on the Earth, yet an important one because that very thing would cause a ripple of inventions to emerge from curiosity. Nanoparticles can be traced back to colloidal gold usage in ancient civilizations, used by the Damascans to create swords that contained far sharper edges [4]. The Romans used this colloidal gold to create the iridescent glassware. To this day, we praise the Roman Civilization [5].

The modern take in nanotherapeutics was credited to Élie Metchnikoff and Paul Ehrlich, who often take the "modern pioneers of nanomedicine" [6]. Together they were the recipients of The Nobel Prize for Medicine in 1908 and have caused a great shift in the world of medicine. Through their works of phagocytosis, commonly known as "cellular eating", they concluded that through cell-specific diagnostic and therapy, there was a higher yield in patients recovery. Fundamental deals with nanoparticles for nanomedicine were progressively evolved over the most recent 30 years of the twentieth century and included the use of liposomes. Now remains the key to the puzzling issues that arise in the 21st century. The use of nanoparticles in nanotherapeutics bloomed after the experiments of Metchnikoff and Ehrlich, and the knowledge that was acquired in the last century has changed the face of nanomedicine. Modern treatments for many debilitating diseases have now found it beneficial to use nanoparticles, and this science will be developed further in the future. The development of this science thus far has led to an improvement in the quality of life and advanced societal planted interests. Welfare concerns have been met with the interest of living longer, developed in trials of the use of this new technological science.

2.1. Economic Importance of Nanotherapeutics

The strides that nanotherapeutics left in the science field remain easily evident: increasing lifespan, decreasing pain in treatment, overall lower mortality rates in the human population. The hidden economic changes left after the health improvements tend to be the less recounted effect of introducing this new medical practice. The role that nanotherapeutics play on the world stage of economic growth is immense. Rising health costs are one of the biggest concerns facing the medical community worldwide. Patients often cannot afford healthcare with all the tests and treatments needed. When possible, they are left in debt for years, commonly the person's lifespan and through future generations. Nanomedicine, as a whole, yields a positive economic mark on the output of jobs for people. The new field has opened the gates for the development of new businesses, jobs, and trade markets. The National Nanomedicine Institute (NNI) remains the leader of this new initiative [12].

While the NNI grows deeper in magnitude and complexity, the nation has been allocating more funds to develop this technology as a step towards proactively lowering healthcare costs in the future. World leaders have seen the potential of this technology in healthcare settings and allocating money as it remains an assurance policy for the future of protecting national interests and health. It is imperative that nations keep monitoring and adapting the funding that is entered into this field; analysis of the funds includes the alignment of the goals nationally, including the strategic plan for nanoscale. Nanotechnology, still in its infancy of development, has shocked the world with the amount of economic impacts. Quantifying the effect of nanotherapeutics in the economy leaves economists baffled, reasoning that the healthcare world is constantly changing and during times of crisis, like the coronavirus pandemic, changes in healthcare-related fields remain elusive to the cause. Economic fluctuations have been common in modern healthcare worlds, and therefore the quantifiable number of changes nanotherapeutics have brought confuses most economists.

As indicated by that report, just a small portion-under $13 billion-of 2004 item incomes originated from deals of developing nanotechnologies, with $12 billion that shows direct benefit to nanotherapy-based businesses [12]. The predicted effect of nanotechnology in the economy has been developed through four unique waves by analyzing past development. Each is categorized by the prediction of consumer or available corporate items and the predicted supply and demand chain. This economic growth model remains the most popular among most of the community and is widely accepted when attempting to gage an understanding of the future hopes of the industry.

The first wave of development of nanotechnology to be perfected is the passive nanostructures and tubes. This was introduced in 2001 and is considered the first generation of products. This includes materials that are nanoparticle-based coatings and bulk materials like nanostructured metals, polymers, and ceramics. The main usage of these in modern society is crafting household appliances, ceramic materials, and the military. The nanostructured metals remain to have stronger properties than those that are naturally occurring. This caused the shift from using metals like steel in weapons to using nanoparticle-based metals. The same concept was applied in the field of ceramics to help make the strongest materials possible the development of altering the molecules on a molecular level, a pillar of nanomedicine was brought into the field.

The second wave of development includes the introduction of active nanoparticles, introduced in 2005. These include transistors, amplifiers, targeted drugs and chemicals, actuators, and adaptive structures. The key focal point of examination for this age of items is novel gadgets and gadget framework designs. Transistors are the amplification point of a semiconductor device that includes rectification, and the usage of nanoparticles increases the efficacy of the amplification speed and capability. The targeted drugs and chemicals explored further in the chapter are used to create specific target sites for drugs to the effect rather than general release, which causes harder treatment turnaround times. Actuators allow machines to work; the addition of nanoparticles increases the amount of work that can be caused by one actuator. The development of the second wave caused great change in the way that tools available to the population work.

The third wave of nanotechnology, introduced around 2010, will involve three-dimensional nanosystems and frameworks of nanosystems equipped for different union and gathering methods. The focal point of exploration will be heterogeneous nanostructures and supramolecular frameworks designing.

The fourth wave of nanotechnology foreseen by 2025 will be founded on heterogeneous sub-atomic nanosystems, every particle of which will have a particular structure and job; the focal point of examination will be controlled at the degree of iotas for the plan of particles and supramolecular frameworks, just as a portrayal of the elements of a solitary atom and the plan of sub-atomic machines. This model is projecting that the growth of the industry development will see an upward trend.

An investigation by Cientifica assessed that limit use in the assembling of one original item-nanotubes-was at close to 50 percent, maybe because of high paces of investments and restricted business requests at present. This often serves as a model that stands for the unpredictability of this market because, when working with nature on the atomic level, it comes with varied risks and benefits economically, as well as safety.

This framework brought on by economics includes all products that fall under the general model of 'systems and technologies for healthcare, aimed at prevention, diagnosis or therapy. This is based on the little market data present for nanomedicine published. The leverage of nanomedicine on the markets is based upon the analysis of market segments of medical devices and drugs and pharmaceuticals. These two market sections spoke to in 2003 an end-client estimation of € 535 billion, of which the portion of the medication is the most significant, with an estimation of € 390 billion. All-inclusive, this market has been developing at a 7 to 9% yearly rate, with varieties as indicated by nation, advances and market fragments.

The worldwide market has opened its arms to this change in medicine; in the years of its initiation, it was able to develop the wings of the nanotherapeutic market in the place it holds on the world stage of economics. The overall market for pharmaceutical medications was developing at a pace of 7% in 2004. The medication market can be divided, with the worldwide market for cutting-edge tranquilize conveyance frameworks representing € 42.9 billion or 11% of the aggregate. Around half of this market is in controlled discharge frameworks, with needleless infusion, injectable/implantable polymer frameworks, transmucosal, rectal, liposomal drug delivery, and cell/gene therapy answerable for the rest and is evaluated to reach € 75 billion of every 2005. Improvements in this market are quick, particularly in the area of options to infused macromolecules, as medication details try to capitalize on the € 6.2 billion overall markets for designed protein and peptide drugs and other organic therapeutics.

Nanomedicine, as it may seem like an innovation that holds a place in our society, is merely a new chapter of nanotherapeutics that has been developed for years. Ancient civilizations have been altering matter at the atomic level far before we can comprehend it in the 21st century. The main effect that hits globally since the reintroduction of nanotherapeutics is the economic growth that has been charted. Healthcare costs have officially lowered and became a part of society to plan for this new industry, increasing jobs, fields, and the business world. The effect that it has on individual people resonates among various societies and societal interests. The quality of living has increased as people have been introduced to new methods of medical interventions. This has caused a ripples effect leading to longer lifespans, better healthcare, and a retouch of societal interests. The societal interests have often led to a sense of nationalistic pride and international competition among nations to be the most dominant and scientifically forward in nanotherapeutics. As for the whole field, controversy often surrounds the development of nanotherapeutics and the extent of development and funding as compared to national interests.

Nanotherapeutics are used in medicine in a variety of ways; the use results in the multitude of developmental features that can ultimately lead to 'systems and technologies for healthcare, aimed at prevention, diagnosis or therapy. Little market data to date can be published about the place of nanomedicine in society due to constant fluctuations of the world's economy. Investigation of the market sections for clinical gadgets and medications and pharmaceuticals gives a thought regarding the influence of Nanomedicine on the business sectors.

Nanotherapeutics as a whole was a practice considered by many physicians as groundbreaking 21st-century innovation, yet the inquisitive nature of our ancestors has proven that this methodology remains to be in one of the most ancient forms. The introduction of this practice into the modern era left the world stage changed in ways that will reminisce forever. The economic bolsters that were seen through markets and the health market field developing at the pace of societal expectations. With the new doors open, the chance of determining illnesses and changing the world of medicine as we know it seems to be right at our reach. But with anything, the leap of faith into new developmental medicine comes with risks that often outweigh the benefits.

2.2. Importance of Nanotherapeutics

The Meningeal neoplasms are small growing tumors in the meninges, the membrane that lines the skull; they often have tumors that press on surrounding tissue and the brain and can be symptomless [7, 8]. The impending treatment of these neoplasms remains to be increasing the lysosomes in the cytarabine [8]. Cytarabine is the chemotherapy medicine given by the needle in the cerebrospinal fluid; with increased lysosomes, it helps with the digestion of the tumor. Lysosomes are naturally found in eukaryotic cells and aid in cellular digestion and apoptosis, programmed cell death. By introducing greater amounts of lysosomes cells can intake the lysosomes through phagocytosis, "cellular eating", and have more lytic enzymes to perform apoptosis , and kill themselves to reduce tumor size exponentially.

Acute lymphoblastic leukemia is cancer that affects the white blood cells of the bone marrow and blood [9]. This cancer is the most common childhood cancer that may develop due to the errors in the DNA of the exons coding for bone marrow proteins. This disease's effect on the body is immense; the pain compares to multiple broken bones, constant infections, and overwhelming fatigue.

The use of nanomedicine in the treatment of acute lymphoblastic leukemia utilizes polymer protein conjugates in pegaspargase [10]. Polymer protein conjugates refer to the modification of proteins by other polymers that result in different protein forms. Pegaspargase is a chemotherapy drug used to treat cancers that affect the white blood cells, like acute lymphoblastic leukemia. The introduction of these polymer protein conjugates allows for the development of cancer to be slowed down and increases the efficiency of the chemotherapy drug, leading to shorter treatment times [10].

Both the lysosomes in Cytarabine and the polymer protein conjugates reside under the topic of nanotherapeutic agents [11]. The nanotherapeutic agents refer exclusively to the term of the actual particles or molecules being changed at the microscopic level to help with the treatment of the illness. In this case, the treatment of Meningeal Neoplasms and Acute lymphoblastic lymphoma, respectively.

3. NANOTHERAPEUTICS IN MEDICINE

Nanotherapeutics use in medicine is often widespread in practice, from early biosensors that may detect antigens, foreign substances that can provoke the natural immune response, to rapid diagnosis and treatment of diseases. Biosensors are the most surface-level use of the nanotherapeutic technology; they aid in finding the antigens in the body [13]. Biosensors consist of three parts: a component that recognizes the analyte and produces a signal, a signal transducer, and a reader device. They are used as a technical approach to the normal immune response; the biosensors can often be more efficient than the body's natural immune system and sometimes allows doctors to catch nosocomial infections before they actually are being fought off by the immune system. The use of biosensors assists with the early detection principle that has become a staple of preventative medicine.

Nanotherapeutics also can assist in the active transport of materials; this refers to getting molecules or substances into a cell against the natural concentration gradient [14]. In the body, we often see this with the use of chemical energy compounds like ATP, adenosine triphosphate. In cell respiration, the proton pump uses energy to transport protons from the matrix of the mitochondrion to the intermembrane space. An active pump generates a proton concentration gradient across the inner mitochondrial membrane because there are more protons outside the matrix than inside. Nanotherapeutics allow special drugs to be altered to go within a cell at bulk and, in the end, reversg the concentration gradient. This is often seen with the hydrolytic enzymes needed for apoptosis or cellular suicide.

This emerging new technology is also used for rapid diagnosis and therapy. This is often seen with the repair of DNA and other genetic material that has undergone damage. Common examples include the thymine dimer caused by prolonged exposure to ultraviolet radiation. Cellular surgery, another use of nanoparticles, refers to the advancement of new strategies and biomaterials is altering careful treatment, diminishing the effect of surgeries, and improving recuperation [15]. Ordinary and restorative surgeries are getting less intrusive, not so much forceful but rather more powerful for patients. And the improvement of natural physiological functions may include more glucose uptake by cells under the GLUT-4 receptor or the efficiency of glycolysis in hard anaerobic exercise conditions for humans. The extensive ways nanotechnology is used in therapy and diagnosis can significantly improve the lifespan of any patient who has used the technology for early detection.

Triggered response is another benefit of nanotherapeutics in medicine. This is one way that the drug molecules can be used most efficiently by the body to produce the most viable output [16]. This relies on the fact that when there is a triggered response or any targeted drug therapy, they have the specific target location of the drug. Nanotherapeutic drugs can pick up on signals or tendencies, so the drug's location can target the needed locations and not be in locations with little therapeutic yield for the patient. When someone takes non-altered cholesterol medication, some of the benefits remain widespread because when taking 12 mg of a drug, not all 12 will be concentrated into the cholesterol targets in the body; this causes an increase in prescription quantities and potential kidney damage.

This technology is often used widely in treating many ailments that affect physiological functions. One of which includes metabolic disorders, abnormal chemical disorders in the body usually related to hormones. These disorders usually have an output of too much or little of a substance vital for the body's function. These include familial hypercholesterolemia, Metachromatic leukodystrophy, Mitochondrial encephalopathy, lactic acidosis, and stroke-like episodes (MELAS). With metabolic disorders, nanotherapeutics can affect the output of hormones by altering the speed, whether it be too fast or slow. Similar cases lie in the works of autoimmune, neurodegenerative, and inflammatory disorders, where promising studies show great improvement and hope for the future.

3.1. Cancer and Nanotherapeutics

Cancer remains one of the main usages of nanotherapeutics in the modern world. Cancer is when the faulty cells, with lack of density-dependent or anchorage inhibition, start dividing uncontrollably, leading to the destruction of healthy body tissue and cells. Cancer spreads from just a few faulty cells to invading and spreading to multiple body tissues and, by extension affecting multiple body systems and functions. When diagnosing cancer, there often is a tumor, an inflamed region generally called by an abnormal growth of tissue. The type of tumor can usually be discovered by a biopsy and then diagnosed if it is malignant or benign. Benign tumors are non-cancerous and cannot rapidly divide and travel to extensive body tissues. Malignant tumors are more serious medically; this is because they are cancerous and in a constant division state and can travel across body systems and tissues.

Signs for cancer usually include thickening lumps (tumors), an unhealing sore, unusual bleeding, persistent cough, or hoarseness. When diagnosed, there are three main methods of treatment: chemotherapy, radiation, and surgery. Most oncologists use some mixture of all three methods to treat various cancers of the body. Chemotherapy uses strong and toxic chemicals to kill the fast-growing cancerous cells in the body. Radiation has high-power rays on the electromagnetic spectrum to kill cancer cells, and surgery removes tumors and surrounding tissue through the operation. Cancer is one of the most versatile physiological body disorders, ; it can truly be omnipresent or anywhere in the body, and the area sometimes affects which of the 3 techniques/methods works the best. The most common types of cancers are skin, lung, colorectal cancers. For males, prostate cancer and females breast cancer are also common, yet males can get breast cancer as well.

Cancer and its relation with nanotherapeutics involve getting the treatment and detection of tumors early before late stages of cancer are diagnosed needing end-stage palliative treatment. Significant breakthroughs that have emerged include, detection of cancer at the earlier stages, diagnosing cancer at a quicker rate, treatment of cancer quicker and more effective, and new promising research holds places in the modern-day society to further cancer treatment development so we can combat the efforts made by cancerous cells. Critics have expressed that nanotechnology has not fulfilled its early promises, specifically communicated worry that progress and interest in the research center have not been reflected by similar advancement by huge clinical achievement in disease treatment. Nevertheless, many scientists believe that nanomedicine is developing at such an astounding pace that nanotherapeutics "are the future of diagnosis and drug delivery with the potential to overcome many of the obstacles that cancer presents [17]."

3.2. Problems with Conventional Cancer Treatment

As successful as a cancer treatment may seem, according to estimates from the International Agency for Research on Cancer (IARC), in 2018, there were 17.0 million new cancer cases and 9.5 million cancer deaths worldwide [18]. These astounding numbers of deaths lie in the number of problems integrated into the cancer treatment that patients receive. The first and most prominent being late detection; cancer symptoms usually tend to lie dormant until reaching stages 3 and beyond; even then, strong definable symptoms might be caught by the patient when entering the late stages of cancer development. Most symptoms appear when multiple bodily functions are affected, meaning that cancer has already attacked different types of body tissue. This late detection is the fundamental cause of the high mortality rates associated with cancer [19]. MRI and PET scans are also widely accepted in the diagnosis of cancer and imaging of the development. Doctors tend to wait to order these until some promising results show they have cancer because of the high associated costs. The machines also are unable to detect any tumors smaller than 1-mm, which hinders early detection methods. This incompetence leaves space for nanotherapeutic developments to detect cancerous tumors earlier, smaller, and cheaper.

The second problem in cancer treatment includes the unspecified results [20], chemotherapy drugs are highly toxic in order to kill the malignant cells. Yet, they attack the tumor at the expense of the rest of the body. The drugs are not altered to specifically target the tumor but rather the entire body cells, which focus on the tumor and the surrounding healthy body tissue and cells. This causes extreme pain and lethargy in patients because the compromised immune system is introduced to toxic chemicals. The weakness that many cancer patients often report is the highest during their times during chemotherapy because of all the healthy body tissue being affected along with the malignant tissues. Due to these symptoms, weakness, and lethargy, causes patients to stray from their treatment and stop fighting. This is often seen in younger and elderly patients as they are in more vulnerable states when sick. The psychological aspect of hope has been proven to help cancer treatment, and hope is stripped from the patient when the pain of chemotherapy is implemented. This position that the patient is put into can be altered by nanotherapeutic-based drugs.

3.3. Nanotherapeutic Solution for Cancer Treatment

The current integration of nanotherapeutics in cancer treatment, includes solutions for the problems outlined above. This provides a promising future for cancer treatment and a hopeful goal to lower the mortality rate and pain imposed on cancer patients. In society, the idea of being a "victim" is frowned upon as the mindset it sets is less desirable than calling cancer patients "fighters". Society has already developed itself to combat the negative mental aspects in the patients, yet medicine has not developed with societal interests in this front until the development of nanotherapeutics in cancer treatment. Through various ways, the integration of different aspects of life causes great changes in the world of oncology.

Nanotherapeutics bring more accurately diagnosing and detection of smaller tumors and symptoms. Promising outcomes in nanoparticle-based specialists to differentiate differentiating in existing imaging advancements, including having the contrasting elements for PET and CT scans that allow for smaller, more minute tumors to be highlighted to the physician for further tests and concerns. Having programmable properties of drugs that can essentially catch the things that regular detection dyes and drugs miss. It may also assist uninvolved/dynamic vehicles in imaging by having gold rods that help with the light frequency targets [21]. The gold rod can draw more clear pictures to smaller aspects. Each gold rod includes a silica center and gold shell that can retain explicit frequencies of light. This new nanotherapeutic technology has extraordinary potential for disease imaging and restorative applications.

Quantum dots are yet another development of cancer nanotherapeutic use. Recognizable quantum dots help with the recognition of unusual substances in blood/tissue tests, also known as a biopsy [22]. Luminescent nanoparticles are used to draw special coloring to these concerned elements and regularly remain to be selenides/sulfides of cadmium or zinc. The light precluded is reliant on the quality of spots; the dabs they make are more extreme and stable than fluorescent partners. These materials are known widely having more noteworthy photostability due to the inorganic shell, which is more stable in the carbon-rich environment of body elements. Significant confinement of quantum dots in imaging is a procedure called "Blinking" [23]. This is because of the change of the quantum dots between the light-transmitting and non-emanating states. This restrains the measure of signals caught at a particular time so doctors can not immediately get a finished picture of what is occurring in the patient's body at one given time.

MRI development has also been proven to be a benefit of nanotherapeutics in cancer treatments. Advancements of nanoparticle frameworks to improve MRI for malignant growth imaging and determination have gained critical ground. Inorganic nanoparticle center and a surface covering that give dependability in fluid scatterings are used to remain stable and functional in the case of aqueous solutions [24]. This surface covering is controlled to encourage focusing on, ongoing observing, or both for the issues that may have some concerns. Improved proton unwinding and profound tissue imaging capacities, non-obtrusiveness, and low poisonousness, give a more promising patient experience.

Super magnetic iron oxide (SPIO) nanoparticles are currently generally utilized as entrail differentiate specialists and have been utilized for quite a while in spleen/liver imaging [25]. SPIO nanoparticles are promptly taken up by macrophages present in the liver parenchyma (Kupffer cells) as liver tumors are normally without macrophages, the macrophage-explicit take-up of SPIOs builds the difference among solid and sick tissue permitting liver tumors or miniaturized scale metastases as little as 2–3 nm to be distinguished [26, 27]. Iron particles discharged into the plasma upon debasement can tie hemoglobin. To maintain a strategic distance from the freedom of the SPIO nanoparticles, they are frequently covered with polyethylene glycol (PEG), which upgrades the flow time during the imaging and treatment of prostate malignancy [28].

Molecular diagnostics refer to an assortment of methods used to examine natural markers in the genome and proteome-the person's hereditary code and how their cells express their qualities as proteins-by applying sub-atomic science to clinical testing. This field has been greatly affected by the development of nanotherapeutics in oncology practices. This is assisted by gold nanoparticles which have a sizable change property and are sensitive and specific to their codes [29]. Aptamer-conjugated NPs can likewise be utilized for the assortment and recognition of various malignancy cells [30]. Gold nanoshells and gold nanorods have been utilized to actuate photothermal treatment; this is a model for a "theragnostic" specialist, as the gold nanorods aid finding of the malignancy yet additionally, help in evacuating the tumor [31].

Perhaps the most significant benefit for nanotherapeutic agents in the development of cancer research is the specific drug targeting. Chemotherapy drugs are more protected and proficient when altered. Documented improvement in conveyance, cellular acceptance of drugs, pharmacokinetic profiles have been seen. The possible capacity of nano medicates conveyance frameworks to defeat the weaknesses of numerous anticancer medications. EPR is another development made to help these drugs be more efficient in the stages of use. The enhanced penetrability and retention (EPR) impact is a controversial idea by which particles of specific sizes (commonly liposomes, nanoparticles, and macromolecular medications) will in general gather in tumor tissue substantially more than they do in ordinary tissues [2]. Tumors have expanded vasculature, permitting the passage of macromolecules and colloidal particles of width up to 600nm.

Furthermore, the lymphatic framework isn't powerful in clearing the interstitial liquid from the tumor tissues; nanoparticles can specifically target tumor tissues diminishing harmful reactions the improved penetration and maintenance properties of the tumor over the ordinary tissues cause the nanoparticle to have delayed contact with the tumor cells. Cell surface receptors collaborate with ligand-covered nanoparticles prompting their take-up by endocytosis, cellular eating. It is proposed that decidedly energized nanoparticles are taken all the more promptly because of electrostatic fascination. Connection with explicit serum proteins brings about the development of a crown, advancing cell passage. Late examinations demonstrate that non-circular particles, such as bar formed structures, are disguised as superior to round structures. The Take-up of bigger nanoparticles upsets the layer surface, subsequently actuating cell passing. Lung epithelial cells and red platelets could cause harmful symptoms. A possibly beat the weaknesses of numerous anticancer medications, for example, low watery solvency and security and high vague harmfulness progressively utilized in light of the fact that their focusing on capacity diminish fundamental dissemination of cytotoxic mixes *in vivo*. Upgrades take-up at the objective site, bringing about viable treatment at lower portions.

Nanodrug delivery systems have been developed to combat the efforts of the anti-specific drug market that only within recent years has started to be the catalyst for change. Nanodrug delivery systems can either utilize passive focusing on systems, for example, the EPR impact, or active systems focusing on components such as ligands. Utilizing ligands coordinated against differentially overexpressed cell surface markers surface on tumor cells, a nanoparticle intended to be 100nm or less in breadth with a hydrophilic surface will have a more extended course time and subsequently a more prominent capacity to focus on the necessary site because of diminished freedom by macrophages.

Liposomes have been being used for a long time and are built up as medication and imaging operator transporters with demonstrated clinical viability. Counterfeit phospholipid vesicles 50 nm to ≥ 1 μm in size, either unilamellar or multilamellar nanocarriers, give insurance from degradation. Polymeric micelles comprise of a hydrophobic center and a hydrophilic shell and are helpful medication transporters because of their tunable size and surface capacities, high monodispersity, and great strength. They can frame hydrogels and are utilized for sedate exemplification or medication conjugation right conditions, pluronic, the most notable thermosensitive polymers, structure a hydrogel at internal heat level however is water dissolvable at 2-4°C. This permits them to be infused as a fluid, yet they structure a hydrogel in situ, bringing about delayed medication arrival of the embodied medication. Inorganic nanoparticles, for example, gold nanoparticles, can be utilized as a payload for drug conveyance. Gold has various engaging surface properties, for example, light dissipating, which makes them alluring inorganic biomaterials for tranquilize conveyance when joined with nanoparticles. Numerous medications can be conjugated to the outside of gold through hydrophobic interactions. Different antibiotics, anticancer specialists, and oligonucleotides are additionally conjugated with gold nanoparticles to yield more reasonable medication delivery agents.

Nanoparticles as therapeutic agents are now of great use in the field of oncology. Through a procedure called "intercrossing" upon excitation by light, their capacity to change the substrate particle is utilized to treat malignancy cells in the photodynamic treatment. This is the property of little inorganic atoms to produce heat upon excitation exploited to instigate apoptosis or corruption of cells.

Drug resistance is a great issue facing the medical community as many pathogens and illness causing factors. Defeating resistance is now being explored to combat the natural evolution and natural selection of which the principles of nature run against. Nanovehicles conveying remedial medication mix that not just objective the tumor cells specifically the focal point of concentrated exploration demonstrated particularly successful in going around multidrug opposition (MDR) in different malignancy models.

Prevention is now a great trend in the medical field, to be more active to prevent before treating the illness if it can be prevented, it saves a lot of pain and money for the patient. The medical community is now transitioning to a more proactive way of treatment and encouraging regular exercise and healthy habits to lessen any risk factors for any illness. It is not deemed possible to totally forestall the development of cancer, its natural course of life. But the understanding to educate and catch early can affect mortality rates. Ano-EGCG had an essentially longer half-life and had in excess of a 10-overlap portion advantage over nonencapsulated EGCG; this is assisting with the cell growth inhibition, proapoptotic, and angiogenic inhibitory effects [32]. A huge number of approaches using nanoparticles to battle these current deficiencies in the chemopreventive systems will re-charm the 'silver bullet' for chemoprevention soon.

Improving compliance is one of the main societal interests when it comes to dealing with cancer treatment. When looking from the outside and hearing stories, society opens its eyes to the actual pain that cancer treatment has caused. Many cancer patients revoke treatment or commit suicide to stop the pain felt during stages of treatment, specifically chemotherapy. Introducing nanotherapeutics into the comfort of patients in cancer situations, prompts shorter recuperation times and a diminished danger of infection and is less intrusive than customary determination and treatment strategies. These favorable circumstances thus should prompt a decrease in cost and improved life expectancy and quality.

4. ETHICAL ISSUES ASSOCIATED WITH NANOTHERAPEUTIC TREATMENT

In its entirety, the use of nanotherapeutics brings great advancements to the medical specialty oncology field but compromising some values that are held deep-rooted in our society. This leaves a deep-rooted debate in a society that spans from engineers, economics, doctors, business professionals, and many other professions. The arguments of both sides leave the end question Is the promise of developing nanotherapeutics the right step for the nation when starting to adapt to this modern age? The two poles provide compelling arguments that leave most of the society confused about where to stand on this difficult topic that may change the face of medicine forever.

Nanotherapeutics bring many benefits to the societal interests pursued by the people. Further exploration leads to more expansion into rapid and sensitive detection of cancer treatments and empowers researchers to recognize atomic changes in any event, when they happen just in a small percentage of cells. The new studies have also shown that nanotherapeutic agents are profoundly restorative operators and can bring the natural balance back to the body.

Nanoscale materials for malignant growth descends to their capacity to be promptly functionalized and effectively tuned, its capacity to convey and/or go about as the remedial, indicative, or both. It leaves it a compelling treatment for many to choose. Also, it allows it to be conveyed across customary organic obstructions in the body, for example, thick stromal tissue of the pancreas or the blood-mind hindrance that exceptionally controls conveyance of biomolecules to/from our focal sensory system. The first catch approach of nanotherapeutics allows the life expectancy to be higher after diagnosis with the help of advanced technology and drugs. The benefit of comfort to the patient is also brought because of the specific nature of drug targeting that they have an overall less painful and positive treatment experience. This development also leaves with the societal interests being pursued and the economic world stage booming with a developmental new industry.

Yet, nanotherapeutics does not remain the haven that it seems on paper; the effects of nanotherapeutics challenge deep-rooted morals, religious beliefs, and safety concerns. The small size, high reactivity, and special pliable and attractive properties of nanomaterials-similar properties that drive enthusiasm for their biomedical and mechanical applications have raised worries about environmental, health, and safety (EHS). However, uncertain discussion as of late about the likely poisonousness of a particular sort of nanomaterial-carbon nanotubes (CNTs)-which has been related to tissue harm in animal testing. Morally, the idea of nanotherapeutics has been challenged. The safety of putting altered human nature into the body at the atomic level is a moral issue that faces many communities of targeting to change the natural beauty of the world we live in. Do people want to put scientifically altered particles in their bodies? Many religious groups have spoken out on this debate about the development of science, from sources like the Bible, Quran, Geeta, Torah from Christianity, Islamism, Hinduism, Judaism respectively have shown proof in the texts of god's creation of the Earth not to be changed and altered by humans. As a result, the development of nanotherapeutics has been seen as looking down on this new developmental technology from the religious communities.

CONCLUSION

Now that leaves us, the future of science, to decide where this technology can go. Should this technology be pursued further, or is it immoral to stand by? Regardless of whether genuine or saw, the potential well-being dangers related to the assembling and utilization of nanomaterials must be deliberately concentrated so as to propel our comprehension of this field of science and to understand the noteworthy advantages that nanotechnology brings to the table society, for example, for malignancy exploration, diagnostics, and treatment. Far less harmful than family unit cleaning items, bug sprays utilized on family pets, and over-th--counter dandruff cures are in the proximity now that the development has spread further into the counter shelf world. One can even go to the local pharmacy and find nanotherapeutic agents in their daily lives. Society leaves itself at a tug of war with this technology. The rope pulling from both sides with captivating arguments and the winner regardless will change the face of not just medicine. The face of the world will be affected with the willingness to pursue this dangerous yet promising technology that can bring unimaginable benefits, with associated drawbacks that will usher the world into the next era and change the world of healthcare as we know it.

CONSENT FOR PUBLICATION

Not applicable.

CONFLICT OF INTEREST

The author declares no conflict of interest, financial or otherwise.

ACKNOWLEDGEMENTS

Declared none.

REFERENCES

[1]   Pelaz B, Alexiou C, Alvarez-Puebla RA, *et al.* Diverse applications of nanomedicine. ACS Nano 2017; 11(3): 2313-81.
[http://dx.doi.org/10.1021/acsnano.6b06040] [PMID: 28290206]

[2]   Shi J, Kantoff PW, Wooster R, Farokhzad OC. Cancer nanomedicine: progress, challenges and opportunities. Nat Rev Cancer 2017; 17(1): 20-37.
[http://dx.doi.org/10.1038/nrc.2016.108] [PMID: 27834398]

[3]   van der Meel R, Sulheim E, Shi Y, Kiessling F, Mulder WJM, Lammers T. Smart cancer nanomedicine. Nat Nanotechnol 2019; 14(11): 1007-17.
[http://dx.doi.org/10.1038/s41565-019-0567-y] [PMID: 31695150]

[4]   Nealon GL, Donnio B, Greget R, Kappler J-P, Terazzi E, Gallani J-L. Magnetism in gold nanoparticles. Nanoscale 2012; 4(17): 5244-58.
[http://dx.doi.org/10.1039/c2nr30640a] [PMID: 22814797]

[5]   Freestone I, Meeks N, Sax M, Higgitt C. The lycurgus cup-A roman nanotechnology. Gold Bull 2007; 40: 270-7.
[http://dx.doi.org/10.1007/BF03215599]

[6]   Schmid SL, Sorkin A, Zerial M. Endocytosis: Past, present, and future. Cold Spring Harb Perspect Biol 2014; 6(12): a022509.
[http://dx.doi.org/10.1101/cshperspect.a022509] [PMID: 25359499]

[7]   Flühmann B, Ntai I, Borchard G, Simoens S, Mühlebach S. Nanomedicines: The magic bullets reaching their target? Eur J Pharm Sci 2019; 128: 73-80.
[http://dx.doi.org/10.1016/j.ejps.2018.11.019] [PMID: 30465818]

[8]   Lamar Z, Lesser GJ. Management of meningeal neoplasms: meningiomas and hemangiopericytomas. Curr Treat Options Oncol 2011; 12(3): 230-9.
[http://dx.doi.org/10.1007/s11864-011-0156-2] [PMID: 21537847]

[9]   Terwilliger T, Abdul-Hay M. Acute lymphoblastic leukemia: a comprehensive review and 2017

update. Blood Cancer J 2017; 7(6): e577-7.
[http://dx.doi.org/10.1038/bcj.2017.53] [PMID: 28665419]

[10]   Rau RE, Dreyer Z, Choi MR, *et al.* Outcome of pediatric patients with acute lymphoblastic leukemia/lymphoblastic lymphoma with hypersensitivity to pegaspargase treated with PEGylated Erwinia asparaginase, pegcrisantaspase: A report from the Children's Oncology Group. Pediatr Blood Cancer 2018; 65(3): e26873.
[http://dx.doi.org/10.1002/pbc.26873] [PMID: 29090524]

[11]   Pola R, Janoušková O, Etrych T. The pH-dependent and enzymatic release of cytarabine from hydrophilic polymer conjugates. Physiol Res 2016; 65 (Suppl. 2): S225-32.
[http://dx.doi.org/10.33549/physiolres.933424] [PMID: 27762588]

[12]   Council NR Matter of Size: Triennial Review of the National Nanotechnology Initiative. National Academies Press 1900.

[13]   Metkar SK, Girigoswami K. Diagnostic biosensors in medicine – A review. Biocatal Agric Biotechnol 2019; 17: 271-83.
[http://dx.doi.org/10.1016/j.bcab.2018.11.029]

[14]   Ye H, Shen Z, Yu L, Wei M, Li Y. Manipulating nanoparticle transport within blood flow through external forces: an exemplar of mechanics in nanomedicine. Proc- Royal Soc, Math Phys Eng Sci 2018; 474(2211): 20170845.
[http://dx.doi.org/10.1098/rspa.2017.0845] [PMID: 29662344]

[15]   Wong KKY, Liu XL. Nanomedicine: a primer for surgeons. Pediatr Surg Int 2012; 28(10): 943-51.
[http://dx.doi.org/10.1007/s00383-012-3162-y] [PMID: 22892910]

[16]   Tran S, DeGiovanni P-J, Piel B, Rai P. Cancer nanomedicine: a review of recent success in drug delivery. Clin Transl Med 2017; 6(1): 44.
[http://dx.doi.org/10.1186/s40169-017-0175-0] [PMID: 29230567]

[17]   Krishnan SR, George SK. Nanotherapeutics in cancer prevention, diagnosis and treatment. Pharmacol Ther 2014; 233.

[18]   Bray F, Ferlay J, Soerjomataram I, Siegel RL, Torre LA, Jemal A. Global cancer statistics 2018: GLOBOCAN estimates of incidence and mortality worldwide for 36 cancers in 185 countries. CA Cancer J Clin 2018; 68(6): 394-424.
[http://dx.doi.org/10.3322/caac.21492] [PMID: 30207593]

[19]   Virnig BA, Baxter NN, Habermann EB, Feldman RD, Bradley CJ. A matter of race: early-versus late-stage cancer diagnosis. Health Aff (Millwood) 2009; 28(1): 160-8.
[http://dx.doi.org/10.1377/hlthaff.28.1.160] [PMID: 19124866]

[20]   Moreau-Bachelard C, Coquan E, Le Tourneau C. Imputability of adverse events to anticancer drugs. N Engl J Med 2019; 380(19): 1873-4.
[http://dx.doi.org/10.1056/NEJMc1900053] [PMID: 31067382]

[21]   Li B, Lane LA. Probing the biological obstacles of nanomedicine with gold nanoparticles. Wiley Interdiscip Rev Nanomed Nanobiotechnol 2019; 11(3): e1542.
[http://dx.doi.org/10.1002/wnan.1542] [PMID: 30084539]

[22]   Devi P, Saini S, Kim K-H. The advanced role of carbon quantum dots in nanomedical applications. Biosens Bioelectron 2019; 141: 111158.
[http://dx.doi.org/10.1016/j.bios.2019.02.059] [PMID: 31323605]

[23]   De CK, Roy D, Mandal S, Mandal PK. Suppressed blinking under normal air atmosphere in toxic-metal-free, small sized, InP-based core/alloy-shell/shell quantum dots. J Phys Chem Lett 2019; 10(15): 4330-8.
[http://dx.doi.org/10.1021/acs.jpclett.9b01157] [PMID: 31294573]

[24]   Choi JH, Lee YJ, Kim D. Image-guided nanomedicine for cancer. J Pharm Investig 2017; 47(1): 51-64.

[http://dx.doi.org/10.1007/s40005-016-0297-1]

[25]　Wáng YXJ, Idée J-M. A comprehensive literatures update of clinical researches of superparamagnetic resonance iron oxide nanoparticles for magnetic resonance imaging. Quant Imaging Med Surg 2017; 7(1): 88-122.
[http://dx.doi.org/10.21037/qims.2017.02.09] [PMID: 28275562]

[26]　Kania G, Sternak M, Jasztal A, *et al.* Uptake and bioreactivity of charged chitosan-coated superparamagnetic nanoparticles as promising contrast agents for magnetic resonance imaging. Nanomedicine 2018; 14(1): 131-40.
[http://dx.doi.org/10.1016/j.nano.2017.09.004] [PMID: 28939490]

[27]　Unterweger H, Janko C, Schwarz M, *et al.* Non-immunogenic dextran-coated superparamagnetic iron oxide nanoparticles: a biocompatible, size-tunable contrast agent for magnetic resonance imaging. Int J Nanomedicine 2017; 12: 5223-38.
[http://dx.doi.org/10.2147/IJN.S138108] [PMID: 28769560]

[28]　Zhou J, Huang L, Wang W, Pang J, Zou Y, Shuai X, *et al.* Prostate cancer targeted MRI nanoprobe based on superparamagnetic iron oxide and copolymer of poly(ethylene glycol) and polyethyleneimin. Chin Sci Bull 2009; 54(18): 3137-46.
[http://dx.doi.org/10.1007/s11434-009-0256-6]

[29]　Singh P, Pandit S, Mokkapati VRSS, Garg A, Ravikumar V, Mijakovic I. Gold Nanoparticles in Diagnostics and Therapeutics for Human Cancer. Int J Mol Sci 2018; 19(7): 1979.
[http://dx.doi.org/10.3390/ijms19071979]

[30]　Das V, Chikkaputtaiah C, Pal M. 14 - Aptamer-conjugated functionalized nano-biomaterials for diagnostic and targeted drug delivery applications. In: Maiti S, Jana SBT-FP for BA, editors. Woodhead Publishing. 2019.

[31]　Kim HS, Lee DY. Photothermal therapy with gold nanoparticles as an anticancer medication. J Pharm Investig 2017; 47(1): 19-26.
[http://dx.doi.org/10.1007/s40005-016-0292-6]

[32]　Negri A, Naponelli V, Rizzi F, Bettuzzi S. Molecular Targets of Epigallocatechin—Gallate (EGCG): A Special Focus on Signal Transduction and Cancer. Nutrients. 1936.

CHAPTER 6

Emerging Nanomaterials for Cancer Therapy

Sibgha Batool[1], Maryam Bibi[1], Abid Mehmood Yousaf[2], Han Gon Choi[3] and Fakhar ud Din[1,*]

[1] *Department of Pharmacy, Faculty of Biological Sciences, Quaid-i-Azam University, 45320 Islamabad, Pakistan*

[2] *Department of Pharmacy COMSATS University Islamabad Lahore Campus, Lahore 54000, Pakistan*

[3] *College of Pharmacy & Institute of Pharmaceutical Science and Technology, Hanyang University, 55 Hanyangdaehak-ro, Sangnok-gu, Ansan, 15588, South Korea*

Abstract: Nanotechnology has gained much interest over the past few years due to its ability to efficiently detect and treat different types of cancers. To overcome the limitations associated with traditional cancer treatment strategies such as lack of specificity, toxic effects, the pre-mature release of the drug, and multidrug resistance, nanomaterials have been widely utilized. Nanomaterials not only enhance the drug accumulation at a specific site but also improve the therapeutic efficacy of anti-cancer drugs. Some other advantages of nanocarriers include targeted and controlled drug delivery, less toxic effects, enhanced solubility and stability, and greater availability of chemotherapeutic agents to the cancer cells due to enhanced permeability and retention effect. The physicochemical properties of nanocarriers can be modified by varying their shapes, sizes, and surface characteristics (PEGylation, ligand, or functional group attachment). Various types of nanomaterials have been utilized for pharmaceutical and medical purposes, most importantly for cancer therapy, depending upon their nature and composition, such as lipid-based, polymeric-based, protein-based, carbon-based, and hybrid nanomaterials. Many of these nanocarrier drug delivery systems have been developed, among which only a few have been clinically approved for anti-cancer drug delivery. The rationale of using nanotechnology for anticancer drugs is to achieve targeted delivery via active or passive targeting and diminish the damages to healthy tissues. So, the ultimate objective of these nanocarriers is to effectively treat the diseases with fewer side effects.

Keywords: Active Targeting, Carbon Nanotubes, Mesoporous Silica Nanomaterials, Nanomaterials, Nanocarriers, Polymeric Nanocarriers, Passive Targeting.

---

* **Corresponding author Fakhar Ud Din:** Department of Pharmacy, Faculty of Biological Sciences, Quaid- i-Azam University, 45320 Islamabad, Pakistan; E-mail: fudin@qau.edu.pk

1. INTRODUCTION OF NANOMATERIALS

Cancer occurrence, prevalence, and mortality rates are increasing day by day, indicating the demand for novel technologies to combat it. According to WHO, cancer is a major health concern in developing countries and is a significant cause of death along with other heart diseases [1]. There are 100 different types of cancers that affect different body parts by uncontrollable cell growth and proliferation [2]. A major reason is its challenging diagnosis and detection. Advanced technologies can help in detecting cancer at earlier stages, thereby decreasing the mortality rate [3].

Nanotechnology is an innovative technology showing advancements in different fields of science and physics. The researchers are transforming human lives by formulating nanoscale things having the ability to work at smaller scales [4]. Remarkably small structures can be studied using nanotechnology. Nanotechnology is also defined as studying, forming, and applying particles and devices by managing their diameter within 1–100 nm size. Nanobiotechnology is the combination of nanotechnology and biotechnology through which conventional technologies can be manipulated and used at the molecular level [5]. Nanotechnology has attained so much attention over the last few years in many fields. National Institute of Health defined nanomedicine as the use of nanotechnology for detecting, diagnosing, monitoring, and regulating living systems. The term nanomedicine is referred to the materials having a size in nanometer-scale, which can easily be modified according to pharmaceutical applications [6]. Although the application of basic nanotechnology was started many years ago, the role of nanomedicine in cancer therapy has gained captivating interest over the last few years [7]. Nanomaterials have promising effects in drug delivery [8]. The very small size makes them appropriate for entering the human cells having a size less than 50 nm and circulating easily with the blood flow. Owing to high surface area to volume ratio, nanoparticles are able to modify the characteristics and activities of drugs. They are also capable of identifying minor changes related to tumor cells and transporting the drug moieties to the specific desired site without bothering nearby tissues and cells. Furthermore, the physicochemical properties of nanoparticles can be modified by varying their shapes, sizes and surface characteristics (PEGylation, attachment of ligand or functional groups).

Consequently, nanoparticles drug delivery vehicles can be lipid in nature or polymeric, along with that some are hybrid nanoparticles and some are peptide-based [9]. Some salient features of nanoparticles include targeted and controlled drug delivery, less toxic effects, enhanced solubility and stability, and greater availability of chemotherapeutic agents to the cancer cells due to enhanced permeability and retention effect. The ultimate objective of nanoparticles utilization is to effectively treat the diseases with fewer side effects [10].

Radiotherapy and surgical therapy help in eliminating localized cancers, but advanced stages of cancers are cured using chemotherapy. However, chemotherapy is not much effective because of its limited availability to cancerous cells. Some other limitations of chemotherapy are lack of specificity, potential toxic effects, and multidrug resistance. Therefore, because of the limitation of conventional therapies and their associated challenges, they are not considered effective for treating different types of cancers, so developing novel strategies for targeting cancerous cells is the necessity of time [11]. As the cancer progression is diverse, cancer treatment is complex due to different responses of therapy among different patients [12]. Therefore, along with recent advancements in nanomedicine-based cancer therapy, the pathophysiology of tumors and their microenvironment are supreme factors that should be kept in mind to overcome the hindrances in their production and commercialization [13]. However, chemotherapeutics agents can be effectively delivered to the tumors with the help of nanoparticles-based drug delivery systems showing improved therapeutic effects [14].

Moreover, the conjugation of nanoparticles with targeting ligands helps in targeting the overexpressing factors of tumor cells. The therapeutic efficacy of nanomedicines is also affected by their circulation time in the body and interactions with different types of proteins [15]. A variety of nanoparticles-based drug delivery systems have been approved for treating different types of tumors, and numerous products are in clinical trials [10]. In this chapter, we have discussed different types of nanoparticles and their roles in cancer therapy. Then we have explained the targeting strategies and surface modification of nanoparticles for improving their targeting and circulation time. In the end, we discussed the future aspects of nanomaterials, most particularly for cancer therapy.

2. TYPES OF EMERGING NANOMATERIALS

Various types of nanomaterials are being utilized for pharmaceutical and medical purposes depending upon their nature and composition, and their roles are briefly described in this section. The graphical illustration of these emerging nanomaterials is given in (Figs. **1** and **2**) .

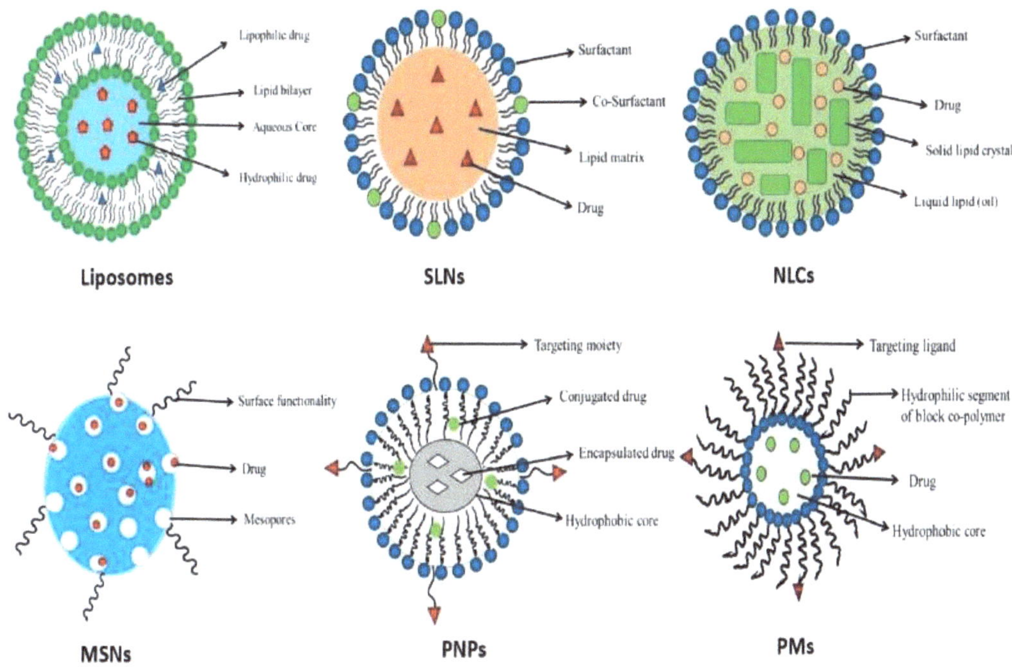

Fig. (1). Graphical illustration of Liposomes, SLNs, NLCs, MSNs, PNPs and PMs.

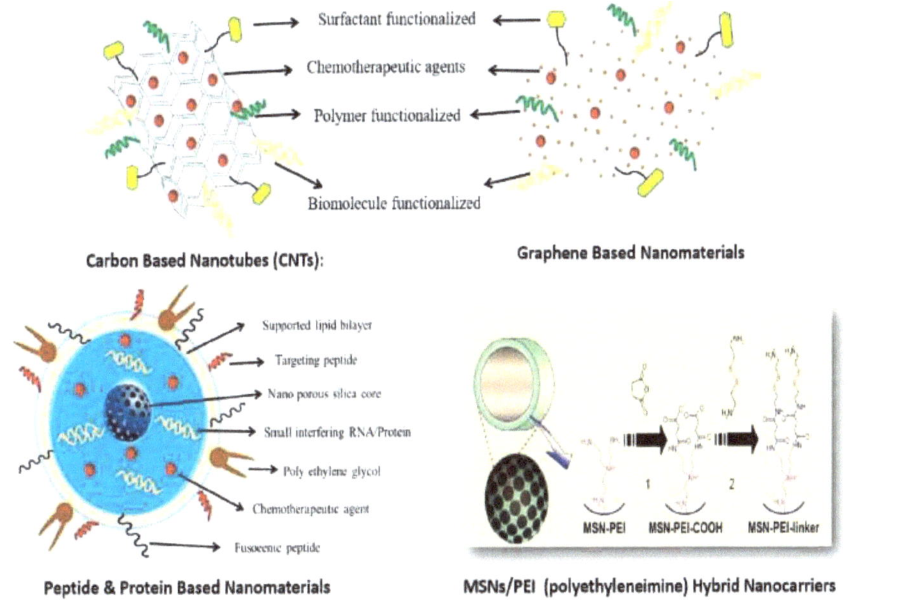

Fig. (2). Graphical illustration of CNTs, Graphene, peptide and protein and MSNs/PEI based nanomaterials.

2.1. Emerging Lipid-Based Nanomaterials

2.1.1 Liposomes

Liposomes are spherical concentric bilayer vesicles that are composed of phospholipids [16]. Liposomes can encapsulate both hydrophilic and hydrophobic drugs because of both hydrophilic core and hydrophobic shell. The charge present on the surface of liposomes depends on the nature of phospholipids [17]. The hydrophilic drug is present in the aqueous core, while the hydrophobic drug is in lipophilic layers. When chemotherapeutic agents are loaded in liposomes, it offers greater encapsulation of drugs with high stability, biocompatibility, controlled release of the drug, and fewer toxic effects [18]. Moreover, they are potential candidates for delivering chemotherapeutic agents and have been approved to treat different types of cancers due to their increased targeting properties. Liposomes can be coated with polymers like polyethylene glycol (PEG) and poly(lactic-*co*-glycolic acid) (PLGA) for prolonging their circulation time in blood [19].

Breast cancer, ovarian cancer, and Kaposi sarcoma have been treated using liposomes as a vehicle for anti-cancerous drugs [20, 21]. Marketed liposomal products include AmBisome® (amphotericin B) and Doxil® (doxorubicin hydrochloride). They either block the P-glycoprotein efflux or bypass it through endocytosis. Liposomes have the potential to modify the structural and chemical properties of drugs, thereby decreasing the mortality rate [22]. Currently, liposomes are used to target CD 45 or CD 90 T-cells for biological response immune therapy [23]. Doxorubicin with polymethacrylate-loaded liposomes was prepared, and their effects on MCF7 and liver cancer H22 cells were studied. It was shown that these doxorubicin-loaded liposomes caused increased cancerous cells death [24].

The pharmacokinetic properties of drugs can be improved by regulating their distribution in plasma by drug-loaded liposomes. When doxorubicin is loaded in PEGylated liposomes, its volume of distribution reduces from from 1000 to 3 L/m^2 [14]. Furthermore, it increases accumulation of drugs inside cancer cells with less damage to nearby healthy cells. Target specificity of liposomes can be enhanced by conjugating them with ligands and antibodies [25].

2.1.2. Solid Lipid Nanoparticles (SLNs)

Solid lipid nanocarriers (SLNs) are colloidal drug delivery systems having size between 50- 1000 nm. These nanoscale particles were developed in the 1990s and are considered as a promising technology for drug delivery due to their safety profile. SLNs are composed of different types of lipids, including fatty acids, fatty alcohols, glycerides (mono, di, and tri-diglycerides), steroids, and waxes. All the lipids are solid at room temperature. However, emulsions with particle size in the nanometer range are closely related to SLNs with the only difference of lipids, *i.e.*, liquid lipids are used for their preparation. SLNs are prepared by two techniques; micro-emulsification and high-pressure homogenization [25]. During its preparation, lipids are added in water with a specific amount of surfactant to stabilize the colloidal suspension. SLNs are suitable vehicles for highly hydrophobic drugs [26].

SLNs are biocompatible, have high drug encapsulating capacity, and have better-releasing properties. Subsequently, after SLNs production, many anti-cancerous drugs have been incorporated into them. These potential nanocarriers are capable of overcoming the limitations of conventional treatment strategies. Moreover, some significant hindrances limit the use of these nanocarriers in cancer therapy, like rapid clearance of SLNs by RES, ability to carry both hydrophilic and ionic moieties, and controlled release of drug from the carrier.

Curcumin loaded SLNs were prepared, and their effect was determined on breast cell lines MCF-7. It was observed that the drug was released slowly over the period of 12 hrs and was more effective against cancerous cells as compared to curcumin [27]. Cytotoxic effects of iron oxide and heparin loaded SLNs were studied through lymphatic system to mimic the interstitial absorption in CaCo-2 cells when given through oral route which portrayed the utilization of SLN as significant for oral route administration [28]. Furthermore, irinotecan has been encapsulated in SLN which was further entrapped in hydrogel for cancer therapy [29]. This study demonstrated a significantly enhanced antitumor effect and demonstrated reduced toxicity towards normal cells.

2.1.3. Nanostructured Lipid Carriers (NLCs)

Nanostructured lipid carriers (NLCs) are the newer generations of solid lipid nanoparticles. It is composed of both solid and liquid lipids that induce deformity in the crystalline structure for encapsulation of more drug, therefore, have enhanced drug encapsulation efficiency. It has the same advantages as SLNs, sustained release pattern of drug moieties, and compatibility. Moreover, it overcomes the issues related to SLNs like drug leakage and less drug encapsulation efficiency, so NLCs are potential candidates for carrying chemotherapeutic drugs and prolonging their half-life [30]. It also improves the accumulation of chemotherapeutics to the cancer cells due to increased leaky vasculature, thereby increasing the effectiveness of drugs [31].

According to a study, Disulfiram-loaded NLCs modified with D- α-tocopheryl polyethylene glycol 1000 succinate (Vitamin E TPGS) were prepared. It was observed that these nanocarriers had greater encapsulating efficiency due to the presence of TPGS. Moreover, it also had a greater cytotoxic effect and increased cell line uptake compared to disulfiram solution alone [32]. Some other examples of NLC loaded drugs for cancer therapy include albumin – paclitaxel loaded NLCs for breast cancer approved in the 2000s, topotecan NLCs for lungs and ovarian cancer, and NLCs loaded with etoposide found effective for lungs cancer. Yang *et al.* reported that coating NLCs improved paclitaxel's circulation and residence time with hyaluronic acid. The anti-cancerous activity of paclitaxel loaded NLCs coated with hyaluronic acid was found to be greater [33].

2.2. Emerging Polymeric Nanomaterial

2.2.1. Polymeric Nanoparticles (PNPs)

Polymers have achieved greater interest of scientists in drug development for the last few years because of their striking characteristics. Biodegradable polymers have been used in the preparation of PNPs. The polymers can be natural or synthetic in nature. Some natural polymers are albumin, chitosan, dextran and heparin, while synthetic polymers include; PEG, polylactic acid (PLA), PLGA, polyglycolic acid (PGA), and polyglutamic acid [34]. PNPs are promising carriers for treating and diagnosing cancers. Like other nanoparticles, they also share the same benefits as cheaper, biocompatible, stable, and sustained release. Therefore, they are suitable for cancer therapy. Functionalization of nanoparticles with targeting moieties leads to their better accumulation at the target site. PNPs are of two types; either they are nanocapsules, or they are nanospheres. PNPs carrying chemotherapeutic drugs show their action by passively targeting drugs to the cancerous cells by increasing their circulation and targeting cancers with ligands coated surfaces. PNPs have the ability to target the healthy cells that help in cancer progression. Moreover, versatile PNPs can be prepared to have different sizes, shapes, and modifiable surfaces for targeting cancers. pH-sensitive polymers can be used to prepare pH-responsive PNPs that can change their characteristics according to the environment, resulting in more significant effects in cancer therapy [35].

2.2.2. Polymeric Nano Micelles (PMs)

In 1990, Kataoka's group produced PMs as drug carriers by producing doxorubicin conjugated block copolymer micelles [36]. PMs are composed of amphiphilic copolymers, thus containing both hydrophobic and hydrophilic parts

[37]. They have a core and shell in their structure; the internal core is a lipophilic part in which the lipophilic drug is loaded while the outer hydrophilic shell shields the drug moiety from the external environment and protects PMs from recognition of RES. Solid tumors have been targeted using liposomes and other lipids nanoparticles, but their use is limited due to resistance and lack of specificity. As the cancerous cells are heterogeneous, there is a crucial need for a suitable drug delivery system. PMs are unique systems capable of overcoming multidrug resistance utilizing different techniques passive targeting, pH-responsive, and folate mediated systems [36].

PMs have already been used for chemotherapeutics delivery. As chemotherapeutics are lipophilic in nature, they can easily be encapsulated within the polymeric core and enhance its hydrophilic properties. The hydrophilic part of PMs, helps in their greater circulation and prevents them from recognizing by RES. Nanoscale size range and extended circulation in the blood cause PMs to accumulate in tumor cells due to enhanced leaky vasculature (EPR). Along with passive targeting, active targeting of cancerous cells can be done using PMs by modifying their properties. Many chemotherapeutic-loaded PMs are in different phases of clinical trials [38]. Paclitaxel, doxorubicin, and cisplatin-loaded PMs have been prepared effectively. It is reported that PEG – PLA micelles, PEG-PAA micelles, and poloxamer-based nano micelles have been prepared for cancer treatment [39].

2.3. Emerging Protein and Peptide-Based Nanomaterials

2.3.1. Protein Based Nanomaterials (PBNs)

Along with other nanocarriers, PBNs are attracting the attention of researchers as they are biocompatible and undergo structural modifications [40]. There are fewer chances of proteins opsonization by RES due to aqueous steric barrier along with their properties such as the capability to bind with water molecules, emulsification, and gelation. Proteins nanocarriers can be prepared easily. Due to the presence of multiple functional groups in polypeptides, proteins nanocarriers can develop 3D networking with different therapeutic molecules to protect drug molecules and make them target specific. Owing to natural occurrence, protein nanoparticles can easily be metabolized. These factors are appealing for encapsulation of anti-cancerous drugs having potential toxic effects. They can be prepared using both hydrophilic proteins such as albumin and gelatin and hydrophobic proteins like gliadin [41].

Human serum albumin (HSA) is a common blood protein composed of 585 amino acids. It is a temperature and pH-sensitive protein. The preparation of nanocarriers using albumin has achieved so much attention in the field of cancer. Carboxylic and amino groups are responsible for modifying nanocarrier surfaces. Chemotherapeutic agents with less solubility can be delivered through the intravenous route using albumin-bound nanocarriers [42]. *In-vivo* studies showed that chemotherapeutic drugs in albumin nanocarriers have a greater therapeutic effect as compared to the drugs alone. This potential effect was due to increased water solubility of poorly soluble drugs and higher drug concentration in cancerous cells.

Abraxane® (paclitaxel- albumin bounded nanocarrier), having size 130 nm, is FDA approved protein-based nanocarrier with significant effects in breast cancer. It was reported that albumin-bound paclitaxel produced no hypersensitivity reaction when administered rapidly. A higher amount of Abraxane can be administered using PBN without higher toxic effects and greater therapeutic efficacy against breast cancer [43]. Gelatin is another denatured protein mostly used in drug production. Hydrophilic and lipophilic chemotherapeutic drugs can be delivered using gelatin-bound nanocarriers. They can also be used for gene delivery in cancer treatment [44]. Another protein that can be used to delivers anti-cancerous drugs is casein, an appropriate carrier for hydrophobic chemotherapeutics [45].

2.3.2. Peptide Based Nanomaterials

Peptides are composed of amino acids monomers that are linked by a peptide linkage. They can also self-assemble to form different structures by van der Waals interactions. Different forms of peptides like amphiphilic peptides and aromatic dipeptides can be used to develop peptide- based nanomaterials [46]. The peptide-based nanomaterials have gained much interest because of their stability against enzymes and ability to encapsulate lipophilic drugs with fewer chances of drug leakage. Therefore, these nanocarriers have been widely used in the cancer for the past few years [47]. Different peptide-based nanocarriers have been reported for cancer therapy. These particles easily permeate into the cancerous cells due to EPR effect. Moreover, peptide-based nanocarriers help in the detection of cancers at the initial stages.

FDA approved sipuleucel-T peptide vaccine for prostate tumors, and clinical trials have been done for different types of cancers [48]. Lung cancer was treated using peptides of natural origin. Oleic acid soybean peptides exhibited cytotoxic effects in cancerous cells [49]. Furthermore, peptides of eastern green mamba venom have poisonous effects on NSCLC cell lines [50]. Recent advancements in technology allow better conjugation of peptides with nanocarriers that have promising effects in cancer therapy. It was reported that a formulation (LFC131-

DOX nanocarriers) containing doxorubicin, PLGA nanocarriers, and LFC131 peptide (CXCR4 inhibitor) could interact to A549 human lung cancer cell line, showing that the product could be used for treating lung cancer [51].

VEGF, an angiogenesis stimulator, is over-expressed in tumor vessels. VEGFR2 binds with VEGF, enhancing permeability and angiogenesis. However, VEGFR1 inhibits the binding of VEGF to VEGFR2, thus inhibiting the functions of VEGF. Peptide-based vaccine targets VEGFR1 and is successful in retarding tumor formation. So, both VEGFR1 and VEGFR2 are important factors that can be targeted. Masuzawa *et al.* reported that peptide-based vaccination containing VEGFR1, VEGFR2, and cisplatin exhibited enhanced therapeutic effects with less toxic effects in patients with gastrointestinal cancers [52].

2.4. Emerging Carbon Based Nanomaterials

2.4.1. Carbon Nanotubes (CNTs)

In 1990s, tube-shaped structures of carbon of fullerenes family known as CNTs were discovered by Iijama [53]. CNTs are composed of single or multiple graphene sheets. CNTs can be single walled (SWCNTs) or multi walled (MWCNTs). Important characters of CNTs include optical properties, stability, flexibility, surface modification ability, and high surface area. CNTs can be used as a drug carrier and in the imaging of tumors [54]. CNTs easily permeate cell membranes due to their needle like structure [55]. CNTs are generally poorly soluble and have toxic effects. However, surface modification capability overcomes the limitations of CNTs. CNTs are considered suitable candidates for cancer therapeutics and have been studies for the last few years for cancer treatment.

Chemotherapeutic agents can be covalently or non-covalently attached to CNTs surface or can be loaded into the inner core of these nanotubes. Moreover, targeting ligands can be attached to the surface of CNTs to make them target-specific. Methotrexate, cisplatin, paclitaxel and doxorubicin can be delivered using CNTs as nanocarriers [56, 57].

2.4.2. Mesoporous Silica Nanoparticles (MSNs)

In the medical field, silica has gained much attention because of its easy production and accessibility. MSNs have many pores in the honeycomb structure and is widely used for drug delivery. Due to their biocompatibility, high surface-to-volume ratio, greater encapsulation efficiency, manageable pore size, ability to load both hydrophilic and lipophilic drugs, and high stability against environmental changes make them potential candidates for nanoscale drug delivery [35].

The attractive structural and functional characteristics of MSNs make them suitable for cytotoxic drugs delivery. Moreover, its porous structures allow a greater amount of drug to be loaded into it, and the nanometer size range helps in the accumulation of drugs within tumors due to EPR effect. Different types of ligands can be attached to MSNs surface to make them site-specific by active targeting mechanism. Chemotherapeutic agents such as doxorubicin, methotrexate, and paclitaxel can be delivered successfully by MSNs [58].

2.4.3. Graphene Based Nanomaterials

As cancer cases and mortality rates are increasing day by day, so effective approaches are highly required for its treatment. Conventional therapies were not so effective in treating cancers. With recent advancements in the biomedical field, new approaches have been developed, such as carbon-based, lipid-based and polymeric-based nanomaterials for cancer therapy. Recently, graphene-based nanomaterials have been widely used for treating cancers. Graphene was firstly extracted from graphite. Graphene-based nanomaterials can be of different types like graphene oxide, graphene in reduced form and graphene with multiple layers. Graphene oxide and their reduced form are most commonly used due to their adjustable characteristics [59].

Graphene-based nanomaterials are capable of targeting the tumor and its environment. Along with that, they are able to react to the signals like magnetic fields, light, and ultrasound rays. These features help control the release of drug from the nanomaterials by external stimulation and help in diagnosing and detecting cancers by using different techniques like photothermal therapy, photodynamic therapy, radiation, and hyperthermia therapy [60]. These nanomaterials are capable of absorbing infrared radiations, so they have been utilized in photothermal therapy. Furthermore, graphene nanomaterials behave as heating material to increase the localized body temperature with external stimuli of ultrasound radiations, so they play a vital role in ultrasound-based hyperthermia therapy [61, 62].

According to studies, it has reported that doxorubicin effects on tumor cells can be increased by photothermal therapy because of the increased susceptibility of tumor cells [63]. It is also reported that photothermal therapy helps in increasing the effectiveness of anti- cancer drugs. So, photothermal therapy and chemotherapy can be given simultaneously to produce the additive therapeutic effect [64].

2.5. Emerging Hybrid Nanomaterials

2.5.1. MSNs/PEI (polyethyleneimine) Hybrid Nanocarriers

Along with the ability to deliver chemotherapeutic drugs to the site of action, the surface of MSNs can be modified by using organic and inorganic linkers, which work as a nucleic acid vehicle so can be used to deliver siRNAs effectively [65]. MSNs permit the nucleic acids binding to its surface and the loading of drugs inside the porous structure, so it is practical to deliver both drugs and nucleic acids simultaneously. To bind these nanoparticles to siRNA and increase the transport of nucleic acid (anionic in nature), the positive charge has to be induced to their surface. The positive charge can be introduced on silica by chemical bonding or electrostatic interactions [66].

The binding of organic molecules with inorganic produces the effects of both materials. This hybrid combination is used to increase the targeting and effectiveness of anti-cancer drugs. Surface modification of MSNs with cationic polymer polyethyleneimine (PEI) aids in the effective delivery of nucleic acids and increases MSNs uptake. It is reported that MSN with PEI developed a sustained pattern of siRNA release. These hybrid nanocarriers effectively delivered drugs to the tumor microenvironment at the same time exuding to the extracellular matrix [67]. Furthermore, the special structure of these nanocarriers with lipidic layers has gained attention in the medical field. Lipid layers are present over MSNs to control the burst release of drugs and avoid drug resistance. In a reported study, MSNs and lipids hybrid nanocarriers have been used for the delivery of zoledronic acid in breast carcinoma [68]. Han *et al.* reported the development of doxorubicin-loaded hybrid MSNs with pH-sensitive drug release. These hybrid nanocarriers manifested greater release and cumulation of the drug in tumor cells and higher toxicity [69].

2.5.2. Metal Oxides onto Multiwall Carbon Nanotubes (MWNT)

CNTs and magnetic iron oxide nanoparticles can be combined to develop a new drug delivery system in the pharmaceutical field. As iron oxides have fewer toxic effects, so they have been utilized in magnetic resonance imaging techniques. In a study, Khandare *et al.* developed hybrid system containing MWCNTs and iron oxide nanoparticles with PEG and FITC contrast agent. The study indicated the fast, controlled and time-based uptake of hybrid nanocarriers by MCF7 cancer cells with no specific toxic effects making it a suitable nominee for imaging purposes. Moreover, Fe_3O_4 and CNT hybrid systems displayed positive outcomes generating caspase-mediated cancer cell death by photothermal therapy and magnetism-induced therapy.

In tumor cells, over-expressed folate receptors have been targeted using folic acid-mediated chemotherapy. CNT and folic acid passively deliver active moieties to the target site. In the presence of a magnetic field, CNTs can target cancer cells by active targeting procedures. Magnetite nanoparticles can be attached to CNTs for drug delivery to the lymphatic system. Therefore, CNTs nanoparticles must carry plenty of anti-cancerous drugs with site-specificity and release the drug in a sustained fashion [70].

3. TARGETING MECHANISMS AND SURFACE FUNCTION-ALIZATION ON NANOCARRIERS

3.1. Active Tumor Targeting

For active targeting, the nanocarriers are modulated with the ligands that selectively bind to their targets expressed onto the surface of tumor tissues [71]. Nano carriers owing to their small size and tunable surfaces, have large surface areas allowing the space for multiple ligands to be conjugated onto their surface and hence paving the way towards more specificity (Fig. **3**). The choice of ligand depends on its targeting capabilities, molecular weight, valence, and compatibility within the body. The ligands may be the antibodies, peptides, nucleic acids, glycoproteins, vitamins and growth factors [35]. Generally, the drugs that are unable to pass through plasma membranes and profound damaging effects are favored for active tumoral targeting and the consideration of other tumoral features. Active tumor targeting has been executed by targeting the tumor features like cell lines, tumor vasculature, acidic tumoral environment, and cell nucleus. Direct targeting of the cell lines with the receptor-directed ligands results in the formation of an endosome by a plasma membrane and the subsequent release of the drug and receptor for further actions. For efficient achievement of ligand-directed active targeting, there are few considerations:

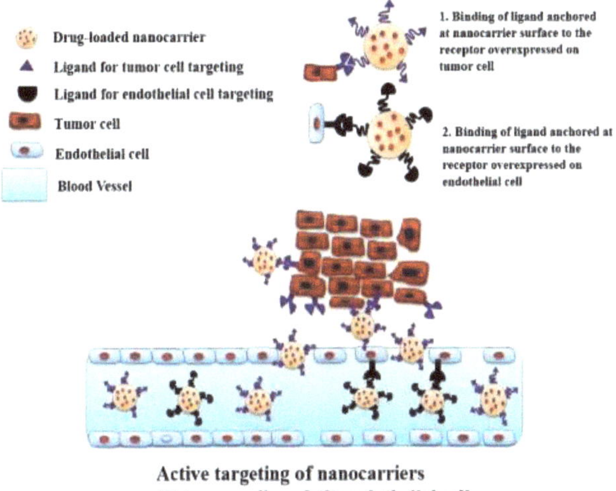

Fig. (3). Active targeting of anticancer nanomaterials.

- There should be a high density of receptors on the target site for efficient binding.
- The ligands should have a high surface density for better targeting.
- Nano carriers may encounter opsonization due to ligand.
- Hepatic affinity of a certain ligand may lead to its uptake. For example, folic acid, modulated nano carriers undergo hepatic uptake due to their special affinity [72].

The basic mechanism underlying the active targeting is to achieve a greater cellular concentration of the anticancer drug rather than its accumulation in tumor tissues. For this purpose, the receptors that have higher expression on the tumor tissues and are capable of delivering the drug into cells are targeted [71] (Table **1**).

Table 1. A brief description of target receptors.

Target Receptors	Brief Description	Ligands	Examples
Transferrin receptors	Responsible for delivering iron to neoplastic cells after binding to a respective ligand. Higher expression in neoplastic cells is about 100 times more than the normal cells	Transferrin	Gold nanoparticles and Nano composites of graphene oxide having surface modified with transferrin.
Folate receptors	Vital role in DNA synthesis after binding to its ligand Important tumor indicator having greater expression in neoplastic cells especially when it advances.	Folic acid, antibodies, folate	Folate grafted micelles containing paclitaxel

(Table 1) contd.....

Target Receptors	Brief Description	Ligands	Examples
Epidermal growth factor receptor	Its stimulation regulates key processes involved in the growth and development of neoplastic cells. Higher expression at advanced stages of cancer. Human epidermal receptor (HER 2) having up to 91% expression in breast cancer	Epidermal growth factors. Epiregulin Betacellulin, Amphiregulin	Tanstuzumab (antagonizing HER 2 receptor)
CD44-receptor	Glycoprotein receptors having higher expression in breast, colorectal, liver, and cervical cancers. Important bioindicator for malignant stem cells.	Hyaluronic acid	Liposomes and micelles conjugated with Hyaluronic acid

Besides cell surface receptors (peptide, folate, transferrin receptors), proteins or antigens (erb B2), as well as the lipoid constituents of the membranes, have been targeted by the ligands [73]. The effect of transferrin ligand targeting nanocrystals loaded with docetaxel has been analyzed for cytotoxic effects on cancerous A549 cell lines. The ligand conjugation enhanced the nanocrystal's targeting and hence the effectiveness of docetaxel compared to unconjugated docetaxel nanocrystals [74]. Furthermore, Apatinib bearing liposomes and paclitaxel-bearing micelles were surface modified with cyclic arginyl-glycyl-aspartic acid (RGD) peptide and folate ligand, respectively, for better antitumor efficacy [75].

In active vascular targeting (*i.e.* targeting the vascular endothelium), the receptors that have a vital role in the angiogenesis of tumoral endothelium are targeted. These include vascular endothelial growth factor (VEGF), vascular cell adhesion molecule (VCAM), matrix metalloproteinase (MMPs), and $\alpha v \beta 3$ integrin. Targeting the angiogenic factors of the tumoral endothelium, which is the basic phenomena responsible for tumor progression of tumor will diminish the supply of oxygen and basic nutrients for growth and development and ultimately result in cell death [76]. Vascular targeting not only overcome drug resistance and drug delivery challenges since it does not require permeability across blood vessel walls, but it can also be utilized to target different types of tumors [77 - 79]. For example, single-walled carbon nanotubes grafted with RGD linked poly ethylene glycol (PEG) for $\alpha v \beta 3$ integrin targeting on vascular endothelium resulted in efficient tumor targeting [80].

Table 2. A brief description of vascular targets.

Vascular Targets	Brief Description
Vascular Endothelial Growth Factor Receptor (VEGFR)	Important vascular target involved in tumor growth by angiogenesis after stimulation by certain genes and hypoxic conditions.
αvβ3 Integrin	Involved in the generation of new blood vessels involving cell transfer through Ca signaling networks.
Vascular Cell Adhesion Molecule (VCAM)	Present on endothelial cells responsible for the adhesion of integrin to matrix proteins leading to cancer metastasis.
Matrix Metalloproteinase	Responsible for the generation of extracellular matrix promoting the recruitment and development of new vessels.

Tumor cells possess distinguishing features *i.e.* the development of an acidic extracellular environment that has been utilized for targeted drug delivery [81]. It is noteworthy that rapidly growing tumors were tuned to high metabolic rates to meet the energy demand of rapidly growing cells and hence undergo increased glycolysis giving rise to the formation of the increased amount of lactic acid [82]. This lactic acid, when accumulated in cells, is troublesome and even causes death [83]. Cancerous cells tackle this problem by utilizing the Warburg effect i;e the pumping of protons out of the cells by means of various transporters into the extracellular fluid [84, 85]. Recent studies using pH responsive doxorubicin liposomes exhibited better efficacy in breast cancer as compared to doxorubicin liposomes alone [86].

Many anti-cancer drugs target cancerous cell nucleus, and their efficacy is dependent on the delivery of therapeutic moiety to the site of action. Delivering the drugs to the nucleus is a challenging task since it requires efficient passage of the drug through many physiological barriers. It has been demonstrated that nano-carriers are best suited for the targeted delivery of therapeutic and diagnostics agents. Active nuclear targeting will arrest cell division and ultimately results in apoptotic cell death [72]. It has been documented in a study that nuclear targeting was executed with gold nanoparticles having a surface modified with peptides along with PEG coating. Deposition of gold nanoparticles onto the nucleus resulted in cell death [87]. Recently, targeting moieties like nuclear location sequence (NLS) conjugated with nanocarriers are being utilized for active tumor targeting [88]. Examples include NLS conjugated PLGA nanoparticles, and NLS conjugated quantum dots for Hela cell nucleus [89].

Active targeting mechanisms are preferred for site-oriented delivery, thus avoiding the side effects, improved affinity, increased amount of drug reaching target site and hence better efficacy of the drug [72], suppression of multi drug resistance and capability of bypassing the blood-brain barrier [90]. Yet, it has a constraint that clinically it is feasible for the tumors that possess required cell surface receptors [91].

3.2. Passive Tumor Targeting

Passive targeting is the passive diffusion of nanocarriers into the tumor interstitium using spacing present in endothelial cell linings of tumor blood vessels (Fig. **4**). Passive diffusion appears to be the major underlying phenomenon since convection has been ruled out due to high interstitial pressure in solid tumors [71]. Additionally, it does not require any ligand for organ or tissue targeting [92]. Furthermore, it has been utilized for drugs with good cell permeation like doxorubicin [72]. Successful passive targeting is based on optimal execution of enhanced permeability and retention effect (EPR) by the tumors along with tumor characteristics (pH, microenvironment, extent of angiogenesis) [76]. The development of distinguishing features by the tumors vasculature leads to the exhibition of EPR effect. Physiologically tumor hypoxia initiates angiogenesis that led to the formation of irregular blood vessel networks having enhanced permeability due to large gaps developed between endothelial cells with a size up to 600 nm. Additionally, accompanied by reduced lymphatic drainage in tumor interstitium. The EPR effect is recognized as a gold standard and has been the focus of interest for passive antitumor targeting [72]. Examples of nanoparticles approved for clinical use based on EPR effect include Feridex, Doxil, Abraxane, Zevalin, Oncospar, Mylotarg, and Ontac [76]. The EPR effect can be well utilized if nanocarriers are designed to escape the reticuloendothelial system and have a long circulation time. For this purpose, the size should be above 10 nm and below 100 nm to avoid elimination by kidney and liver, respectively. Moreover, neutral nanoparticles are able to withstand renal clearance [71].

Furthermore, certain mediators like nitric oxide (NO), bradykinin, angiotensin II modulate the EPR effect by causing vasoconstriction resulting in increased extravasation of nanocarriers into tumor vicinity allowing for targeted delivery of anticancer loaded nanocarriers [93]. Passive targeting based on EPR effect have few constraints like high interstitial pressure of solid tumors [94], absence of EPR effect in certain tumors having decreased blood vessels [95, 96], failure to prolong the circulation time of nanocarriers, and difficulty in development of nanocarriers with enhanced retention due to physiological differences in blood vessels of animal models and humans. The development of nanoparticles that can alter tumor environment is the focus of interest; this includes different strategies like the blockage of angiogenesis and growth factors and the modulation of immune response [76].

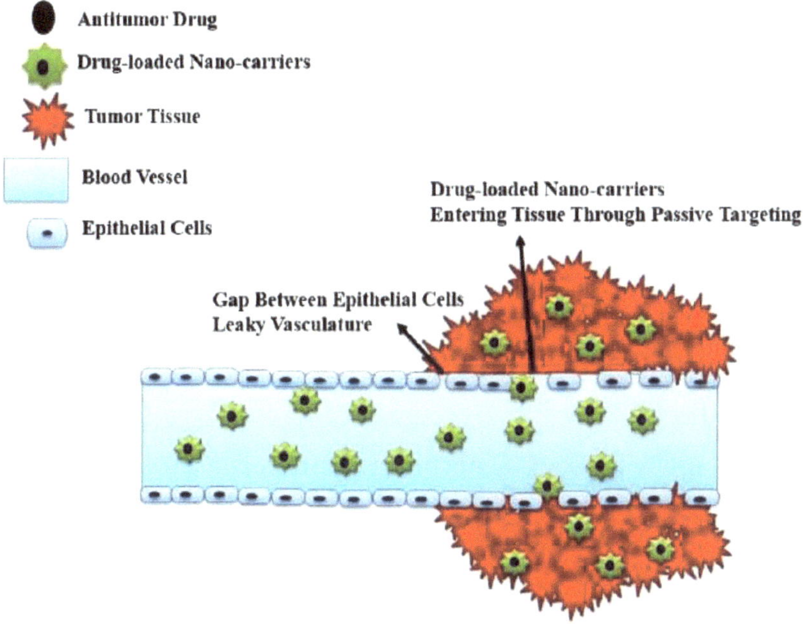

Fig. (4). Passive targeting of anticancer nanomaterials.

4. POTENTIAL APPLICATIONS OF EMERGING NANOMATERIALS IN CANCER THERAPY

4.1. High Drug Loading, Better Stability

Biocompatible lipid-based nano particles like liposomes have the advantage of increased drug loading capacity such that they can hold the bulk of drug entities in them [97]. In a study, Pei kan *et al*. demonstrated the high loading capacity and the anti-cancer efficacy of paclitaxel-loaded liposomes for human colon cancer c 26 cell lines [98]. The commercial application of the high loading capacity of the nanoparticle can be viewed in Doxil, a Dox-bearing liposomal formulation. The nanocarrier showed high loading of doxorubicin prepared to utilize ammonium sulfate transmembrane [22]. Nanomaterials like carbon nanotubes also possess the potential feature of high drug loading as discussed in a review on carbon nanotubes for anti-cancer therapy [99].

4.2. Rapid Release Effective Internalization

For efficient active targeting, the intracellular accumulation of drugs is important compared to drug accumulation in tumors. Hence, the internalization capable receptors like transferrin and folate receptors are targeted, giving rise to prompt release [71]. A doxorubicin bound liposomal formulation exhibited enhanced cellular internalization via CD 44 receptors resulting in greater anti-tumor activity. Furthermore, antigen modified immuno liposome showed effective cellular internalization and cytotoxic activity as described in a number of studies [100].

4.3. Extended Circulation Time

The successful application of nanotechnology depends on their escape from reticuloendothelial systems favoring long circulation time and, hence, greater drug accumulation at the tumor site. PEGylation is one of the strategies that help protect the nanoparticles from early uptake. It involves the coating of nanoparticle surfaces with polymers like Polyethylene glycol (PEG). The surface modification not only enhanced the circulation time but also resulted in targeted delivery of anticancer drug into the tumor interstitium. The synthetic approach of nanocarriers along with PEG coating helps in both efficient active targeting along with prolonged circulation potential. Currently this strategy is being utilized for tumor targeting purposes. Moreover, it could benefit optimal active targeting if nanocarriers with prolonged circulation time are grafted with targeting ligands [101]. Other applications include polymeric micelles loaded with anti-cancer drugs that showed prolong circulation time, increased localization and anti-tumor efficacy, as demonstrated in a number of studies [102 - 105]. Moreover, the surface PEGylating virus-based nano particles (VNPs) also increased their systemic circulation time in breast, colon, and lung cancers [12, 106 - 109]. Metal nano particles like Gold nanoparticles have been reported to have high drug loading and prolong circulation time [110].

4.4. Targeted Delivery of Anti-Cancer Agents

The rationale of using nanotechnology for anticancer drugs is to achieve targeted delivery via active or passive targeting and diminishing the damages to healthy tissues. The applications of targeted delivery of anticancer drugs have been demonstrated in the work of Verdun *et al.*, and Bibbly *et al.*, Verdun and coauthors reported the design of nanospheres loaded with doxorubicin. The prepared nanospheres showed targeted delivery in mice as depicted by their higher concentrations in the liver, spleen and lungs. The study of Bibbly *et al.*

deals with the special issue of mononuclear phagocytic systems (MPS) that on one side is challenging for tumor targeting while on the other side it could be utilized for targeting MPS bearing tumors like hepatic tumors, Bronchopulmonary carcinomas, primitive tumors and metastasis, small cell tumors and myelomas. The prepared RGD conjugated nanoparticles containing doxorubicin showed increased distribution to the liver as compared to tumor, demonstrating the key role of MPS. The beneficial effect of MPS was manifested in the hepatic metastasis model in mice utilizing doxorubicin-loaded nanoparticles. Liu *et al.* reported targeted delivery of 5-fluorouracil (5 FU) for the treatment of colon cancer. The hyaluronic acid-based silica-based nanoparticles of sizes up to 130 nm were developed and checked for their anti-tumor activity. The prepared nanoparticles exhibited increased cytotoxic effects in comparison to untargeted nanoparticles. Furthermore, it was demonstrated in a study that targeted liposomes possess better potential as compared to non-targeted liposomes for the desired anti-cancer effect [101].

4.5. Reduced Side Effects

Conventional chemotherapeutic agents have a drawback of reduced specificity resulting in increased side effects. The potential benefit of nanotechnology in chemotherapy is avoided the off-target side effects. Examples of such applications include targeted liposomal formulation containing anticancer drugs like doxorubicin and cisplatin showed enhanced therapeutic efficacy in breast cancer along with suppression of major side effects, including cardiac toxicity [111]. Additionally, reduced side effects have been demonstrated by chitosan nano particles containing cisplatin, showing better anti-tumor results in comparison to cisplatin alone [112]. Likewise, gelatin nanoparticles loaded with anti-cancer drugs like cisplatin [113], curcumin [114], and methotrexate [115] demonstrated enhanced anti-tumor efficacy and reduced adverse effects. Similarly, nanoparticles containing doxorubicin were reported to attain targeted delivery to the lungs and diminished delivery to other tissues, hence reducing side effects .Similarly, nanocarriers like dendrimers were loaded with docetaxel for reduced toxicity in the treatment of colon cancer. Docetaxel-based dendrimers showed promising cytotoxic effects as compared to docetaxel alone [34]. Furthermore, Cohen *et al.* incorporated two drugs in conjugated nano carriers for breast cancer. The prepared nano particles demonstrated increased cancer cell killing and decreased side effects [111].

4.6. siRNA and RNA Interference

RNA interference (RNAi) is a knockout or silencing strategy for cancer-related genes when applied to oncology. RNAi showed promising results in preventing tumors, overcoming the multi drugs resistance, and improving the proficiency of chemotherapy. Nanotechnology is being applied to RNAi for cancer therapy as it improves RNAi's response by preventing degradation, capturing by the immune system, renal excretion, and improved penetration across plasma membranes [116]. A study by Kim *et al.* reported the careful designing of PEG complexes grafted with vascular endothelial growth factors (VEGF) directed siRNA. Their successful application gives rise to inhibition of neovascular synthesis and tumor growth [117]. Likewise, Li and co-authors highlight the suppression of VSGF expression by delivering siRNA-based mesoporous silica nanoparticles (MSN) [118]. The *in-vitro* and *in-vivo* investigation of cationic nanoparticles bearing indoleamine 2, 3-dioxygenase (IDO), siRNA and tyrosine related protein 2 (Trp 2) was performed by Liu *et al.* The nanoparticles thus prepared promoted T cell immune response. Furthermore, it triggered the release of various cytokines and prevented the expression of IDO, and subsequently, these events resulted in the suppression of tumor growth [119]. Anionic polymers like poly lactic-co-glycolic acids had a promising role in the delivery of siRNA. A study documented paclitaxel's targeted delivery and siRNA for focal adhesion kinase (FAK) using both PLGA and hyaluronic acid for CD44 targets [120]. Magnetic hyperthermia-based cellular killing is a topic of review that sheds light into the use of magnetic field for the delivery of magnetic nanoparticles (MNPs) loaded with siRNA and anti-cancer drug, to the tumor cells [121, 122]. Gold nanoparticles (AuNPs) have certain characteristics like decreased toxicity, high drug loading, increased circulation time, and suppression of certain genes and triggering of the immune response, making them suitable for siRNA transport. AuNPs loaded with Bcl-2 (B- cell lymphoma) or VEGF-based siRNAs have been reported for silencing of Enhanced green fluorescent protein (EGFP) and Luciferase genes exhibited by cervical and glioma cell lines. Recently, DNA scaffolds have been successfully employed for transfection by siRNA. These scaffolds, along with targeting ligands and anti-cancer drugs resulted in improved response along with high specificity [123, 124].

4.7. Photodynamic Therapy

Nanotechnology emerged as an advancing field in photodynamic therapy (PDT) as it addresses the challenges of previously used photosensitizers of organic origin [125]. Nanomaterials like Superparamagnetic iron oxide nanoparticles (SPIONS), AuNPs and quantum dots (QDs) have applications in cancer therapy and diagnosis [126]. SPIONS have been successfully used as a contrast agent in cancer diagnosis, magnetic hyperthermia, and chemotherapy. The work of Lei *et al.*, [127] and Zeng *et al.* [128] reported the applications of SPIONS in cancer therapy. Lei *et al.* demonstrated the development of PGE functionalized iron oxide nanoparticles bearing chlorin e6 (for targeting purpose) for photodynamic therapy-based delivery of porphyrin drugs. The communication by Zeng *et al.*, reported the targeted tumor delivery of non-porphyrin drugs. Additionally, Zeng *et al.* developed multifunctional nano particles for serving both cancer imaging and therapeutic purposes. Jang and co-authors discussed the role of gold nano rods as carriers for anti-cancer drugs. These nanoparticles exhibited photo thermal therapy *in vivo* along with imaging [129]. The role played by QDs in photodynamic therapy could be attributed to their unique features like excellent optical and light absorption properties, resistance to photo bleaching, large surface area and differing sizes [126]. QDs have vast applications in cancer diagnosis [130]. The surface of QDs has been modified with targeting ligands to indicate tumor localization in the body [126].

Nanoparticles like liposomes successfully augmented the PDT by acting as a carrier for photosensitizer i:e photofrin, in two different models [131, 132]. Likewise, the cationic liposomes have been reported to enhance the tumor excision effect of chlorin e6 [133]. The tumor ablation effect of chlorin e6 based PDT was reported to be enhanced by the conjugation of hyperbranched poly ether-ester (HPEE) [134]. Lymphatic vessels undergo lymphangiogenesis that further promote tumor metastasis. Liposomes have been used as an efficient carrier of Benzoporphyrin derivative monoacid ring A (BPD) for PDT based on lymphatic vessels' ablation, hence arresting tumor metastasis [135].

4.8. Nanomaterials for Diagnostic Purposes

4.8.1. Radionuclide Scanning

To detect the specific biomarkers in the surrounding areas, a special type of targeted contrast agentis required, as it is impossible to visualize nano molecules without invasive procedures. In this type of scanning, the expressed proteins are labelled using different radio labelled agents, which are further traced *in vivo*. 99m tetrofosmin and sestamibi are employed in positron emission tomography scanning for the detection of multidrug resistance in cancer patients [136]. Different types of nanocarriers can be used for imaging, such as polymeric nanoparticles, liposomes, and dendrimers. These nanocarriers can load a number of radioactive and optical active agents for detection and scanning purposes using imaging machines. Actin filaments present in the plasma membranes have been visualized using boron dipyrromethene labelled jasplakinolide (BODIPY) dye [137]. Furthermore, the utilization of advanced imaging techniques with PET/CT and nanocarriers for theranostics provides greater sensitivity along with higher resolution imaging and accurate detection [138].

4.8.2. Biosensors

Biosensor technology is the most recent advancement in the field of nanotechnology from the past few years. Biosensors perform their functions by detecting certain molecules in the body. This recognition is dependent on the structure of molecules and their interactions like antigen-antibody, hormone receptor and substrate enzyme linkage. Nanocarriers like magnetic nanoparticles, quantum dots, gold nanoparticles (GNPs) and carbon nanotubes (CNTs) are used in biosensors [139, 140]. The sensitivity and specificity of biosensors depend upon these nanocarriers' physical, chemical, and mechanical properties. The most commonly used biosensors are GNPs based. For the detection of human gonadotrophin (HCG) amount, glassy carbon electrode (GCE) films are formed by the combination of methylene blue and GNPs through layer-by-layer technique [141].

Moreover, CNTs have an emerging role in biosensing. DNA detection can be done by using multi-walled carbon tubes (MWNT) bionanocomposites. Moreover, due to the magnetic properties, magnetic nanomaterials have numerous roles in the biotechnology field including, immunoassays, tissue engineering, cell culturing and MRI. Biosensor devices can also be employed for the detection of DNA oligonucleotides through CNT-SsDNA probes. Likewise, liposomes based biosensors are used in determining the concentration of organophosphate pesticides like paraoxon and dichlorvos [142].

4.8.3. Nanodiamonds (ND)

Nanodiamonds have gained a lot of attention for the past few years because of their mechanical, optical, and thermal properties. NDs are biocompatible and less cytotoxic as compared to CNTs. NDs applications include biosensors, magnetic and electrical sensors, bio-imaging through cell monitoring, bio-probes, and nanoelectromechanical systems (NEMS) [143]. For the improvement of optical detection methods, theranostics medicine has been used. Theranostics drugs allow the observation of *in vitro* and *in vivo* drug pharmacokinetics and efficacy studies. The optical properties of NDs, are enhanced by combining them with liposomes and this conjugation allows detection which is the theranostics application of liposomes. Liposomes also have the ability to conjugate with other agents, thus increasing their site-specific behaviour and physiological stability.

NDs have the ability to overcome the multidrug resistance observed in cancer therapy [144]. Additionally, NDs are used in the suppression of resistance due to chemotherapy and topical delivery of anti-cancer drugs. They are considered appropriate nanocarriers due to their adjustable surface and biocompatibility which offers tumor specificity and greater circulation time in the body.

NDs loaded with doxorubicin showed inhibition of cancerous growth with increased drug uptake. Now-a-days new techniques have been evolving for the treatment of cancer with lesser side effects to the healthy cells compared to the cancerous cells. The combination of photothermal therapy (conversion of light to heat energy) and photodynamic therapy (producing ROS), leads to the destruction of cancerous cells. These nanocarriers have potential applications in photodynamic therapy. Moreover, NDs are also capable of the eradication of cancerous cells through photothermal therapy [145]. Furthermore, targeting agent's addition and utilization of nanoparticles produce much better results. Maziukiewicz *et al.* studied the NDs coated with polydopamine and indocyanine green for determining their photochemical behaviour [146].

4.8.4. Quantum Dots (QD)

Quantum dots are nanocrystals that are semiconductors in nature with optical and mechanical properties. These nanocrystals are used for labeling the biological cells *in vivo* and *in vitro* due to their surface modification and biocompatibility. The imaging properties of QDs change as a function of their size and shape [147]. Graphene quantum dots (GQDs) are found to be promising candidates for imaging properties. QDs have an outer shell and inner core, which is metallic in nature [148]. The inner core is commonly made of cadmium selenide and cadmium sulfide. In order to preserve the optical properties of QDs, the shell is assembled on the core with a greater band energy gap providing better insulation. These QDs with variable shapes and sizes are used as promising biomarkers. The surface modification of QDs with different ligands leads to their site specific binding to receptors. QDs linked with tumor specific binding agents are used for visualizing the prostate cancer studies in mice. QDs have remarkable dominancy over the conventional fluorescent agents with increased stability and higher spectrum for absorption.

Metal sulfide QDs with thiol groups have greater circulation time in the body due to their aqueous nature and produce greater fluorescence. The fluorescent properties of QDs make them appropriate for imaging cancer cells. QDs conjugated with A10RNA and doxorubicin have been used for tumor cell imaging. In the *in vivo* imaging, there is restricted use of QDs because of their increased toxicity imparted by the heavy metals incorporated in them. However, recent advancements focus on reducing the toxicity profile and trying to improve the compatibility of QDs with the biological fluids and cells [142]. Copper indium sulfide and zinc sulfide QDs without cadmium were used for the lymph node cells imaging resulted in reduced toxicity and increased stability in the biological fluid [149].

5. FUTURE ASPECTS OF NANOMATERIALS IN CANCER THERAPY

It is reported that nanomaterials have been successfully used for the diagnosis and treatment in the field of oncology. Still, only a few nanoparticles loaded with chemotherapeutic agents have been clinically translated. It could be attributed to the fact that the research and development of nanoparticles are expensive and time-consuming. Moreover, the major breakthroughs of cancer nanotherapeutics are relevant to the initial stages and based on basic research in academia with no clinical connection. Furthermore, along with regulatory hurdles, miscommunication between academia and industries also limited the clinical translation. To cope up with these obstacles in nanotechnology design, more tactical approaches will be required. The clinical implementation of cancer nano medicines requires integrated research, which involves collaboration between industries and academia and must include experts from different disciplines like physicians and engineers.

Although the line extension of nano medicines endorse benefits like the -oriented delivery of nanomedicines, it proposes certain impediments (including the consideration of pharmacoeconomics, regulatory challenges, and poor expertise) that need to be addressed. In the context of recent clinical trials, the amalgam of treatments appears as a future research area though it has the limitation of clinical translation, requiring deep insight into toxicities. Moreover, it is reported that nanoparticle toxicology has devastating effects, which need to be further explored. Since targeting cancer nanomedicines is relevant to cancer pathophysiology, a thorough understanding of pathophysiological conditions is required for better insight into potential nanomedicines. This will promote the development of more accurate cancer therapeutics. Furthermore, the interplay of nanoparticles with the cellular components like proteins, lipids and the immune system is an important consideration, which needs to be inquired. The *in vivo* evaluation of nanotherapeutics for anti-tumor targeting is of prime importance and needs to be pursued further in relatable models to improve safety and efficacy. Future studies should focus on recognizing the best combination of nanoparticle and anti-cancer drugs to achieve better results.

CONSENT FOR PUBLICATION

Not applicable.

CONFLICT OF INTEREST

The author declares no conflict of interest, financial or otherwise.

ACKNOWLEDGEMENTS

Declared none.

REFERENCES

[1]   Ferlay J, Soerjomataram I, Dikshit R, *et al.* Cancer incidence and mortality worldwide: sources, methods and major patterns in GLOBOCAN 2012. Int J Cancer 2015; 136(5): E359-86.
[http://dx.doi.org/10.1002/ijc.29210] [PMID: 25220842]

[2]   Kaliberov SA, Buchsbaum DJ. Cancer treatment with gene therapy and radiation therapy. Advances in cancer research. 115. Elsevier 2012; pp. 221-63.

[3]   Etzioni R, Urban N, Ramsey S, *et al.* The case for early detection. Nat Rev Cancer 2003; 3(4): 243-52.
[http://dx.doi.org/10.1038/nrc1041] [PMID: 12671663]

[4]   Arora S, Rajwade JM, Paknikar KM. Nanotoxicology and *in vitro* studies: the need of the hour. Toxicol Appl Pharmacol 2012; 258(2): 151-65.
[http://dx.doi.org/10.1016/j.taap.2011.11.010] [PMID: 22178382]

[5]   Fakruddin M, Hossain Z, Afroz H. Prospects and applications of nanobiotechnology: a medical perspective. J Nanobiotechnology 2012; 10(1): 31.
[http://dx.doi.org/10.1186/1477-3155-10-31] [PMID: 22817658]

[6]   Moghimi SM, Hunter AC, Murray JC. Nanomedicine: current status and future prospects. FASEB J 2005; 19(3): 311-30.
[http://dx.doi.org/10.1096/fj.04-2747rev] [PMID: 15746175]

[7]   Kim BY, Rutka JT, Chan WC. Nanomedicine. N Engl J Med 2010; 363(25): 2434-43.
[http://dx.doi.org/10.1056/NEJMra0912273] [PMID: 21158659]

[8]   Prow TW, Grice JE, Lin LL, *et al.* Nanoparticles and microparticles for skin drug delivery. Adv Drug Deliv Rev 2011; 63(6): 470-91.
[http://dx.doi.org/10.1016/j.addr.2011.01.012] [PMID: 21315122]

[9]   Lavik E, von Recum H. The role of nanomaterials in translational medicine. ACS Nano 2011; 5(5): 3419-24.
[http://dx.doi.org/10.1021/nn201371a] [PMID: 21604811]

[10]   Sun T, Zhang YS, Pang B, Hyun DC, Yang M, Xia Y. Engineered nanoparticles for drug delivery in cancer therapy. Angew Chem Int Ed Engl 2014; 53(46): 12320-64.
[http://dx.doi.org/10.1002/anie.201403036] [PMID: 25294565]

[11]   Bor G, Mat Azmi ID, Yaghmur A. Nanomedicines for cancer therapy: current status, challenges and future prospects. Ther Deliv 2019; 10(2): 113-32.
[http://dx.doi.org/10.4155/tde-2018-0062] [PMID: 30678550]

[12]   Jabir NR, Tabrez S, Ashraf GM, Shakil S, Damanhouri GA, Kamal MA. Nanotechnology-based approaches in anticancer research. Int J Nanomedicine 2012; 7: 4391-408.
[PMID: 22927757]

[13]   Shi J, Kantoff PW, Wooster R, Farokhzad OC. Cancer nanomedicine: progress, challenges and opportunities. Nat Rev Cancer 2017; 17(1): 20-37.
[http://dx.doi.org/10.1038/nrc.2016.108] [PMID: 27834398]

[14]   Wang AZ, Langer R, Farokhzad OC. Nanoparticle delivery of cancer drugs. Annu Rev Med 2012; 63: 185-98.

[http://dx.doi.org/10.1146/annurev-med-040210-162544] [PMID: 21888516]

[15]   Wang L, Huo M, Chen Y, Shi J. Tumor microenvironment-enabled nanotherapy. Adv Healthc Mater 2018; 7(8): e1701156.
[http://dx.doi.org/10.1002/adhm.201701156] [PMID: 29283221]

[16]   Bozzuto G, Molinari A. Liposomes as nanomedical devices. Int J Nanomedicine 2015; 10: 975-99.
[http://dx.doi.org/10.2147/IJN.S68861] [PMID: 25678787]

[17]   Motomura M, Ichihara H, Matsumoto Y. Nano-chemotherapy using cationic liposome that strategically targets the cell membrane potential of pancreatic cancer cells with negative charge. Bioorg Med Chem Lett 2018; 28(7): 1161-5.
[http://dx.doi.org/10.1016/j.bmcl.2018.03.013] [PMID: 29534927]

[18]   Zhang Y, Xuan S, Owoseni O, *et al.* Amphiphilic polypeptoids serve as the connective glue to transform liposomes into multilamellar structures with closely spaced bilayers. Langmuir 2017; 33(11): 2780-9.
[http://dx.doi.org/10.1021/acs.langmuir.6b04190] [PMID: 28248521]

[19]   Qu M-H, Zeng R-F, Fang S, Dai Q-S, Li H-P, Long J-T. Liposome-based co-delivery of siRNA and docetaxel for the synergistic treatment of lung cancer. Int J Pharm 2014; 474(1-2): 112-22.
[http://dx.doi.org/10.1016/j.ijpharm.2014.08.019] [PMID: 25138252]

[20]   Allen TM, Cullis PR. Liposomal drug delivery systems: from concept to clinical applications. Adv Drug Deliv Rev 2013; 65(1): 36-48.
[http://dx.doi.org/10.1016/j.addr.2012.09.037] [PMID: 23036225]

[21]   Yang F, Jin C, Jiang Y, *et al.* Liposome based delivery systems in pancreatic cancer treatment: from bench to bedside. Cancer Treat Rev 2011; 37(8): 633-42.
[http://dx.doi.org/10.1016/j.ctrv.2011.01.006] [PMID: 21330062]

[22]   Barenholz Y. Doxil®--the first FDA-approved nano-drug: lessons learned. J Control Release 2012; 160(2): 117-34.
[http://dx.doi.org/10.1016/j.jconrel.2012.03.020] [PMID: 22484195]

[23]   Zheng Y, Tang L, Mabardi L, Kumari S, Irvine DJ. Enhancing adoptive cell therapy of cancer through targeted delivery of small-molecule immunomodulators to internalizing or noninternalizing receptors. ACS Nano 2017; 11(3): 3089-100.
[http://dx.doi.org/10.1021/acsnano.7b00078] [PMID: 28231431]

[24]   Wang W, Shao A, Zhang N, Fang J, Ruan JJ, Ruan BH. Cationic polymethacrylate-modified liposomes significantly enhanced doxorubicin delivery and antitumor activity. Sci Rep 2017; 7(1): 43036.
[http://dx.doi.org/10.1038/srep43036] [PMID: 28225062]

[25]   Torchilin VP. Recent advances with liposomes as pharmaceutical carriers. Nat Rev Drug Discov 2005; 4(2): 145-60.
[http://dx.doi.org/10.1038/nrd1632] [PMID: 15688077]

[26]   Weber S, Zimmer A, Pardeike J. Solid Lipid Nanoparticles (SLN) and Nanostructured Lipid Carriers (NLC) for pulmonary application: a review of the state of the art. Eur J Pharm Biopharm 2014; 86(1): 7-22.
[http://dx.doi.org/10.1016/j.ejpb.2013.08.013] [PMID: 24007657]

[27]   Mulik RS, Mönkkönen J, Juvonen RO, Mahadik KR, Paradkar AR. Transferrin mediated solid lipid nanoparticles containing curcumin: enhanced *in vitro* anticancer activity by induction of apoptosis. Int J Pharm 2010; 398(1-2): 190-203.
[http://dx.doi.org/10.1016/j.ijpharm.2010.07.021] [PMID: 20655375]

[28]   Truzzi E, Bongio C, Sacchetti F, *et al.* Self-assembled lipid nanoparticles for oral delivery of heparin-coated iron oxide nanoparticles for theranostic purposes. Mol 2017; 22(6): 963.
[http://dx.doi.org/10.3390/molecules22060963] [PMID: 28598368]

[29]   Patel MN, Lakkadwala S, Majrad MS, *et al.* Characterization and evaluation of 5-fluorouracil-loaded solid lipid nanoparticles prepared *via* a temperature-modulated solidification technique. AAPS PharmSciTech 2014; 15(6): 1498-508.
[http://dx.doi.org/10.1208/s12249-014-0168-x] [PMID: 25035070]

[30]   Müller RH, Radtke M, Wissing SA. Solid lipid nanoparticles (SLN) and nanostructured lipid carriers (NLC) in cosmetic and dermatological preparations. Adv Drug Deliv Rev 2002; 54 (Suppl. 1): S131-55.
[http://dx.doi.org/10.1016/S0169-409X(02)00118-7] [PMID: 12460720]

[31]   Maeda H, Wu J, Sawa T, Matsumura Y, Hori K. Tumor vascular permeability and the EPR effect in macromolecular therapeutics: a review. J Control Release 2000; 65(1-2): 271-84.
[http://dx.doi.org/10.1016/S0168-3659(99)00248-5] [PMID: 10699287]

[32]   Banerjee P, Geng T, Mahanty A, Li T, Zong L, Wang B. Integrating the drug, disulfiram into the vitamin E-TPGS-modified PEGylated nanostructured lipid carriers to synergize its repurposing for anti-cancer therapy of solid tumors. Int J Pharm 2019; 557: 374-89.
[http://dx.doi.org/10.1016/j.ijpharm.2018.12.051] [PMID: 30610896]

[33]   Yang XY, Li YX, Li M, Zhang L, Feng LX, Zhang N. Hyaluronic acid-coated nanostructured lipid carriers for targeting paclitaxel to cancer. Cancer Lett 2013; 334(2): 338-45.
[http://dx.doi.org/10.1016/j.canlet.2012.07.002] [PMID: 22776563]

[34]   Rao JP, Geckeler KE. Polymer nanoparticles: preparation techniques and size-control parameters. Prog Polym Sci 2011; 36(7): 887-913.
[http://dx.doi.org/10.1016/j.progpolymsci.2011.01.001]

[35]   ud Din F, Aman W, Ullah I, Qureshi OS, Mustapha O, Shafique S, *et al.* Effective use of nanocarriers as drug delivery systems for the treatment of selected tumors. Int J Nanomed 2017; 12: 7291.

[36]   Kedar U, Phutane P, Shidhaye S, Kadam V. Advances in polymeric micelles for drug delivery and tumor targeting. Nanomed 2010; 6(6): 714-29.
[http://dx.doi.org/10.1016/j.nano.2010.05.005] [PMID: 20542144]

[37]   Zhu Y, Liao L. Applications of nanoparticles for anticancer drug delivery: a review. J Nanosci Nanotechnol 2015; 15(7): 4753-73.
[http://dx.doi.org/10.1166/jnn.2015.10298] [PMID: 26373036]

[38]   Talelli M, Rijcken CJ, Hennink WE, Lammers T. Polymeric micelles for cancer therapy: 3 C's to enhance efficacy. Curr Opin Solid State Mater Sci 2012; 16(6): 302-9.
[http://dx.doi.org/10.1016/j.cossms.2012.10.003]

[39]   Ren J, Fang Z, Yao L, *et al.* A micelle-like structure of poloxamer-methotrexate conjugates as nanocarrier for methotrexate delivery. Int J Pharm 2015; 487(1-2): 177-86.
[http://dx.doi.org/10.1016/j.ijpharm.2015.04.014] [PMID: 25865570]

[40]   Weber C, Coester C, Kreuter J, Langer K. Desolvation process and surface characterisation of protein nanoparticles. Int J Pharm 2000; 194(1): 91-102.
[http://dx.doi.org/10.1016/S0378-5173(99)00370-1] [PMID: 10601688]

[41]   Elzoghby AO, Helmy MW, Samy WM, Elgindy NA. Spray-dried casein-based micelles as a vehicle for solubilization and controlled delivery of flutamide: formulation, characterization, and *in vivo* pharmacokinetics. Eur J Pharm Biopharm 2013; 84(3): 487-96.
[http://dx.doi.org/10.1016/j.ejpb.2013.01.005] [PMID: 23403015]

[42]   Elzoghby AO, Samy WM, Elgindy NA. Albumin-based nanoparticles as potential controlled release drug delivery systems. J Control Release 2012; 157(2): 168-82.
[http://dx.doi.org/10.1016/j.jconrel.2011.07.031] [PMID: 21839127]

[43]   Gradishar WJ, Tjulandin S, Davidson N, *et al.* Phase III trial of nanoparticle albumin-bound paclitaxel compared with polyethylated castor oil-based paclitaxel in women with breast cancer. J Clin Oncol 2005; 23(31): 7794-803.

[http://dx.doi.org/10.1200/JCO.2005.04.937] [PMID: 16172456]

[44]   Karthikeyan S, Prasad NR, Ganamani A, Balamurugan E. Anticancer activity of resveratrol-loaded gelatin nanoparticles on NCI-H460 non-small cell lung cancer cells. Biomedicine & Preventive Nutrition 2013; 3(1): 64-73.
[http://dx.doi.org/10.1016/j.bionut.2012.10.009]

[45]   Elzoghby AO, El-Fotoh WSA, Elgindy NA. Casein-based formulations as promising controlled release drug delivery systems. J Control Release 2011; 153(3): 206-16.
[http://dx.doi.org/10.1016/j.jconrel.2011.02.010] [PMID: 21338636]

[46]   De Santis E, Ryadnov MG. Peptide self-assembly for nanomaterials: the old new kid on the block. Chem Soc Rev 2015; 44(22): 8288-300.
[http://dx.doi.org/10.1039/C5CS00470E] [PMID: 26272066]

[47]   Rudra JS, Tian YF, Jung JP. A self-assembling peptide acting as an immune adjuvant. Proc Natl Acad Sci USA 2010; 107: 622.
[http://dx.doi.org/10.1073/pnas.0912124107] [PMID: 20080728]

[48]   Cheever MA, Higano CS. PROVENGE (Sipuleucel-T) in prostate cancer: the first FDA-approved therapeutic cancer vaccine. Clin Cancer Res 2011; 17(11): 3520-6.
[http://dx.doi.org/10.1158/1078-0432.CCR-10-3126] [PMID: 21471425]

[49]   Rayaprolu SJ, Hettiarachchy NS, Chen P, Kannan A, Mauromostakos A. Peptides derived from high oleic acid soybean meals inhibit colon, liver and lung cancer cell growth. Food Res Int 2013; 50(1): 282-8.
[http://dx.doi.org/10.1016/j.foodres.2012.10.021]

[50]   Conlon JM, Prajeep M, Mechkarska M, *et al.* Peptides with *in vitro* anti-tumor activity from the venom of the Eastern green mamba, Dendroaspis angusticeps (Elapidae). J Venom Res 2014; 5: 16-21.
[PMID: 25035794]

[51]   Chittasupho C, Lirdprapamongkol K, Kewsuwan P, Sarisuta N. Targeted delivery of doxorubicin to A549 lung cancer cells by CXCR4 antagonist conjugated PLGA nanoparticles. Eur J Pharm Biopharm 2014; 88(2): 529-38.
[http://dx.doi.org/10.1016/j.ejpb.2014.06.020] [PMID: 25119723]

[52]   Masuzawa T, Fujiwara Y, Okada K, *et al.* Phase I/II study of S-1 plus cisplatin combined with peptide vaccines for human vascular endothelial growth factor receptor 1 and 2 in patients with advanced gastric cancer. Int J Oncol 2012; 41(4): 1297-304.
[http://dx.doi.org/10.3892/ijo.2012.1573] [PMID: 22842485]

[53]   Iijima S. Helical microtubules of graphitic carbon. Nature. 1991; 354(6348): 56-8.

[54]   Eatemadi A, Daraee H, Karimkhanloo H, *et al.* Carbon nanotubes: properties, synthesis, purification, and medical applications. Nanoscale Res Lett 2014; 9(1): 393.
[http://dx.doi.org/10.1186/1556-276X-9-393] [PMID: 25170330]

[55]   Vardharajula S, Ali SZ, Tiwari PM, *et al.* Functionalized carbon nanotubes: biomedical applications. Int J Nanomed 2012; 7: 5361-74.
[PMID: 23091380]

[56]   Das M, Datir SR, Singh RP, Jain S. Augmented anticancer activity of a targeted, intracellularly activatable, theranostic nanomedicine based on fluorescent and radiolabeled, methotrexate-folic Acid-multiwalled carbon nanotube conjugate. Mol Pharm 2013; 10(7): 2543-57.
[http://dx.doi.org/10.1021/mp300701e] [PMID: 23683251]

[57]   Lay CL, Liu HQ, Tan HR, Liu Y. Delivery of paclitaxel by physically loading onto poly(ethylene glycol) (PEG)-graft-carbon nanotubes for potent cancer therapeutics. Nanotechnology 2010; 21(6): 065101.
[http://dx.doi.org/10.1088/0957-4484/21/6/065101] [PMID: 20057024]

[58]   Lu J, Liong M, Zink JI, Tamanoi F. Mesoporous silica nanoparticles as a delivery system for

hydrophobic anticancer drugs. Small 2007; 3(8): 1341-6.

[59]   Nejabat M, Charbgoo F, Ramezani M. Graphene as multifunctional delivery platform in cancer therapy. J Biomed Mater Res A 2017; 105(8): 2355-67.
[http://dx.doi.org/10.1002/jbm.a.36080] [PMID: 28371194]

[60]   Chen Y-W, Liu T-Y, Chang P-H, *et al.* A theranostic nrGO@MSN-ION nanocarrier developed to enhance the combination effect of sonodynamic therapy and ultrasound hyperthermia for treating tumor. Nanoscale 2016; 8(25): 12648-57.
[http://dx.doi.org/10.1039/C5NR07782F] [PMID: 26838477]

[61]   Ganguly S, Ray D, Das P, *et al.* Mechanically robust dual responsive water dispersible-graphene based conductive elastomeric hydrogel for tunable pulsatile drug release. Ultrason Sonochem 2018; 42: 212-27.
[http://dx.doi.org/10.1016/j.ultsonch.2017.11.028] [PMID: 29429663]

[62]   He L, Sarkar S, Barras A, Boukherroub R, Szunerits S, Mandler D. Electrochemically stimulated drug release from flexible electrodes coated electrophoretically with doxorubicin loaded reduced graphene oxide. Chem Commun (Camb) 2017; 53(28): 4022-5.
[http://dx.doi.org/10.1039/C7CC00381A] [PMID: 28338701]

[63]   Schaaf L, Schwab M, Ulmer C, *et al.* Hyperthermia synergizes with chemotherapy by inhibiting PARP1-dependent DNA replication arrest. Cancer Res 2016; 76(10): 2868-75.
[http://dx.doi.org/10.1158/0008-5472.CAN-15-2908] [PMID: 27013194]

[64]   Wang Y, Wang K, Zhao J, *et al.* Multifunctional mesoporous silica-coated graphene nanosheet used for chemo-photothermal synergistic targeted therapy of glioma. J Am Chem Soc 2013; 135(12): 4799-804.
[http://dx.doi.org/10.1021/ja312221g] [PMID: 23495667]

[65]   Park IY, Kim IY, Yoo MK, Choi YJ, Cho M-H, Cho CS. Mannosylated polyethylenimine coupled mesoporous silica nanoparticles for receptor-mediated gene delivery. Int J Pharm 2008; 359(1-2): 280-7.
[http://dx.doi.org/10.1016/j.ijpharm.2008.04.010] [PMID: 18490119]

[66]   Bharali DJ, Klejbor I, Stachowiak EK, *et al.* Organically modified silica nanoparticles: a nonviral vector for *in vivo* gene delivery and expression in the brain. Proc Natl Acad Sci USA 2005; 102(32): 11539-44.
[http://dx.doi.org/10.1073/pnas.0504926102] [PMID: 16051701]

[67]   Prabhakar N, Zhang J, Desai D, *et al.* Stimuli-responsive hybrid nanocarriers developed by controllable integration of hyperbranched PEI with mesoporous silica nanoparticles for sustained intracellular siRNA delivery. Int J Nanomedicine 2016; 11: 6591-608.
[http://dx.doi.org/10.2147/IJN.S120611] [PMID: 27994460]

[68]   Desai D, Zhang J, Sandholm J, *et al.* Lipid bilayer-gated mesoporous silica nanocarriers for tumor-targeted delivery of zoledronic acid *in vivo.* Mol Pharm 2017; 14(9): 3218-27.
[http://dx.doi.org/10.1021/acs.molpharmaceut.7b00519] [PMID: 28737925]

[69]   Han N, Zhao Q, Wan L, *et al.* Hybrid lipid-capped mesoporous silica for stimuli-responsive drug release and overcoming multidrug resistance. ACS Appl Mater Interfaces 2015; 7(5): 3342-51.
[http://dx.doi.org/10.1021/am5082793] [PMID: 25584634]

[70]   Yang D, Yang F, Hu J, *et al.* Hydrophilic multi-walled carbon nanotubes decorated with magnetite nanoparticles as lymphatic targeted drug delivery vehicles. Chem Commun (Camb) 2009; (29): 4447-9.
[http://dx.doi.org/10.1039/b908012k] [PMID: 19597621]

[71]   Danhier F, Feron O, Préat V. o exploit the tumor microenvironment: Passive and active tumor targeting of nanocarriers for anti-cancer drug delivery. J Cont Rel 2010; 148(2): 135-46.

[72]   Attia MF, Anton N, Wallyn J, Omran Z, Vandamme TF. An overview of active and passive targeting

strategies to improve the nanocarriers efficiency to tumour sites. J Pharm Pharmacol 2019; 71(8): 1185-98.
[http://dx.doi.org/10.1111/jphp.13098] [PMID: 31049986]

[73] Kumar Khanna V. Targeted delivery of nanomedicines. ISRN pharmacology 2012.
[http://dx.doi.org/10.5402/2012/571394]

[74] Choi J-S, Park J-S. Development of docetaxel nanocrystals surface modified with transferrin for tumor targeting. Drug Des Devel Ther 2016; 11: 17-26.
[http://dx.doi.org/10.2147/DDDT.S122984] [PMID: 28031702]

[75] Song Z, Lin Y, Zhang X, *et al.* Cyclic RGD peptide-modified liposomal drug delivery system for targeted oral apatinib administration: enhanced cellular uptake and improved therapeutic effects. Int J Nanomedicine 2017; 12: 1941-58.
[http://dx.doi.org/10.2147/IJN.S125573] [PMID: 28331317]

[76] Jani RK, Krupa G. Active targeting of nanoparticles: An innovative technology for drug delivery in cancer therapeutics. J Drug Deliv Ther 2019; 9(1-s): 408-15.
[http://dx.doi.org/10.22270/jddt.v9i1-s.2356]

[77] Shi S, Yang K, Hong H, *et al.* Tumor vasculature targeting and imaging in living mice with reduced graphene oxide. Biomaterials 2013; 34(12): 3002-9.
[http://dx.doi.org/10.1016/j.biomaterials.2013.01.047] [PMID: 23374706]

[78] Hong H, Yang K, Zhang Y, *et al. in vivo* targeting and imaging of tumor vasculature with radiolabeled, antibody-conjugated nanographene. ACS Nano 2012; 6(3): 2361-70.
[http://dx.doi.org/10.1021/nn204625e] [PMID: 22339280]

[79] Seon BK, Haba A, Matsuno F, *et al.* Endoglin-targeted cancer therapy. Curr Drug Deliv 2011; 8(1): 135-43.
[http://dx.doi.org/10.2174/156720111793663570] [PMID: 21034418]

[80] Liu Z, Cai W, He L, *et al. in vivo* biodistribution and highly efficient tumour targeting of carbon nanotubes in mice. Nat Nanotechnol 2007; 2(1): 47-52.
[http://dx.doi.org/10.1038/nnano.2006.170] [PMID: 18654207]

[81] Omran Z, Rauch C. Acid-mediated Lipinski's second rule: application to drug design and targeting in cancer. Eur Biophys J 2014; 43(4-5): 199-206.
[http://dx.doi.org/10.1007/s00249-014-0953-1] [PMID: 24687685]

[82] Xu RH, Pelicano H, Zhou Y, *et al.* Inhibition of glycolysis in cancer cells: a novel strategy to overcome drug resistance associated with mitochondrial respiratory defect and hypoxia. Cancer Res 2005; 65(2): 613-21.
[PMID: 15695406]

[83] Schornack PA, Gillies RJ. Contributions of cell metabolism and H+ diffusion to the acidic pH of tumors. Neoplasia 2003; 5(2): 135-45.
[http://dx.doi.org/10.1016/S1476-5586(03)80005-2] [PMID: 12659686]

[84] Mahon BP, Pinard MA, McKenna R. Targeting carbonic anhydrase IX activity and expression. Molecules 2015; 20(2): 2323-48.
[http://dx.doi.org/10.3390/molecules20022323] [PMID: 25647573]

[85] Walsh M, Fais S, Spugnini EP, *et al.* Proton pump inhibitors for the treatment of cancer in companion animals. J Exp Clin Cancer Res 2015; 34(1): 93.
[http://dx.doi.org/10.1186/s13046-015-0204-z] [PMID: 26337905]

[86] Paliwal SR, Paliwal R, Pal HC, *et al.* Estrogen-anchored pH-sensitive liposomes as nanomodule designed for site-specific delivery of doxorubicin in breast cancer therapy. Mol Pharm 2012; 9(1): 176-86.
[http://dx.doi.org/10.1021/mp200439z] [PMID: 22091702]

[87] Tkachenko AG, Xie H, Coleman D, *et al.* Multifunctional gold nanoparticle-peptide complexes for

nuclear targeting. J Am Chem Soc 2003; 125(16): 4700-1.
[http://dx.doi.org/10.1021/ja0296935] [PMID: 12696875]

[88] Derfus AM, Chan WC, Bhatia SN. Intracellular delivery of quantum dots for live cell labeling and organelle tracking. Adv Mater 2004; 16(12): 961-6.
[http://dx.doi.org/10.1002/adma.200306111]

[89] Cheng F-Y, Wang SP-H, Su C-H, *et al.* Stabilizer-free poly(lactide-co-glycolide) nanoparticles for multimodal biomedical probes. Biomaterials 2008; 29(13): 2104-12.
[http://dx.doi.org/10.1016/j.biomaterials.2008.01.010] [PMID: 18276001]

[90] Bazak R, Houri M, El Achy S, Kamel S, Refaat T. Cancer active targeting by nanoparticles: a comprehensive review of literature. J Cancer Res Clin Oncol 2015; 141(5): 769-84.
[http://dx.doi.org/10.1007/s00432-014-1767-3] [PMID: 25005786]

[91] Muhamad N, Plengsuriyakarn T, Na-Bangchang K. Application of active targeting nanoparticle delivery system for chemotherapeutic drugs and traditional/herbal medicines in cancer therapy: a systematic review. Int J Nanomedicine 2018; 13: 3921-35.
[http://dx.doi.org/10.2147/IJN.S165210] [PMID: 30013345]

[92] Maeda H. The enhanced permeability and retention (EPR) effect in tumor vasculature: the key role of tumor-selective macromolecular drug targeting. Adv Enzyme Regul 2001; 41: 189-207.
[http://dx.doi.org/10.1016/S0065-2571(00)00013-3] [PMID: 11384745]

[93] Bae KH, Chung HJ, Park TG. Nanomaterials for cancer therapy and imaging. Mol Cells 2011; 31(4): 295-302.
[http://dx.doi.org/10.1007/s10059-011-0051-5] [PMID: 21360197]

[94] Heldin C-H, Rubin K, Pietras K, Östman A. High interstitial fluid pressure - an obstacle in cancer therapy. Nat Rev Cancer 2004; 4(10): 806-13.
[http://dx.doi.org/10.1038/nrc1456] [PMID: 15510161]

[95] Maeda H, Sawa T, Konno T. Mechanism of tumor-targeted delivery of macromolecular drugs, including the EPR effect in solid tumor and clinical overview of the prototype polymeric drug SMANCS. J Control Release 2001; 74(1-3): 47-61.
[http://dx.doi.org/10.1016/S0168-3659(01)00309-1] [PMID: 11489482]

[96] Unezaki S, Maruyama K, Hosoda J-I, Nagae I, Koyanagi Y, Nakata M, *et al.* Direct measurement of the extravasation of polyethyleneglycol-coated liposomes into solid tumor tissue by *in vivo* fluorescence microscopy. Int J Pharm 1996; 144(1): 11-7.
[http://dx.doi.org/10.1016/S0378-5173(96)04674-1]

[97] Allen TM, Cullis PR. Drug delivery systems: entering the mainstream. Science 2004; 303(5665): 1818-22.
[http://dx.doi.org/10.1126/science.1095833] [PMID: 15031496]

[98] Kan P, Tsao C-W, Wang A-J, Su W-C, Liang H-F. A liposomal formulation able to incorporate a high content of Paclitaxel and exert promising anticancer effect. Journal of drug delivery 2011.
[http://dx.doi.org/10.1155/2011/629234]

[99] Kushwaha SKS, Ghoshal S, Rai AK, Singh S. Carbon nanotubes as a novel drug delivery system for anticancer therapy: a review. Braz J Pharm Sci 2013; 49(4): 629-43.
[http://dx.doi.org/10.1590/S1984-82502013000400002]

[100] Wang X, Yang L, Chen ZG, Shin DM. Application of nanotechnology in cancer therapy and imaging. CA Cancer J Clin 2008; 58(2): 97-110.
[http://dx.doi.org/10.3322/CA.2007.0003] [PMID: 18227410]

[101] Mohanraj V, Chen Y. Nanoparticles-a review. Tropical journal of pharmaceutical research 2006; 5(1): 561-73.

[102] Wang H, Zhao Y, Wu Y, *et al.* Enhanced anti-tumor efficacy by co-delivery of doxorubicin and paclitaxel with amphiphilic methoxy PEG-PLGA copolymer nanoparticles. Biomaterials 2011; 32(32):

8281-90.
[http://dx.doi.org/10.1016/j.biomaterials.2011.07.032] [PMID: 21807411]

[103]   Biswas S, Kumari P, Lakhani PM, Ghosh B. Recent advances in polymeric micelles for anti-cancer drug delivery. Eur J Pharm Sci 2016; 83: 184-202.
[http://dx.doi.org/10.1016/j.ejps.2015.12.031] [PMID: 26747018]

[104]   Rapoport N. Physical stimuli-responsive polymeric micelles for anti-cancer drug delivery. Prog Polym Sci 2007; 32(8-9): 962-90.
[http://dx.doi.org/10.1016/j.progpolymsci.2007.05.009]

[105]   Li X, Yang Z, Yang K, *et al.* Self-assembled polymeric micellar nanoparticles as nanocarriers for poorly soluble anticancer drug ethaselen. Nanoscale Res Lett 2009; 4(12): 1502-11.
[http://dx.doi.org/10.1007/s11671-009-9427-2] [PMID: 20652138]

[106]   Wendelsdorf KV, Alam M, Bassaganya-Riera J, *et al.* ENteric Immunity SImulator: a tool for *in silico* study of gastroenteric infections. IEEE Trans NanoBiosci 2012; 11(3): 273-88.
[http://dx.doi.org/10.1109/TNB.2012.2211891] [PMID: 22987134]

[107]   Cao J, Guenther RH, Sit TL, Opperman CH, Lommel SA, Willoughby JA. Loading and release mechanism of red clover necrotic mosaic virus derived plant viral nanoparticles for drug delivery of doxorubicin. Small 2014; 10(24): 5126-36.
[http://dx.doi.org/10.1002/smll.201400558] [PMID: 25098668]

[108]   Honarbakhsh S, Guenther RH, Willoughby JA, Lommel SA, Pourdeyhimi B. Polymeric systems incorporating plant viral nanoparticles for tailored release of therapeutics. Adv Healthc Mater 2013; 2(7): 1001-7.
[http://dx.doi.org/10.1002/adhm.201200434] [PMID: 23335438]

[109]   Singh P, Destito G, Schneemann A, Manchester M. Canine parvovirus-like particles, a novel nanomaterial for tumor targeting. J Nanobiotechnology 2006; 4(1): 2.
[http://dx.doi.org/10.1186/1477-3155-4-2] [PMID: 16476163]

[110]   Mahmoodi Chalbatani G, Dana H, Gharagouzloo E, *et al.* Small interfering RNAs (siRNAs) in cancer therapy: a nano-based approach. Int J Nanomedicine 2019; 14: 3111-28.
[http://dx.doi.org/10.2147/IJN.S200253] [PMID: 31118626]

[111]   Cohen SM, Mukerji R, Cai S, Damjanov I, Forrest ML, Cohen MS. Subcutaneous delivery of nanoconjugated doxorubicin and cisplatin for locally advanced breast cancer demonstrates improved efficacy and decreased toxicity at lower doses than standard systemic combination therapy *in vivo*. Am J Surg 2011; 202(6): 646-52.
[http://dx.doi.org/10.1016/j.amjsurg.2011.06.027] [PMID: 21982998]

[112]   Wang W, Chen S, Zhang L, *et al.* Poly(lactic acid)/chitosan hybrid nanoparticles for controlled release of anticancer drug. Mater Sci Eng C 2015; 46: 514-20.
[http://dx.doi.org/10.1016/j.msec.2014.10.048] [PMID: 25492016]

[113]   Tseng C-L, Su W-Y, Yen K-C, Yang K-C, Lin F-H. The use of biotinylated-EGF-modified gelatin nanoparticle carrier to enhance cisplatin accumulation in cancerous lungs *via* inhalation. Biomaterials 2009; 30(20): 3476-85.
[http://dx.doi.org/10.1016/j.biomaterials.2009.03.010] [PMID: 19345990]

[114]   Cao F, Ding B, Sun M, Guo C, Zhang L, Zhai G. Lung-targeted delivery system of curcumin loaded gelatin microspheres. Drug Deliv 2011; 18(8): 545-54.
[http://dx.doi.org/10.3109/10717544.2011.595842] [PMID: 21812751]

[115]   Cascone MG, Lazzeri L, Carmignani C, Zhu Z. Gelatin nanoparticles produced by a simple W/O emulsion as delivery system for methotrexate. J Mater Sci Mater Med 2002; 13(5): 523-6.
[http://dx.doi.org/10.1023/A:1014791327253] [PMID: 15348607]

[116]   Xin Y, Huang M, Guo WW, Huang Q. zhen Zhang L, Jiang G. Nano-based delivery of RNAi in cancer therapy. Mol Cancer 2017; 16(1): 1-9.

[http://dx.doi.org/10.1186/s12943-017-0683-y] [PMID: 28093071]

[117] Kim SH, Jeong JH, Lee SH, Kim SW, Park TG. LHRH receptor-mediated delivery of siRNA using polyelectrolyte complex micelles self-assembled from siRNA-PEG-LHRH conjugate and PEI. Bioconjug Chem 2008; 19(11): 2156-62.
[http://dx.doi.org/10.1021/bc800249n] [PMID: 18850733]

[118] Jing C, Zhang H. Inhibition of VEGF expression and SMMC 7721 cell growth by VEGFsiRNA. Chinese Journal of Pathophysiology 1986.

[119] Liu DQ, Lu S, Zhang LX, *et al.* An indoleamine 2, 3-dioxygenase siRNA nanoparticle-coated and Trp2-displayed recombinant yeast vaccine inhibits melanoma tumor growth in mice. J Control Release 2018; 273: 1-12.
[http://dx.doi.org/10.1016/j.jconrel.2018.01.013] [PMID: 29355622]

[120] Byeon Y, Lee J-W, Choi WS, *et al.* CD44-targeting PLGA nanoparticles incorporating paclitaxel and FAK siRNA overcome chemoresistance in epithelial ovarian cancer. Cancer Res 2018; 78(21): 6247-56.
[PMID: 30115698]

[121] Long R-M, Dai Q-L, Zhou X, *et al.* Bacterial magnetosomes-based nanocarriers for co-delivery of cancer therapeutics *in vitro*. Int J Nanomedicine 2018; 13: 8269-79.
[http://dx.doi.org/10.2147/IJN.S180503] [PMID: 30584299]

[122] Wu Z, Xu X-L, Zhang J-Z, *et al.* Magnetic cationic amylose nanoparticles used to deliver survivin-small interfering RNA for gene therapy of hepatocellular carcinoma *in vitro*. Nanomaterials (Basel) 2017; 7(5): 110.
[http://dx.doi.org/10.3390/nano7050110] [PMID: 28492491]

[123] Mendes R, Fernandes AR, Baptista PV. Gold nanoparticle approach to the selective delivery of gene silencing in cancer—the case for combined delivery? Genes (Basel) 2017; 8(3): 94.
[http://dx.doi.org/10.3390/genes8030094] [PMID: 28257109]

[124] Hou W, Wei P, Kong L, Guo R, Wang S, Shi X. Partially PEGylated dendrimer-entrapped gold nanoparticles: a promising nanoplatform for highly efficient DNA and siRNA delivery. J Mater Chem B Mater Biol Med 2016; 4(17): 2933-43.
[http://dx.doi.org/10.1039/C6TB00710D] [PMID: 32262971]

[125] Chen J, Fan T, Xie Z, *et al.* Advances in nanomaterials for photodynamic therapy applications: Status and challenges. Biomaterials 2020; 237: 119827.
[http://dx.doi.org/10.1016/j.biomaterials.2020.119827] [PMID: 32036302]

[126] Fakayode OJ, Tsolekile N, Songca SP, Oluwafemi OS. Applications of functionalized nanomaterials in photodynamic therapy. Biophys Rev 2018; 10(1): 49-67.
[http://dx.doi.org/10.1007/s12551-017-0383-2] [PMID: 29294258]

[127] Li Z, Wang C, Cheng L, *et al.* PEG-functionalized iron oxide nanoclusters loaded with chlorin e6 for targeted, NIR light induced, photodynamic therapy. Biomaterials 2013; 34(36): 9160-70.
[http://dx.doi.org/10.1016/j.biomaterials.2013.08.041] [PMID: 24008045]

[128] Zeng L, Xiang L, Ren W, Zheng J, Li T, Chen B, *et al.* Multifunctional photosensitizer-conjugated core–shell Fe 3 O 4@ NaYF 4: Yb/Er nanocomplexes and their applications in T 2-weighted magnetic resonance/upconversion luminescence imaging and photodynamic therapy of cancer cells. RSC Advances 2013; 3(33): 13915-25.
[http://dx.doi.org/10.1039/c3ra41916a]

[129] Jang B, Park J-Y, Tung C-H, Kim I-H, Choi Y. Gold nanorod-photosensitizer complex for near-infrared fluorescence imaging and photodynamic/photothermal therapy *in vivo*. ACS Nano 2011; 5(2): 1086-94.
[http://dx.doi.org/10.1021/nn102722z] [PMID: 21244012]

[130] Malik P, Gulia S, Kakkar R. Quantum dots for diagnosis of cancers. Adv Mater Lett 2013; 4: 811-22.

[131]   Jiang F, Lilge L, Grenier J, Li Y, Wilson MD, Chopp M. Photodynamic therapy of U87 human glioma in nude rat using liposome-delivered photofrin. Lasers Surg Med 1998; 22(2): 74-80.
[http://dx.doi.org/10.1002/(SICI)1096-9101(1998)22:2<74::AID-LSM>3.0.CO;2T] [PMID: 9484699]

[132]   Jiang F, Lilge L, Logie B, Li Y, Chopp M. Photodynamic therapy of 9L gliosarcoma with liposome-delivered photofrin. Photochem Photobiol 1997; 65(4): 701-6.
[http://dx.doi.org/10.1111/j.1751-1097.1997.tb01913.x] [PMID: 9114747]

[133]   Shim G, Lee S, Kim YB, Kim C-W, Oh Y-K. Enhanced tumor localization and retention of chlorin e6 in cationic nanolipoplexes potentiate the tumor ablation effects of photodynamic therapy. Nanotechnology 2011; 22(36): 365101.
[http://dx.doi.org/10.1088/0957-4484/22/36/365101] [PMID: 21841215]

[134]   Li P, Zhou G, Zhu X, *et al.* Photodynamic therapy with hyperbranched poly(ether-ester) chlorin(e6) nanoparticles on human tongue carcinoma CAL-27 cells. Photodiagn Photodyn Ther 2012; 9(1): 76-82.
[http://dx.doi.org/10.1016/j.pdpdt.2011.08.001] [PMID: 22369732]

[135]   Tammela T, Saaristo A, Holopainen T, Ylä-Herttuala S, Andersson LC, Virolainen S, *et al.* Photodynamic ablation of lymphatic vessels and intralymphatic cancer cells prevents metastasis. Science translational medicine 2011; 3(69) 69ra11-69ra11
[http://dx.doi.org/10.1126/scitranslmed.3001699]

[136]   Ballinger JR. 99mTc-tetrofosmin for functional imaging of P-glycoprotein modulation *in vivo*. J Clin Pharmacol 2001; 41(S7): 39S-47S.
[http://dx.doi.org/10.1177/009127001773744143] [PMID: 11452727]

[137]   Kowada T, Maeda H, Kikuchi K. BODIPY-based probes for the fluorescence imaging of biomolecules in living cells. Chem Soc Rev 2015; 44(14): 4953-72.
[http://dx.doi.org/10.1039/C5CS00030K] [PMID: 25801415]

[138]   Mitra A, Nan A, Line BR, Ghandehari H. Nanocarriers for nuclear imaging and radiotherapy of cancer. Curr Pharm Des 2006; 12(36): 4729-49.
[http://dx.doi.org/10.2174/138161206779026317] [PMID: 17168775]

[139]   You X, He R, Gao F, Shao J, Pan B, Cui D. Hydrophilic high-luminescent magnetic nanocomposites. Nanotechnology 2007; 18(3): 035701.
[http://dx.doi.org/10.1088/0957-4484/18/3/035701] [PMID: 19636132]

[140]   Pan B, Cui D, Xu P, Li Q, Huang T, He R, *et al.* Study on interaction between gold nanorod and bovine serum albumin. Colloids Surf A Physicochem Eng Asp 2007; 295(1-3): 217-22.
[http://dx.doi.org/10.1016/j.colsurfa.2006.09.002]

[141]   Chai R, Yuan R, Chai Y, Ou C, Cao S, Li X. Amperometric immunosensors based on layer-by-layer assembly of gold nanoparticles and methylene blue on thiourea modified glassy carbon electrode for determination of human chorionic gonadotrophin. Talanta 2008; 74(5): 1330-6.
[http://dx.doi.org/10.1016/j.talanta.2007.08.046] [PMID: 18371786]

[142]   Mir M, Ishtiaq S, Rabia S, *et al.* Nanotechnology: from *in vivo* imaging system to controlled drug delivery. Nanoscale Res Lett 2017; 12(1): 500.
[http://dx.doi.org/10.1186/s11671-017-2249-8] [PMID: 28819800]

[143]   Tinwala H, Wairkar S. Production, surface modification and biomedical applications of nanodiamonds: A sparkling tool for theranostics. Mater Sci Eng C 2019; 97: 913-31.
[http://dx.doi.org/10.1016/j.msec.2018.12.073] [PMID: 30678981]

[144]   Douda J, González-Vargas C, Mota-Díaz I, Basiuk E, Hernández-Contreras X, Fuentes-García J, *et al.* Photoluminescent properties of liposome-encapsulated amine-functionalized nanodiamonds. Nano Express 2020; 1(3): 030009.
[http://dx.doi.org/10.1088/2632-959X/abc1c5]

[145]   Gao G, Guo Q, Zhi J. Nanodiamond-based theranostic platform for drug delivery and bioimaging.

Small 2019; 15(48): e1902238.
[http://dx.doi.org/10.1002/smll.201902238] [PMID: 31304686]

[146] Bondon N, Raehm L, Charnay C, Boukherroub R, Durand J-O. Nanodiamonds for bioapplications, recent developments. J Mater Chem B Mater Biol Med 2020; 8(48): 10878-96.
[http://dx.doi.org/10.1039/D0TB02221G] [PMID: 33156316]

[147] Mohs AM, Provenzale JM. Applications of nanotechnology to imaging and therapy of brain tumors. Neuroimaging Clinics 2010; 20(3): 283-92.
[http://dx.doi.org/10.1016/j.nic.2010.04.002] [PMID: 20708547]

[148] Wang L, Zhu S-J, Wang H-Y, *et al.* Common origin of green luminescence in carbon nanodots and graphene quantum dots. ACS Nano 2014; 8(3): 2541-7.
[http://dx.doi.org/10.1021/nn500368m] [PMID: 24517361]

[149] Pons T, Pic E, Lequeux N, *et al.* Cadmium-free CuInS2/ZnS quantum dots for sentinel lymph node imaging with reduced toxicity. ACS Nano 2010; 4(5): 2531-8.
[http://dx.doi.org/10.1021/nn901421v] [PMID: 20387796]

CHAPTER 7

Toxicity of Silver Nanoparticles

Adeel Hassan[1,#], Sawara Sajal[1,#], Laiba Zakir[1,#], Sakina Munir[1,#], Fahad Hassan Shah[2,#], Song Ja Kim[2,*], Kashif Iqbal[1] and Saad Salman[1,*,*]

[1] *The University of Lahore, Islamabad Campus, Islamabad-44000, Pakistan*

[2] *Department of Biological Sciences, College of Natural Sciences, Kongju National University, Gongju, 32588, Republic of Korea*

Abstract: Silver nanoparticles (AgNPs) are metallic nanoparticles that are used for different biological purposes. Few toxic traits of Silver nanoparticles (AgNPs) producing plants are expressed; however, lesser is known about their genotoxic properties. This work discovered the cytotoxic and genotoxic risks of the entire concentrate from AgNPs of ethereal parts. Few studies had demonstrated that exaggerated reactions were not emerged by the four strains of Salmonella typhimurium, presented to fixations up to 5 mg/plate, with or without mammalian metabolic actuation (liver microsomal S9 division from Wistar rodents). In cytogenic cells and culture studies, higher doses (25–100 µg/mL) demonstrated a significant decrease in cell viability. In sister chromatids, chromosome distortions portrayed that AgNPs are genotoxic at the most noteworthy fixation utilized when clear cytotoxic impacts were also observed. Though, no expansion in micronuclei recurrence in bone marrow cells was identified when the extract was administered orally to mice (100, 500, and 2000 mg/kg dosages). The information was acquired to set up the most far-reaching extract on the genotoxic capability of AgNPs. Furthermore, it is noteworthy that the plant extracts plus AgNPs can cause *in-vitro* DNA hindrance at cytotoxic doses.

Keywords: Biological Properties, Chemical Properties, Physiochemical Properties, Plant Extract, Silver Nanoparticles.

1. INTRODUCTION

Silver nanoparticles (AgNPs) are prepared from different plants obtained from Brazil, North America, Malaysia, China, India, and Pakistan [1 - 4]. It is routinely

---

* **Corresponding author Song Ja Kim and Saad Salman:** Department of Biological Sciences, College of Natural Sciences, Kongju National University, Gongju, 32588, Republic of Korea and The University of Lahore, Islamabad Campus, Islamabad-44000, Pakistan; E-mails: ksj85@kongju.ac.kr and saad.salman@pharm.uol.edu.pk
# These authors have equal contribution.

Shahid Ali Khan, Saad Salman, Youssef O. Al-Ghamd (Eds.)

utilized as a solution for some sicknesses and accounted for by the decoctions and colors acquired from the leaves and underlying foundations of the plant, for instance, antirheumatic, ant syphilitic, hors d'oeuvre, diaphoretic, diuretic, emollient, purgative, and narcotic exercises [5 - 7]. Different properties have been guaranteed by trial pharmacology: mitigating, antimalarial, pain-relieving, antifungal, antibacterial, anticancer, antimitotic, anti-trypanosomal, and diuretics [8 - 11]. The toxic analysis of the AgNPs *in-vivo* ought to be studied [12, 13]. Genetic toxicity is one of the major poisonous impacts and its centrality is plentiful as we are thinking about the sublethal dosages prompting long haul impacts, for example, malignancy and degenerative infections [14 - 18]. Different techniques used in the synthesis of AgNPs are briefly discussed in Table **1**. While, the characterization and behaviors of AgNPs in the biological and environmental samples are briefly discussed in Table **2**. This book chapter focuses on the assessment of the normal genotoxic and cytotoxic danger of AgNPs and the extract in which it was prepared. The diverse hereditary results were examined to evaluate DNA harm at various hereditary articulation degrees. We assessed the viability of cells of AgNPs on CHO cells utilizing the MTT examination. The mutagenicity of the AgNPs on different bacterial strains. The Ames test was used for quality transformation, cytogenetic measures on cytogenic cells, culture study for chromosomal harm outside the body, andclastogenic and aneugenic impacts inside the body. The micronucleus test, in the bone marrow of mouse, is performed and the comet test was used for the assessment of DNA harm.

Table 1. Techniques used in synthesis of AgNPs adapted from Pryshchepa *et al.*, 2020 [19].

Modes	Precursor	Synthesis Condition	Preservation System	Result
Physico-chemical	$AgNO_3$	2 mm cathode and 99.9% titanium anode dipped into silver nitrate solution	Citrate	AgNPs $\approx$ 18 nm
	$Ag_2C_2O_4$	$AgNO_3$ decomposed at 125 centigrade for 100 h Anode is platinum and cathode made up of stainless steel capillary tube immersed in silver nitrate along with fructose solution	-	AgNPs 5–20 nm
	$AgNO_3$	Laser excision of 99.9% purity silicon target	Fructose	Polydisperse irregular AgNPs
	$AgNO_3$	Solution of Silver nitrate, Nd:YAG laser, having wavelength of 355 nm and pulses less than 40 ns, power density per pulse less than 40 J/cm^2 with 5 Hz frequency.	Silica	Polydisperse irregular AgNPs
Physical	AgNPs 99.9%	Electrodes of Silver (Ø 2 milimetre with length forty milimetre), disclosed in a distinct media (distilled water and glucose 10% and 25% w/w, glycerin/distilled water 10% and 25% w/w, phenol/distilled water 5% w/w, Mg(NO3)2•6H2O/distilled water 0.01% w/w and 0,05% w/w, xylene, ethylene glycol, ethyl acetate, and phenol/toluene 5% w/w) with pulses of 5–10 A/cm2, the cathode-anode gap was$\approx$1 mm, the NPs were separated by entrifugation and dried at 70 °C for 24 h	-	Ag@SiO_2 NPs with shell of 1-2 nm and core of 11 $\pm$ 4 nm

(Table 1) contd.....

Biological	AgNO₃	Filtrate of cell of fungus of 1. C. indicum, 2. Alternaria species, 3. Phoma, 4. F. oxysporum, 5. Curvularia species were cultivated on broth of potato dextrosefor almost 72 hours at 28 degree Celsius and combined with the mixture ofsilver nitrate.	Fungal cell filtrate mixture	AgNPs of 1. 7–20 n, 3. 5–23 nm, 5. 7–20 nm 2. 4–13 nm, 4. 10–31nm
		Solution of AgNO3 mixed with phosphate buffer having 7 pH contained O. limnetica homogenate were placed under fluorescence for 48 hours at 35 °C.	Composite of O. limnetica Homogenate	Quasi-spherical AgNPs having size of 3–18 nm.
		Solution of Silver nitrate combined with chrysin, 3-hydroxylflavone, galangin, flavone, kaempferol, tricetin, quercetin, apigenin, myricetin, luteolin, pH ranges from 7.2 to 10.1, the reaction was carried at 40, 23 and 70 °C.	Flavonoids	Depending on flavonoid use AgNPs ranges from size 12–39 nm.
		At 37 °C the solution of Bacillus licheniformis biomass along with silver nitrate was held for 24-h on shaker 200 rpm, then sonication and centrifugation was used to remove biomass	Compounds of Bacillus licheniformis biomass	AgNPs 40 -50 nm
		AgNPs were refined along dialysis with twelve thousand Da break-off and sucrose gradient (200.000×g for nearly 16-h at 4°C via HEPES buffer by using ultracentrifugation. Silver nitrate combined with orange peel essential oil and agitated for 48 hrs at 70°C.	Compounds of essential oil	AgNPs≈ 3 nm
		ultracentrifugation	Betanin	Spherical, shortened and triangualr AgNPs, = 15 nm
		Silver nitrate combined with orange peel essential oil and agitated for 48 hrs at 70°C.	Powdered Zingiber officinale composite	Average sizes of 11, 16, 20, 24nm that depends upon amount of silver nitrate

(Table 1) contd.....

Chemical	$AgNO_3$	In Mueller-hinton broth incubate L. lactisthat is isolated from milk at 26 °C for 5d. Centrifugation (9000 rpm) of culture and then supernatant.	Casein	4-100 nm size range of Casein-conjugated AgNPs.
	$AgNO_3$	The culturemedium along with solution of silver nitrate was retained at 26°C for 7 days. Then segregated by the process of centrifugation for 30 minutes at 14,000 rpm.	Supernatant of Lactococcus lactis compound	Biocomposite along AgNPs = 19 nm
	$AgNO_3$ $AuCl_4$	In heated silver nitrate solution, $HAuCl_4$ was added. Sodium citrate was added when mixture starts boiling. Continue boiling for 30 mins.	citrate	50 ± 9 nm of Au0.5 and Ag 0.5 nano particles commonly silver in the shell.
	$AgNO_3$	Premixed solution of sodium chloride, sodium citrate and silver nitrate quickly added in water (boiled) NaCl and $AgNO_3$ and sodium citrate mixture was added in presence of ascorbic acid. Stirred, heated for 1 h continually.	citrate	23 nm AgNPs seeds
	$AgNO_3$	Almost 12 similar mixtures with sodium citrate H_2O_2 were added with continuous stirring in solution of silver nitrate. $NaBH_4$ solution of different amounts for one and all solution were used.	citrate	Sphere, triangle and rod like structures of AgNPs ranges out of 3 to 30 nannometer.
	$AgNO_3$	Polyvinylpyrrolidone (PVP) with EG solution was heated at 160 °C and added in to the solution of sodium bromide and EG. Silver nitrate was introduced later. Solution was kept for 35 minutes and product was sisolated and washed by water.	Glutathione	Hollow, average silver nanoparticles, Empty AgNPs, hollow silver bromide/AgNPs
	$AgNO_3$	EG was heated at 140 °C temperature and then solutions of PVP/EG, HCL/EG and $AgNO_3$ were added, solution was heated for 8-h and then removed, tightened the vial.	PVP	silver nanowires =20 nm in diameter
	AgCl	Test was performed by adding different quantity of AgCl, NaCl and HCl.	PVP	Asymmetrical AgNPs, nanowires, truncated Octahedral and non-uniform nanocubes, shortened cubes And cuboctahedral shape.
	$CF_3\text{-}CO_2Ag$	Ag trifluoroacetate was dispersed in solution of isoamyl ethereal along with oleic corrosive mix at 160 degree celsius. below the N_2 environment, at which time it rains performed by sonication in ethanol and emerged centrifugation (3000 per minute).	Oleic acid	Hydrophobic AgNPs = 5.2 nm
	$[Ag(NH_3)_2]^+$	Ag trifluoroacetate was dispersed in isoamyl ether / oleic corrosive mix at 155 °C below the N_2 environment, at which time it rains performed by sonication in ethanol and emerged centrifugation (3000 per minute). Quantity 2:16:16 M DNA: silver⁺: sodium BH_4 used.	immersed in Silica	Silica☐Ag nanocomposite
	$AgNO_3$	The DNA was already assembled in clear sequence prepared with phosphate cushion saline at thirty seven ° C for 3 h, at that time silver + particles were added and stored at 3 ° C for one hour, accordingly sodiumBH4 added, the answer is reserved five hour dull at four ° C.	Deoxyribonucleic acid	Deoxyribonucleic acid-harbored Silver clusters with = 4 nm size
	$AgNO_3$	Silver nitrate (molar 4: 3 ratio) were included to pot under a stream of nitrogen with warm ethylene (134 °C) glycol, stored at 145 °C for one minute to prevent vapid formation, at that time the temperature rose by 165 °C at room temperature 16 °C/min. The mixture has dropped in the ice water shower on various time focus (12, 14, 16 18, 24, 30 min).	Deoxyribonucleic acid	3–08 nm Ag_2S NPs, depends on time of reaction
	$[Silver(NH_3)_2]^+$	At different temperature Different levels of silver NPs are added to water , at the same time complex alkali arrangement ascorbic corrosive added, mixed one hour, silvernitrate are separated by centrifugation and reconstituted in sodium citrate system.	Citrate	30–290 nm silver NPs, depends on amount of silver nitrate seeds

Table 2. The characterization of AgNPs for the purpose to study its behavior and for their presence in the biological and Environmental samples.

Purpose	Method	Data	Complications
To study features of AgNPs	Dark field microscopy	Distinctive shapes of nanoparticles were analyzed when single nanoparticle splitting LSPR	Need of fierce or high source of light and prolonged exposure
Interlinkage of green algae with AgNPs		Algae cells processed with AgNPs have shown scattering light intensification	
Activity of AgNPs dissolution		Color change and LSPR scattering were observed due to the potentiality exposure	
Impact of neighboring media on LSPR	Fluorescent microscopy	Due to the increase of refractive index of media change in red wavelength in AgNPs LSPR were identified	Misconception can occur related to less affinity of molecules with nanoparticles and small spatial elucidation
Movement of AgNPs in leafs		Place of nanoparticles distribution discovered in Stevia rebaudiana B.	
Surface attachment of bacteria	Scanning electron microscopy	Change in color and constancy was observed when BALB/3 and MB49 T3 cells marked with ethidium bromide or acridine orange. Programmed cell death and necrosis were revealed.	Nonconductivty of charges present on surface of sample and change in size, shape, sample damage and assemblage
Cell toxic activity of AgNPs with α-Ag$_2$WO$_4$		Bacterial adherence with AgNPs surface was observed	
Biological activity of AgNPs	Transmission electron microscopy	S. aureus, B. subtilis and E. coli showed injury in the cells of bacteria. C. elegans showed splits in the skin.	Nonconductivity of charges present on surface of sample and change in size, shape, sample damage and assemblage during the preparation process of sample and technique needs exceedingly high vacuum and fine sample less than 100 nm
Changes in surface structure		On the surface of spheres and silica rods, AgNPs shells formed and accumulation of AgNPs on fibers of linen and polyester	
Fine surface morphology	Cryogenic transmission electron microscopy	Images revealed AgNPs exposure with R. subcapitata by showing more sensitivity with SE Images observed by using SEM showed AgNPs in round shape 3138 ± 722 AgNPs were found in macrophage. Shape, distribution of size, structure space of the lattice in crystals were determined and calculated.	The change in cantilever motion can occur due to electrostatic charges.
Surface/structure of AgNPs		Liquid phase TEM identified silver nanorod development due to the ingathering of round nanoparticles	
Consumption of AgNPs by SEM and focused ion beam		Assimilation and dispensation of Ag+ on the surface of bacteria following AgNPs development was identified.	
Characteristics of AgNPs		Aggregation of AgNPs forming chain was described.	
Growth of AgNPs		The size of AgNPs made by glucose was 10.3nm and other made by dialdehydenanofibrilllated cellulose was 19-37 nm in diameter placed beside fiber site.	
Restoration of Ag$^+$		22 ± 6 nm size of AgNPs was determined by TEM and while for 100 nanoparticles it was 20 ± 6 nm.	

(Table 2) contd.....

Characteristics of AgNPs	Atomic force microscopy	22 ± 6 nm size of AgNPs was determined by TEM and while for 100 nanoparticles it was 20 ± 6 nm.	Favored direction of non-round NPs, low sign power for NPs under 10 nm, 2% affectability limit for composites
Growth of AgNPs		Red shift was observed by performing LSPR on AgNPs in contrast to ultraviolet visible spectroscopy	
Restoration of Ag$^+$		Size measured in medium of cell was 71 ± 0.2 nm while in water was 79 ± 0.5 nm.	
Ag nanoparticles congregation		The citrate potential was -23.4 $\pm$ 6 by making ready with the extract of green tea that was -36.2 $\pm$ 5 and radii of hydrodynamic was 87.7nm (TEM $-$ 8.3 $\pm$ 3.6 nm).	
Form and structure of surface		When AgNPs were made from extract of green tea they potrayed more strength of accumulation in solution of several PH, glucosamine, sodium chloride and constitutes of cell culture.	
Size of AgNPs		Au @Ag nancocuboids longitudinal band $\approx$552 nm, transverse $\approx$461 nm Spherical Au0.5Ag0.5 band $\approx$ 460 nanometre Silver NPs LSPR band $\approx$ 480 nm	
AgNPs		Triangular Silver NPs, out-of-plane foursided band 228 nanometre, plane out dipolar band 324 nanometre, plane in dipolar resonance 530–590 nanometre	
Size of AgNPs		The newly blended NPs LSPR $\approx$ 399 nm, the NPs presented to daylight for 25 days get another groups (480, 585 nm)	
Accumulation of AgNPs		1.32 ± 0.6 nm AgNPs covered with polymethacrylic corrosive uncovered straight fluorescent charm contingent upon Pb2+ focus in range from 0.2 to 1.2 μM	
Silver nanocomposite		Fluorescent AgNPs $\approx$ 10 nm covered with 4-mercapto phenylboronic corrosive and 30-aminobenzo-18-crown-6 uncovered straight extinguishing relying upon dopamine content (0.01–0.2 mM) because of NPs total	

(Table 2) contd.....

Stability of AgNPs	Atomic force microscopy	Au @Ag nancocuboids longitudinal band ≈552 nm, transverse ≈461 nm Spherical Au0.5Ag0.5 band ≈ 460 nanometre Silver NPs LSPR band ≈ 480 nm Triangular Silver NPs, out-of-plane foursided band 228 nanometre, plane out dipolar band 324 nanometre, plane in dipolar resonance 530–590 nm The newly blended NPs LSPR ≈ 399 nm, the NPs presented to daylight for 25 days get another groups (480, 585 nm) 1.32 ± 0.6 nm AgNPs covered with polymethacrylic corrosive uncovered straight fluorescent charm contingent upon Pb^{2+} focus in range from 0.2 to 1.2 µM	Heating and black body thermal emission can occur. Polyatomic and Atomic interferences, samples usually requires mineralization Test charging, requires super high vacuum, the example change and harm
Measurementof Pb^{2+}		Fluorescent AgNPs ≈ 10 nm covered with 4-mercapto phenylboronic corrosive and 30-aminobenzo-18-crown-6 uncovered straight extinguishing relying upon dopamine content (0.01–0.2 mM) because of NPs total	
Evaluation of dopamine		1213.6 cm^{-1}, 3234.4 cm^{-1} groups appearance, expansion in 1455.7 cm^{-1}, shift 1234.7 cm^{-1} → 1627 cm^{-1} after ampicillin restricting 1.32 ± 0.6 nm AgNPs covered with polymethacrylic corrosive uncovered straight fluorescent charm contingent upon Pb2+ focus in range from 0.2 to 1.2 µM. Fluorescent AgNPs ≈ 10 nm covered with 4-mercapto phenylboronic corrosive and 30-aminobenzo--8-crown-6 uncovered straight extinguishing relying upon dopamine content (0.01–0.2 mM) because of NPs total. 1213.6 cm−1 , 3234.4 cm−1 groups appearance, expansion in 1455.7 cm−1 , shift 1234.7 cm^{-1} → 1627 cm−1 after ampicillin restricting	
Development and functionalization of AgNPs		Presence of 3425 cm^{-1} extending band of C-O bunch and 756 cm^{-1} of frail S - S vibration uncovered alpha-lipoic corrosive restricting.	
Functionalization evaluation of AgNPs		The AgNPs development and restricting to lactoferrin influenced the infrared spectra in range 1650–1400 cm The vibration between Ag° surface and pyridine nitrogen was observed by appearance of 241 cm^{-1} on spectra	
SERS study Method of AgNPs development		All SERS spectra of AgNPs with lyzozyme, BSA, cytochrome-C and hemoglobin has band ≈ 240 cm−1 attributed to Ag=N and Ag=S, band ≈ 1630 cm^{-1} , which replaces the amide-I band at 1655 cm−1 , the shifts near 1375 cm^{-1} in cytochrome and hemoglobin can be assigned to hem bands Presence of 3425 cm−1 extending band of C_O bunch and 756 cm−1 of frail S- - S vibration uncovered alpha-lipoic corrosive restricting The AgNPs development and restricting to lactoferrin influenced the infrared spectra in range 1650–1400 cm The vibration between Ag(0) surface and pyridine nitrogen was observed by appearance of 241 cm−1 on spectra All SERS spectra of AgNPs with lyzozyme, BSA, cytochrome-C and hemoglobin has band ≈ 240 cm−1 attributed to Ag=N and Ag=S, band ≈ 1630 cm−1 , which replaces the amide I band at 1655 cm−1 , the shifts near 1375 cm−1 in cytochrome and hemoglobin can be assigned to hem bands The hydride intermediates s ([Ag7(H){Se2P(Oi Pr)2}6] and [Ag7 (H) {S2 P(OEt)2}6]) formation was revealed by appearance of doublets 1125.ppm (d, JagH + 39.7 Hz) and 1116.7 ppm (d, JAgH = 41.1 Hz) at 298 K as well as octet at 3.50 ppm (1 JH−Ag = 39.4 Hz) at 293 K and broad peak 5.65 ppm, (1 JH−Ag = 39.6 Hz) at 223 K	

(Table 2) contd.....

Reducing agent and stabilizer part in AgNPs development	Near field scanning optical microscopy	In the NPs the electron energy loses corresponding to Ag particles was recognized, presence of C, N and Ca was noticed.	Coupling effect due to conducting tip and scattered by tip light causing interference.
Quantitative binding affinity of taurine	Dynamic light scattering	Significant changes in chemical shifts of sodium dodecyl sulfate protons 4.086 ppm → 4.037 ppm, 1.360 ppm → 1.320 ppm, 0.952 ppm → 0.900 ppm after AgNPs formation in the mixture with trisodium citrate, the decreased intensities of signals from trisodium citrate protons After treatment of AgNPs, the glutathione signals completely diminshed and disappeared. $\approx$2% of Ag as in unbound (elemental) state, Ag=O, Ag=S and Ag=N bounds were found to be ~71%, 16%,11% respectively, that shows binding of sulphonate group to Ag Doped with $\approx$ 4.5 nm AgNPs hydrogen-terminated Si (111) show the photoelectron yield with p-polarization: 2.8•106 , while that without AgNPs has 1.4•104	Due to remarkable shifts and conjoining the bands are difficult to distinguish and depends on molecular structure
Photoelectron emission yield	X-ray photoelectron spectroscopy	LSPR advances relying upon electron portion from 2.1•106 e–å–2 to 18.7 •106 e–å–2 , under most minimal portion no LSPR shift was noticed, with expanding of electron portion blue-shifts were seen from 2.8 to 3.2 eV (for NP $\approx$ 7 nm)	Accumulation, lower size limit (20 nm), difficult to recognize diverse Ag structure
Morphology of Ag sprouting on Fe_3O_4	ICP-MS SAED	Cells treated with 2 µg/mL of AgNPs with sizes 50 and 75 nm uncovered the take-up of 1662 and 605 number/cell separately, while treated with 10 µg/mL of AgNPs uncovered the take-up 1989 and 1740 number/cell	
Changes in Fe, Ag, Mg and N content in Stevia rebaudiana B. treated with AgNPs	UPS AES	By changing frequencies of laser fluence from 15-80 ml/cm2, ordinary particle powers for Au nanoparticles were 0 to 21.104 check/mm^2 and for Ag nanoparticles from 5 to 35x104 tally/mm^2.	Test charging, the example change (for example decrease), test can be inspected uniquely on 2 nm profundity, requires super high vacuum
Investigation of AgNPs crystalline phase in situ toughening conduct of Ag2S NPs	Fluorescence FTIR Raman NMR Ultraviolet – visible spectroscopy	In sure mode silver-amine particles were noticed AgC2H6NO⁺, AgC3H4NO⁺, AgC4NO2H$_3$⁺ at 167, 177, 203.9 mass and Ag fortified with sulfur AgSC$_2$H$_3$N+, AgSC$_3$H$_6$N⁺ at 179.90 and 194.93, mass. In adverse mode AgCOOHCNH$_2$–, C$_3$H$_2$NO$_2$Ag–, C$_4$N$_3$O$_2$Ag⁻ at 179.91, 192, 241 and AgC$_2$H$_3$SN–, C$_3$H$_2$SNAg⁻, C3H7SNO$_2$Ag⁻ at 179.89, 190.89, and 227.92 mass were noticed	Need super high vacuum due to test charging and harm
			Adsorption by matrix, fluorescence caused by sample and adulteration can overload the studies
Distribution of elements over the NPs			Accumulation and calculation depends on the neighboring media.
LSPR modes for AgNPs inserted in SiO_2	XRD EEL SP-ICP-MS MALDI-TOF MS TO F-SIMS	51.77, 51.8, 52.61, 52.19 and 59.52 were the upsides of glass change controlled by DSC for films and the rate upsides of TiO2-Ag were 0, 1, 2, 3, and 4.	Absorbance by contaminations and quencher in fluorescent band and presence of fluorescent pollutants.
Uptake of AgNPs Cellular by Neuro-2a cells		958±21 s, 1048± 15 s, 958 ± 32 s and 1275 ± 115 s were the standard qualities for polyethlylenimine PVP, polyethylene glycol and citrate consecutively when broke down with 40nm covered.	NPs aggregation, analyte fragmentation
MALDI analysis of benzpyridinium		Polyethyleneglicol was isolated in two part blend while citrate was isolated from PVP. Au @Ag nancocuboids longitudinal band $\approx$552 nm, transverse $\approx$461 nm Spherical Au0.5Ag0.5 band $\approx$ 460 nanometre Silver NPs LSPR band $\approx$ 480 nm Triangular Silver NPs, out-of-plane foursided band 228 nanometre, plane out dipolar band 324 nanometre, plane in dipolar resonance 530–590 nanometre	Test charging, little assessment profundity, requires super high vacuum, the example change and harm

(Table 2) contd.....

Modifications and interactions of AgNPs in municipal wastewater	Capillary electrophoresis	Four part blend was hard to isolate. According to observations on the basis of hemispherical cap model, Fe3O4 absorbed Ag gas atoms shows separate layers of AgNPs and no Ag layer. When AgNPs concentration changes in culture media from 0 to 200 mg/L the changes in Mg,N, and Ag content (calculated on dried weigh) were shown Measured d-spacing (nm) were 0.233, 0.203, 0.141, 0.121 which are in good correspondence with Ag (0) hkl(nm) 0.236, 0.204, 0.145, 0.123, and AgOhkl (nm) 0.237 and 0.143. For NPs warmed in air the 2θ signs at ≈29°, 31.5°, 38°, 41°, relating to monoclinic acanthine α-Ag2S vanished, and the 2θ signs 39° and 43° of unadulterated silver showed up. For NPs warmed in argon, the XRD design changed to more perplexing, which might be credited to monoclinic non-stochiometric acanthine α-Ag1.95–1.98S	Significantly low affectability, requires the center absorption of large NPs,Ag has low gyromagnetic proportion and huge T1 esteem, which requires exceptional gadgets and long haul investigation
Gelatin films of doped TiO$_2$-AgNPs stability	AF4	As per UV-apparent, indicator more noteworthy outcomes were deciphered. PVE covered nanoparticles were recuperated with sizes 90, 30, 60 nm for influent, stream water, tape water, treatment plant with 69.4,90.2,55.6 and 78.6 % separately	Spatial goal is restricted by distance across of essential particle shaft, which is regularly greater than NPs size
Detachment of AgNPs	Differential scanning Calorimetry	Established on DLC identifier, emanating and faucet water showed consistency among unique and estimated sizes.	Accumulation, adherence of nanoparticles to capillary walls, low selectivity
Identification of AgNPs in environmental samples		In faucet water ICP-MS showed better partition. The newly blended NPs LSPR ≈ 399 nm, the NPs presented to daylight for 25 days get another groups (480, 585 nm)	Membrane fouling by irreversibly bonded NPs, NPs accumulation, non-selective upon size detectors (UV-Vis/MALS)

2. EVALUATION OF SILVER NANOPARTICLE TOXICITY

For the preparation of AgNPs, different plant materials are used for capping and stabilizing the nanoparticles. The plant extracts are prepared through extraction; fluid is extracted from the dry material of plants. Four rounds of percolation are done before fluid extraction. The raw material is acquired under reduced pressure and stored at 4°C in closed containers. Qualitative evaluation was done for the chemical categorization of the extract which depicts flavonoids, saponins, polysaccharides, terpenes, steroids, sesquiterpenes, and coumarin. Methanol/ethanol was considered the most suitable solvent for the dissolution of plant extract. Dimethyl sulfoxide is used for *in-vitro,* and ethanol was used for *in-vivo* analysis. Positive control: aminoflourine, sodium azide, cyclophosphamide, 9-aminoacridine, and chlorogenic acid are used as positive control in the Ames test. In chromosome anomalies assay, mitomycin-C and X-ray are used; Hydrogen peroxide in alkaline comet assay and CP in mouse bone marrow micronucleus.

3. *IN-VITRO* ASSAYS

Maron and Ames performed plate incorporation mutagenicity assay using strains of salmonella tester TA 1535, TA 153, TA100. Five concentrations were analyzed under a single experiment from 50 to 500 µg solid /plate. After treatment of Wister rats with phenobarbital and benzoflavone liver microsomal S9 fraction was formulated. 4% S9 fraction out of S9 mix is present in the solution of cofactors. After 72-h, the colonies were calculated at 37 °C temperature.

3.1. Cytogenic and Cell Culture Studies in CHO Cells

CHO cells were grown in Ham F10 nutrient medium with 10% FBS (Fetal Bovine Serum), 100 IU/mL penicillin, and 2 mL glutamine. CHO cells were grown at temperature 37 °C and in humidity that contains 5% carbon dioxide.

3.2. The MTT Cytotoxicity Assay

Nearly 1×10^4 CHO cells were added to each well of the culture microplate. For extraction, it was treated for 24-h and incubated with 5 mg/ml MTT for 4-h. Microplate spectrophotometer was used to read plates at 550 nm. Total 5 different concentrations are used and IC_{50} was accessed from the dose-response curve.

3.3. Sister Chromatid Exchanges (SCE) Assay

For almost 3-h, cells were exposed to AgNPs with recovery time of at least 24 or 27 h. During the last 24-h of incubation, cultures were obtained with final concentration of 1.5 µg/ml. The 2h before fixation 5×10 colchicine was always augmented. Sister chromatids were stained and 20 metaphases per experiment were evaluated.

3.4. Chromosomal Aberration Assay

It was performed according to international guidelines. CHO cells growing at an exponential rate were used in the experiment. These were treated under 2 methods. Treatment was done for 3h with a 15-h recovery time. Continues treatment was done until harvesting 5×10^{-7} M for 18-h .2h before harvesting, colchicine was added. Cells were treated with carboxylic acid and methanol solution then stained. For each dose, almost 150 metaphases were scored.

3.5. Alkaline Comet Assay

CHO cells of different concentrations (5,15,45) were treated for 3h. After that, in 5 mL trypan blue 40 µL of suspension was mixed for 3 min. By the use of a pipette, the cell suspension was put on a glass slide and viewed under a microscope. Non-stained cells were calculated under a microscope.180ul of agarose was mixed with 20 μL of cells at 37 °C. It was then put on the slide precoated with 1% agarose. The agarose was set at +4 °C and slides were incubated in the lysis solution. Slides were then put-on horizontal electrophoresis for 20 min. Slides already contain a fresh buffer to carry out DNA unwinding. Electrophoresis was done at 4 °C for 15 min. Slides were stained with ethidium bromide after washing with neutral buffer solution for 5 min and methanol for 3 min. Fluorescent microscopy was done after the chromosomes were attained using the software automatic image analysis system.

3.6. *In-Vivo* Assay

Swiss adult mice of weight 25-30 g and 8-10 weeks old were raised in the laboratory and used for experiments. Each group contains 5 mice.

3.7. Studies of Mouse Micronucleus and Bone Marrow

The plant extract was processed through the oral route in 10 mL/kg. Dose groups of 500,1000 and 2000 mg/kg were investigated in both genders. Bone marrow was separated from every animal for each dose. May Grunewald and Giemsa stains were used to stain the smears. Polychromatic erythrocytes were calculated and cytotoxicity index was calculated from 250 erythrocytes per slide.

4. STATISTICAL ANALYSIS

By using the Kolmogorov-Smirnov test, means and standard deviations were ascertained. The two-way ANOVA, the Dunnett's test, Mann-Whitney U test, the bifactorial and trifactorial ANOVA, Fthe Fisher test and the student's t-test based on the assay, were used to differentiate controls and treated samples. It is observed that when a statistically substantial increase in total alterations frequency surpassed the mean values and tested concentration of the extract was discovered positive. The treated samples and controlled samples were analyzed by making use of SALNAL in the Salmonella test.

4.1. Assays for the toxic Evaluation of AgNPs

In the assay, the four standard bacterial strands are used, and it is observed that whether or not introducing external S9 metabolic activation, the number of reverent did not grow per plate. Comparatively extended concentrations were interrogated (50 to 5000 µg/plate). Post 24-h of treatment, the result showed cytotoxic effects on CHO cells processed with Ag-NPs presenting different concentrations of 12.5, 6.25, 50, 25 and 100 µg/mL that were analyzed by spectrophotometer. During the MTT assay, dose and time were dependent. In 25-100, µg/mL effects of cytotoxicity were described while 20.5 µg/mL of Ag-NPs was used in CHO cells.

4.1.1. Sister Chromatid Exchanges Studies

Treatment of CHO cells with three hours extract. After recuperating for 24 hours in a fresh medium, a remarkable increase of sister chromatid exchanges in each cell was noted at 15 µg/mL. Cells treated with DMSO showed frequency 8.95±2.76 while the frequency of ± SD SCE was 15.2 ± 4.01 at 15 µg/mL. In the extract of AgNPs a remarkable increase in sister chromatid at 5 µg/mL was observed when treated for 27-h. Due to the retardation of the spread of cells of the extract, progressive concentrations and mitosis were not inaugurated.

4.1.2. Chromosome Aberration (CA) Assay

Chromosomal aberration percentage shown by AgNPs along with the extract increased about 45 µg/mL when the tested and mitotic ratio was less than 50%, showing cell toxicity from extract treatment. By treating extricate of AgNPs along with the extract and CHO cells for 18-h and exposure of CHO cells for 3hrs, little change in the frequency of chromatic aberration in 25 µg/mL was analyzed.

4.1.3. Comet Assay

In each experiment, the result showed that the nonviable cells did not exceed 20%. In treated samples, DNA breaks were observed due to an increase in dose. In the apoptotic cells, as well as at a high concentration of extract, vivid results were achieved.

4.1.4. Studies of Mouse Micronucleus and Bone Marrow

According to the data acquired, MNPCE had shown that mice medicated with the extricate of AgNPs along with the extract and negatively controlled revealed that there was no considerable difference in the frequency for both genders. The mice after the treatment with cytophosphane in comparison with the negative control showed more increase in the frequency of micronucleated bone marrow polychromatic erythrocytes. Mice assimilated with negative control and treatment with extract of AgNPs along with the extract showed no significant difference in polychromatic and normochromatic erythrocyte. There was no toxicity effect found at a dose of 500-2000 mg/kg based on body weight. The weight change was not observed in any of the animals. There was no death proclaimed in any of the groups.

AgNPs is a popular botanical formula found in the world but lack the basic proof regarding genotoxicity. AgNPs have a broad pharmacological effect, but the ratio of risks involved is much high. Genotoxic evaluation of this plant has been shown by different *in-vivo* and *in-vitro* assays while finding out how much human DNA is vulnerable to this plant's toxic effect. The plant genus has certain sesquiterpenes lactones, majorly including xanthanolides, xanthatin and 8-ep--tomentosin and other certain compounds which are phytochemicals in nature including xanthus-strumarina, hydroquinones and albuminoids, which are poisonous in nature. Apoptotic cell death is caused by these sesquiterpenes lactones by altering mitochondrial membrane and releasing pro-apoptotic mitochondrial proteins. The cytotoxic capability of AgNPs led result was very high *i.e* (25–100 µg/mL).

The optical properties exhibited by AgNPs are strongly dependent on the localized surface plasmon resonance that give origin to their extraordinary and fascinating phenomena. Still, irregularities may lead to phototoxicity as well [20].

Hence the cytotoxic activity of extracts from AgNPs was noticed during *in-vitro* experimental conditions. However, during *in-vivo* experimental conditions, no cytotoxic activity was shown after acute and sub-acute administration of extract of this plant. The *in-vitro* assay showed a different level of genotoxic mediated damage which was the result of maintaining toxicity concentration greater than IC_{50}. Point mutation was caused at the specific loci in Salmonella Typhimurium as a first step. However, no mutation has been detected in DNA due to the adverse effects of genetic testing. Sister chromatid exchange investigation in mammalian Chinese hamster ovary cells was the second step after this. The extract from AgNPs caused a significant propagation of SCE, a tender way for assessment of DNA damage. The final result which we can gather from *in-vitro* assay, is that the extract causes an apoptotic cell which shows that the substance under observation causes primary deoxyribonucleic acid harm. The double bonds found in the α-methylene γ-lactone and cyclopentanone portion give sesquiterpene lactones and thiol group of glutathione an attraction causing oxidative stress in the cell. Aberration in chromosomes done by sesquiterpenes is not verified because of direct cooperation with the structure of chromosomes, or deoxyribonucleic acid however, cytotoxicity has been proposed by an indirect method [30]. These focuses hinder the main enzyme of vigorous digestion (electron transport chain reactions) and replication of nucleic acid (deoxyribonucleic acid polymerase), expressing NFkB and caspase 3, which are liable for apoptosis and deoxyribonucleic acid harm is seen by sesquiterpene lactones. This study also portrays that no death or toxicity was caused in males and females because the *in-vivo* assays showed no genotoxicity in AgNPs. In the study conducted by Diaz [11], the mouse was orally given a specific selection of the above extract at different doses of 500, 1000 and 2000 μg/kg body weight and micro-nucleated erythrocytes showed no increase. A different study was done using chloroform and hexane part of the plant for acute toxicity assessment showed that administration at a very high level *i.e.* 5 μg/kg body weight, did not show any abnormality at gross as well as the histopathological level of an animal being treated. Effects of genetic toxicity weren't ensured *in-vivo* with the micronucleus test in our scenario. So, it certainly proved our point of view that nontoxic substances did not alter the DNA structure or cause any damage to it. Furthermore, we are provided with the explanation of in vivo failed operation of *in-vitro* genetic toxins concerned with pharmacokinetics such as distribution, absorption, metabolism, and excretion.

CONCLUSION

Our chapter emphasizes the genotoxic capability of the AgNPs as well as ototoxicity and chromosomal aberrations that can lead to DNA damage at cytotoxic concentrations. But in the case of mice administered by mouth with extract of this plant at concentration of 500-2000mg/kg, it did not lead to micronucleus in the bone marrow. It means that AgNPs can be safely utilized with the extract from which it has been prepared.

CONSENT FOR PUBLICATION

Not applicable.

CONFLICT OF INTEREST

The author declares no conflict of interest, financial or otherwise.

ACKNOWLEDGEMENTS

This work was supported by the National Research Foundation of Korea (NRF) funded by the Korean Government (MEST) (2020R1I1A3069699).

REFERENCES

[1]   Jain S, Mehata MS. Medicinal plant leaf extract and pure flavonoid mediated green synthesis of silver nanoparticles and their enhanced antibacterial property. Sci Rep 2017; 7(1): 15867.
[http://dx.doi.org/10.1038/s41598-017-15724-8] [PMID: 29158537]

[2]   Allafchian AR, Jalali SAH, Aghaei F, Farhang HR. Green synthesis of silver nanoparticles using Glaucium corniculatum (L.) Curtis extract and evaluation of its antibacterial activity. IET nanobiotechnology 2018; 12(5): 574-8.

[3]   Kumar V, Singh S, Srivastava B, Bhadouria R, Singh R. Green synthesis of silver nanoparticles using leaf extract of Holoptelea integrifolia and preliminary investigation of its antioxidant, anti-inflammatory, antidiabetic and antibacterial activities. J Environ Chem Eng 2019; 7(3): 103094.
[http://dx.doi.org/10.1016/j.jece.2019.103094]

[4]   Beyene HD, Werkneh AA, Bezabh HK, Ambaye TG. Synthesis paradigm and applications of silver nanoparticles (AgNPs), a review. Sustain Mater Technol 2017; 13: 18-23.
[http://dx.doi.org/10.1016/j.susmat.2017.08.001]

[5]   Baghbani-Arani F, Movagharnia R, Sharifian A, Salehi S, Shandiz SAS. Photo-catalytic, anti-bacterial, and anti-cancer properties of phyto-mediated synthesis of silver nanoparticles from Artemisia tournefortiana Rchb extract. J Photochem Photobiol B 2017; 173: 640-9.
[http://dx.doi.org/10.1016/j.jphotobiol.2017.07.003] [PMID: 28711019]

[6]   Siddiqui MN, Redhwi HH, Achilias DS, Kosmidou E, Vakalopoulou E, Ioannidou MD. Green synthesis of silver nanoparticles and study of their antimicrobial properties. J Polym Environ 2018; 26(2): 423-33.
[http://dx.doi.org/10.1007/s10924-017-0962-0]

[7]   Syafiuddin A. Salmiati, Salim MR, Beng Hong Kueh A, Hadibarata T, Nur H. A review of silver nanoparticles: research trends, global consumption, synthesis, properties, and future challenges. J Chin Chem Soc (Taipei) 2017; 64(7): 732-56.
[http://dx.doi.org/10.1002/jccs.201700067]

[8]   Adur AJ, Nandini N, Shilpashree Mayachar K, Ramya R, Srinatha N. Bio-synthesis and antimicrobial activity of silver nanoparticles using anaerobically digested parthenium slurry. J Photochem Photobiol B 2018; 183: 30-4.
[http://dx.doi.org/10.1016/j.jphotobiol.2018.04.020] [PMID: 29684718]

[9]   Mohanta YK, Panda SK, Bastia AK, Mohanta TK. Biosynthesis of silver nanoparticles from *protium serratum* and investigation of their potential impacts on food safety and control. Front Microbiol 2017; 8: 626.
[http://dx.doi.org/10.3389/fmicb.2017.00626] [PMID: 28458659]

[10]   Khorrami S, Zarrabi A, Khaleghi M, Danaei M, Mozafari MR. Selective cytotoxicity of green synthesized silver nanoparticles against the MCF-7 tumor cell line and their enhanced antioxidant and antimicrobial properties. Int J Nanomedicine 2018; 13: 8013-24.
[http://dx.doi.org/10.2147/IJN.S189295] [PMID: 30568442]

[11]   Pallela PNVK, Ummey S, Ruddaraju LK, Pammi SVN, Yoon S-G. Ultra Small, mono dispersed green synthesized silver nanoparticles using aqueous extract of Sida cordifolia plant and investigation of antibacterial activity. Microb Pathog 2018; 124: 63-9.
[http://dx.doi.org/10.1016/j.micpath.2018.08.026] [PMID: 30121359]

[12]   Calderón-Jiménez B, Johnson ME, Montoro Bustos AR, Murphy KE, Winchester MR, Vega Baudrit JR. Silver nanoparticles: technological advances, societal impacts, and metrological challenges. Front Chem 2017; 5: 6.
[http://dx.doi.org/10.3389/fchem.2017.00006] [PMID: 28271059]

[13]   Jorge de Souza TA, Rosa Souza LR, Franchi LP. Silver nanoparticles: An integrated view of green synthesis methods, transformation in the environment, and toxicity. Ecotoxicol Environ Saf 2019; 171: 691-700.
[http://dx.doi.org/10.1016/j.ecoenv.2018.12.095] [PMID: 30658305]

[14]   Wang X, Li T, Su X, *et al.* Genotoxic effects of silver nanoparticles with/without coating in human liver HepG2 cells and in mice. J Appl Toxicol 2019; 39(6): 908-18.
[http://dx.doi.org/10.1002/jat.3779] [PMID: 30701584]

[15]   Galván Márquez I, Ghiyasvand M, Massarsky A, *et al.* Zinc oxide and silver nanoparticles toxicity in the baker's yeast, *Saccharomyces cerevisiae.* PLoS One 2018; 13(3): e0193111.
[http://dx.doi.org/10.1371/journal.pone.0193111] [PMID: 29554091]

[16]   Liu H, Wang X, Wu Y, *et al.* Toxicity responses of different organs of zebrafish (Danio rerio) to silver nanoparticles with different particle sizes and surface coatings. Environ Pollut 2019; 246: 414-22.
[http://dx.doi.org/10.1016/j.envpol.2018.12.034] [PMID: 30579210]

[17]   Sayed AEH, Soliman HAM. Developmental toxicity and DNA damaging properties of silver nanoparticles in the catfish (Clarias gariepinus). Mutat Res Toxicol Environ Mutagen 2017; 822: 34-40.
[http://dx.doi.org/10.1016/j.mrgentox.2017.07.002] [PMID: 28844240]

[18]   Khosravi-Katuli K, Shabani A, Paknejad H, Imanpoor MR. Comparative toxicity of silver nanoparticle and ionic silver in juvenile common carp (Cyprinus carpio): Accumulation, physiology and histopathology. J Hazard Mater 2018; 359: 373-81.
[http://dx.doi.org/10.1016/j.jhazmat.2018.07.064] [PMID: 30048952]

[19]   Pryshchepa O, Pomastowski P, Buszewski B. Silver nanoparticles: Synthesis, investigation techniques, and properties. Adv Colloid Interface Sci 2020; 284: 102246.
[http://dx.doi.org/10.1016/j.cis.2020.102246] [PMID: 32977142]

[20]   Torres-Torres C, Peréa-López N, Reyes-Esqueda JA, *et al.* Ablation and optical third-order nonlinearities in Ag nanoparticles. Int J Nanomedicine 2010; 5: 925-32. [Internet].
[http://dx.doi.org/10.2147/IJN.S12463] [PMID: 21187944]

CHAPTER 8

Boron Nanomaterials for Biomedical Applications

Fayaz Ali[1,*], **Yinghuai Zhu**[1] and **Yi Zhun Zhu**[1,*]

[1] School of Pharmacy and State Key Laboratory of Quality Research in Chinese Medicine, Macau University of Science and Technology, Avenida Wai Long, Taipa 999078, Macau SAR, China

Abstract: Boron belongs to the metalloid group and has an atomic number 11. Boron does have an important role in humans and animals; however, it is not well understood. According to developmental biology, boron is a necessary component of embryonic development and when it is deficient, it causes impaired embryos or necrosis. Different types of boron nanomaterials, such as nanoclusters, nanotubes, nanowires, nanoribbons, nanobelts, nanosheets, and monolayer crystalline sheets, have recently been created experimentally. Boron nanomaterials have a different bonding configuration than three-dimensional bulk boron crystals in icosahedral because of their reduced dimensionality. Furthermore, the wide range of boron nanoparticles available could serve as building blocks for mixing with other existing nanomaterials, atoms, molecules, and/or ions to create new materials with novel properties and functions. Hexagonal boron nitride (h-BN) is a new two-dimensional (2D) nanomaterial that has been employed in biomedical applications. This material exhibits semi-conductive capabilities due to its enlarged band gap, allowing it to be used as a biosensor and disparity agent. BNNs (boron nitride nanotubes) are also being investigated for use in regenerative medicine and medication delivery. Because of its bioactive properties, this particular nanomaterial (BNNs) has a lot of potential in the field of tissue engineering. The advancement of boron nanoparticles during the previous decade has been evaluated, and future directions and guidelines for biomedical applications are discussed.

Keywords: Anticancer, Antimicrobial, Boron Nanoparticles, BNCT, Nanomaterials, Nanotubes, Nanosphere.

1. INTRODUCTION

Nanomaterials are directly related to the technological interest of the peculiar physiognomies that extant in a scale of handling, *i.e.,* the sizes are in nanometers.

---

* **Corresponding author Fayaz Ali and Yi Zhun Zhu:** School of Pharmacy and State Key Laboratory of Quality Research in Chinese Medicine, Macau University of Science and Technology, AvenidaWai Long, Taipa 999078, Macau SAR, China; E-mails: fayazalisabir@gmail.com and yzzhu@must.edu.mo

Shahid Ali Khan, Saad Salman, Youssef O. Al-Ghamd (Eds.)

Nanotechnology is a diverse field of science that is prompting the already existing technical environment like medicine. Therefore, nanomedicine appears to be a new technique that enhances the development of nanomaterial applications in the field of traditional medicine [1]. Implications of nanomedicine mean that outmoded or traditional methodologies and instrumentation of investigation are enhanced with every novel finding. Consequently, a therapeutic and diagnostic technique based on NPs offers early-stage cancer diagnosis and treatment with high sensitivity [2]. The advancement in the imaging techniques which ease cancer and other fatal diseases diagnosis is magnetic resonance imaging (MRI), positron emission tomography (PET), X-ray computed tomography (CT), and optical imaging and power tool. For therapy approaches, different techniques have been applied, such as photodynamic therapy (PDT), photothermal therapy (PTT), chemotherapeutical drug delivery. Therefore, NMs in medicine had multidirectional characteristic applications. Different NMs are investigated with numerous exceptional physiochemical possessions for the development of new nanomaterial-based tactics: pharmacokinetic analysis, fluorescent labels *via* quantum dots, approaches of separation and refinement of cells or single biomolecules, biosensing, recognition of biological samples and pathogens (*e.g.*, proteins, nucleic acid), final drug or gene delivery, tissue engineering, improvement of therapeutic visualization techniques (*e.g.*, magnetic resonance imaging), and cancer treatment *via* hyperthermia method. NMs have appeared as the most fertile areas for biomedical applications. NMs are measured as a therapeutic boon for the prevention, diagnosis, and treatment of cancer [3, 4]. In addition, following the advances in chemistry, nanotechnology, pharmacy, biology, imaging, and medicine in the last decade, various systems have been developed and combined; for instance, therapy and disease diagnosis as shown in (Fig. **1a**) [5, 6]. These developments stimulate the vast range of objects having nanometer-sized for their organization of cancer tissues, empowering tumors imagining, drugs delivery, and/or demolition of cancers by various healing procedures. The providence of the particles inside the body can be well projected by selecting the right shape, size, charge, and coating along with aiming moiety (Fig. **1b**) [7]. New NMs drugs express innovative possessions by virtue of their shape and size and thus gathering cumulative attention as possible multifunctional healing agents [8].

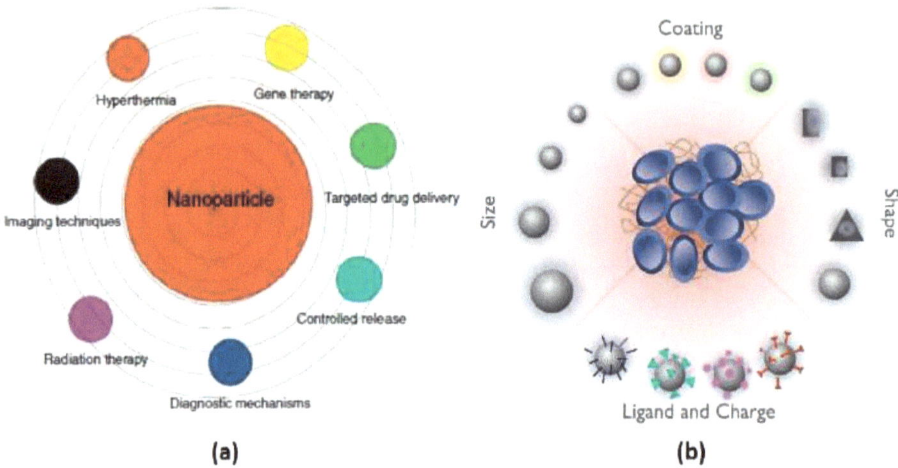

Fig. (1). (a) Theragnostic applications of NPs. Source Ref [6], **(b)** Properties of particles thatinfluence targeting, elimination, and distribution. Source: Ref [7].

Boron element is the first-row neighbor of carbon; however, the study of the boron element is far behind the carbon. For the last two centuries, carbon has been considered a leading element in chemical research. Although boron is rich in nature, it has not been utilized as a building block of its own, despite being used in dealing with carbon [9, 10]. Generally, the amount of boron element in the human body is very minute (*i.e.,* it is not more than 18 mg in an average individual [11]); however, boron compounds are considered vital micronutrients for plants and animals. Boron elements can be used in the drug design of novel pharmaceuticals because they have the potential properties to be considered as a helper in new biological accomplishments. For instance, they can help to strengthen the plant cell walls as well as support bone health in animals. It's reported that the bone lipids in femurs of male pigs were decreased resulted in a higher bending moment by taking boron deficient diet, which suggests the important role of boron in bone metabolism [12]. Therefore, stem cell differentiation could be modulated by boron because it has already been used in biomaterials for medicinal applications and has proven to be vital in bone and cell metabolism. Astonishingly, boron-containing compounds are rarely found in medicine; however, so far, there is no report showing the inherent disadvantages of boron in terms of its incorporation into medicine. Indeed, some boron-containing compounds were recently examined and utilized in clinical applications. Furthermore, more boron-based medicine is predictable due to a new emerging proton boron fusion therapy and the advancement in boron neutron capture therapy (BNCT). This chapter focuses on the biomedical applications of the recently reported novel boron NMs as shown in Fig. (2).

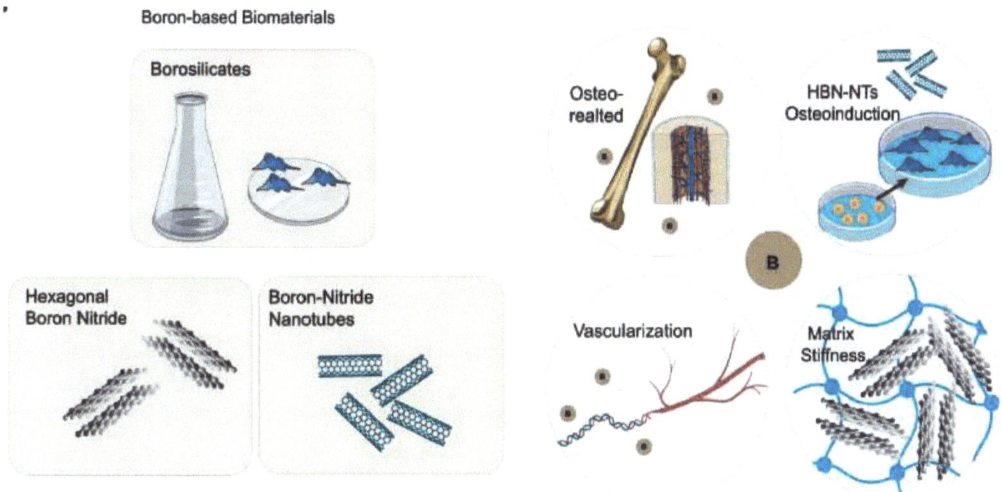

Fig. (2). Boron-based biomaterials to stimulate osteogenesis and angiogenesis. Source: Ref [13].

2. BORON NMS

Two main types of bioactive molecules containing boron: Single boron atom is present in the first kind of molecules, while in the second type, boron is present in the form of cluster. The pure boron NPs having significant boron content is considered to be hypothetically favorable boron carrier agents. Various synthetic approaches are employed to prepare these NPs. The commonly used methods are ball milling, arc discharge, thermal plasma, chemical vapor deposition (CVD), reduction in solution, and pyrolysis [8, 14 - 16]. A ball malling method was recently used by Icten *et al.* [17] to prepared both boron NPs and their magnetic dopamine functionalization. This group also prepared magnetic NCs containing mono- or bis- (ascorbate-borate), Fe_3O_4, and - polyethylene glycol [18] by the method shown in Fig. (3). As ascorbic acid combined with composites are recognized for radical scavenging and antitumor activity; therefore, the prepared materials are reflected as the possible ingredients for magnetic biomedicine.

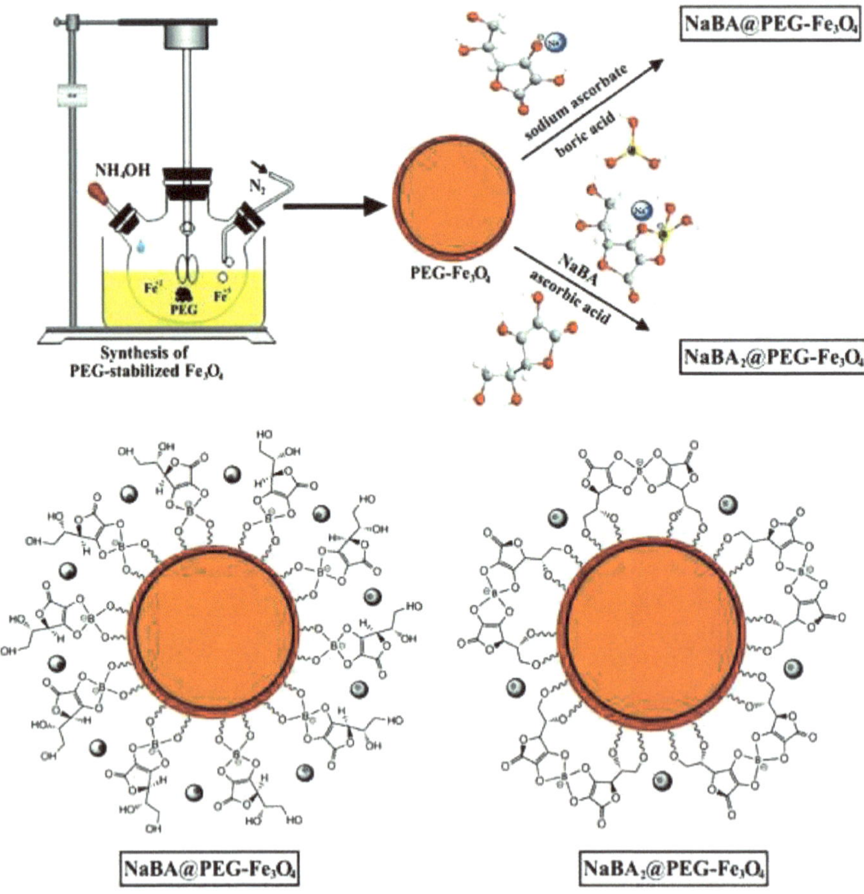

Fig. (3). Schematic description of the preparation route and the proposed structures for NaBA@PEG–Fe$_3$O$_4$ and NaBA$_2$@PEG–Fe$_3$O$_4$ [18].

2.1. Boron NPs

Owing to high boron content in the pure boron NPs, they are the potentially promising boron carrying agents. Recently, several papers have been published on the synthesis of boron nanostructures using different synthetic approaches [14, 15, 19, 20]. Boron NPs were synthesized with metallic reduction of boron compounds [21, 22], ball milling [23, 24], gas-phase boron compounds decomposition/ reduction [25, 26], and BBr$_3$ solution reduction with sodium naphthalenide [27]. Besides, pyrolysis of diborane was used to synthesize the crystalline boron nanoribbons at low pressure and temperature [28]. Single-crystalline boron nanobelts were prepared by using pulsed laser ablation [29], and CVD method was used to prepared single-crystalline boron nanocones [30]. Boron nanowires were also reported by using a cold-wall CVD system using ZrB_2 particles [31]. In addition, raw materials of micro-sized boron powder (~40 μm) were used to synthesized boron NPs by using the pulsed wire discharge method, a simple and low-cost method [32].

2.1.1. Anti-microbial study of Boron NPs

Batalet. al., [33] reported the eco-friendly synthesis of silver boron NPs (AgB NPs) induced by gamma-rays using PVP polymer as a stabilizing agent. The multidrug-resistant microbes were considered to check the antibiofilm and antimicrobial activities of AgB NPs. The data indicates that boric acid and silver nitrate concentrations are dependent on AgB NPs production. As shown in Fig. (**4**), the AgB NPs showed high efficiency against Candida albicans followed by *Escherichia coli* and *Staphylococcus aureus.* In addition, the biofilm inhibition of AgB NPs was observed as 69.4%, 85.3%, and 87.0% against *C. albicans, E. coli* and *S. aureus*, respectively. Accordingly, due to continued-termed stability and antimicrobial properties of AgB NPs; They might be possibly used in medical applications, especially in urinary tract infection treatment.

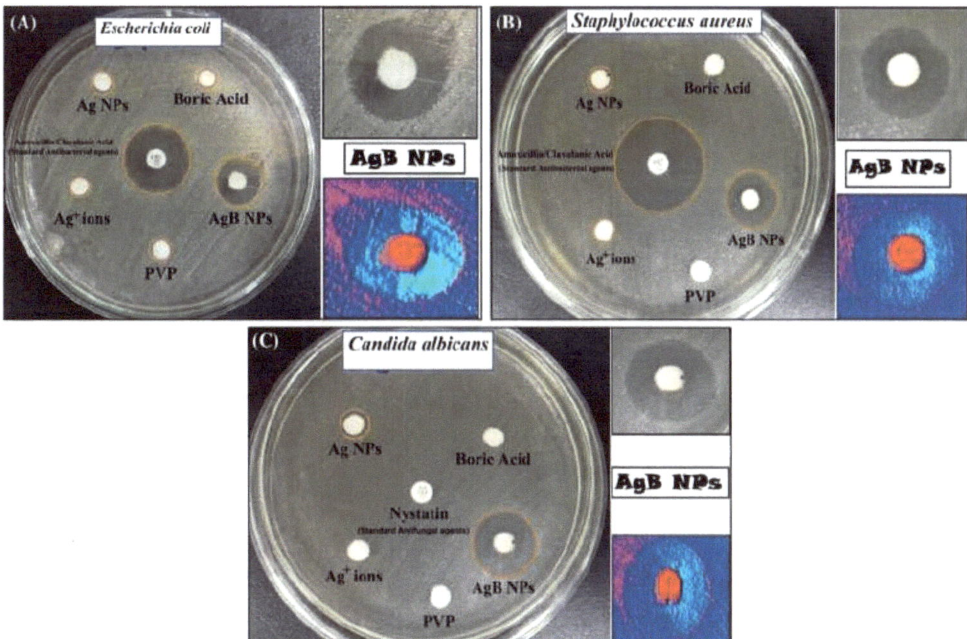

Fig. (4). Antimicrobial activity of the synthesized AgB NPs against (**A**)*E. coli*, (**B**)*S. aureus* and (**C**)*C. Albicans* as ZOI [33].

2.1.2. Boron NPs for Cancer Treatment

Different methods were reported for the production of elemental boron NPs, such as ultrasonic dispersion in a liquid medium defined by Uspenskii *et al.* [34], to synthesize the elemental BNPs in size less than 100 nm. The resulting BNPs were used as a target for BNCT. The results obtained in an experiment of synthesizing BNPs in a preclinical study of BNCT, with the neutron irradiation for 1 h of T98G human glioma cells pre-incubated with BNPs (different concentrations) show noteworthy destruction of cell viability.

2.2. Boron Nitride

A refractory material, boron nitride (BN), is made from boron and nitrogen. Depending on temperature and pressure, it can be crystallized in different forms [35, 36], *i.e.*, (diamond-like cubic, rhombohedral, hexagonal [37], and wurtzite [38]), but at room temperature, the hexagonal form is the most stable form of BN. BN represents a considerable advantage from its structurally similar carbon counterpart because of its unique and specific properties, such as unique mechanical properties [39, 40] and thermal conductivity [41], anti-oxidation capacity [42]. BN can retain the dielectric properties while combining with polymers; however, these properties were compromised in the case of carbon nanostructures to electrical insulation. In addition, BN is white-colored, while its carbon-based counterparts are colored (mostly black). The white color of BN would allow dying and be helpful in the medical field. BN can be easily distinguished from the carbon nanotubes because carbon nanotubes absorb in the IR range, while BN optical properties are applicable in the UV regime. Finally, Piezoelectric properties are also found possesses in the BN compounds, which is a feature that can open new developments for advanced application [43].

Surfactants are often used to improve the dispersibility of BN in aqueous solutions because it is chemically more stable than carbon NMs. Two different ways are followed to use surfactants: (1) direct dispersion and (2) as co-solvents during exfoliation of BN nanosheets [44 - 46]. BN has been used in many different fields for different goals because of these distinctive dispersion parameters: for protective coatings [47, 48], as a lubricant [49], for hydrogen storage [50, 51], in cosmetic products [52], and in composites as a filler to improve both thermal and mechanical properties [53, 54].

In recent years, BN has attracted considerable attention in the biomedical field, considering its similar analogy with carbon structures. However, the use of BN in biomedical applications is exploited in a limited amount as compared to carbon structures. Carbon nanostructures have been vastly examined in imaging, biosensing, and cancer cell targeting, but the cytotoxicity of these NMs has unlocked up sites for an emerging substitute, non-toxic materials, and solutions. The BN's superior chemical inertness compared to carbon nanostructures establishes a strong dispute for replacing carbon nanostructures with BN NMs in biomedical applications [43].

2.2.1. BN for Cancer Treatment

Boron based compounds, which are highly dispersible in water, are advanced and innovative materials that can be used for cancer treatment, especially in BNCT [55]. The highly water dispersible BN nanostructured synthesis at low temperature was reported by Sing *et. al.* [56]. The morphological examinations showed that they were in the transient phase from two-dimensional hexagonal sheets to nanotubes. These nanostructures are useful for BNCT because of their structural deformation due to the ultra-high disperse ability. In addition, the studies of cytotoxicity on different cell lines (human breast adenocarcinoma (MCF-7), Hela (cervical cancer), and human embryonic kidney (HEK-293) presented that these nanostructures could be applied in BNCT [56]. Moreover, it is reported that controlled boron release and crystallinity of hollow BN spheres increases prostate cancer cell apoptosis and decreases cell viability [57]. Also, BN spheres established substantial suppression in tumour growth on subcutaneous tumor mouse models. The *in-vivo* anticancer efficacy of BN spheres was also confirmed by an orthotopic tumor growth model [57].

2.3. Hexagonal Boron Nitride

Hexagonal boron nitride (h-BN) is one of the most exceptional and auspicious layered NMs, which is similar to graphite "white graphene". In the structure of h-BN, the C atoms in graphite are replaced by B and N atoms. The strong covalent bond between boron and nitrogen strongly interlinked them together and formed interlocking hexagonal rings. This material has semi-conductive properties due to an increased bandgap that allows its use in biosensors and contrast agents [13, 58]. Due to the interesting chemical and physical properties of h-BN, these compounds are used in different applications, *e.g.*, in ceramics, plastics, paints, and as an insulator in electronics. In addition, in the cosmetic industry, boron nitride (BN) is considered as a prevalent inorganic compound (*e.g.*, in eye shadow formulation, up to 25% of BN concentration can be found). The use of h-BN in cosmetic formulation suggests the lack of toxicity / cytotoxicity [59]. Besides, it is widely applied for the formation of dental cement (for orthodontic and dental applications) [60]. Therefore, the cytotoxicity in vivo and *in vitrol* of few-layered h-BN-based NCs and novel h-BN nanoplates are still needed because BN appears to be appropriate for biomedical applications. The low cytotoxicity of these compounds is confirmed from the short-time studies that suggest BN as a novel drug delivery system; however, additional verifications from long-term studies are required for medical applications. Thus, some of the new approaches for the synthesis of h-BN or its exfoliated form are expected to study its functionalization and modification to achieve some potentially fascinating NMs.

Recently, h-BN NPs were modified by Hongchao Wu., [61] with polydopamine in a solvent-free aqueous condition, as shown in Fig. (**5**). The h-BN was incorporated with bisphenol E cyanate ester (BECy) in different loading and functionalities to investigate its effect on dynamic-mechanical, thermo-mechanical, thermal conductivity, and dielectric properties. The outstanding performance was shown by their prepared h-BN/BECy NCs in dimensional stability, thermal conductivity, and dynamic-mechanical properties, together with preserved thermal stability for high-temperature applications and controllable dielectric properties.

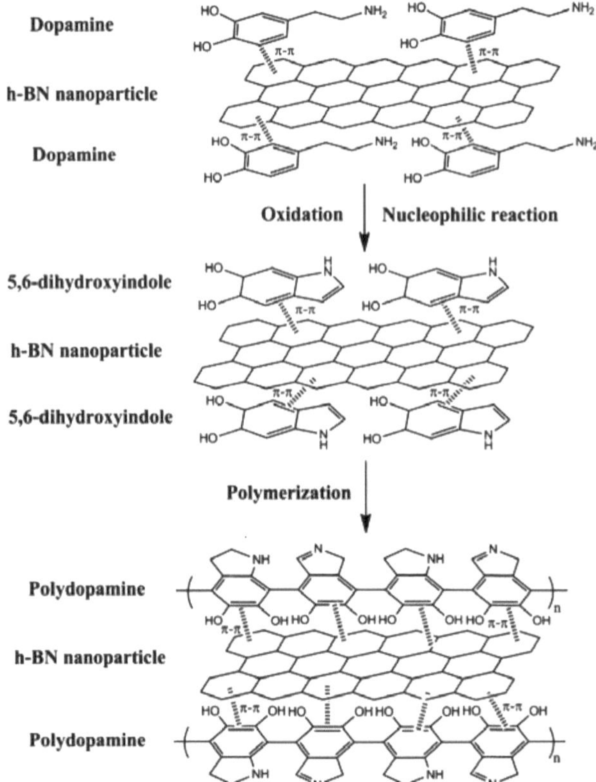

Fig. (5). Schematic Illustration of Noncovalent Functionalization of h-BN NPs *via* Polydopamine (Reprint from Ref [61].)

2.3.1. Antimicrobial Study of h-BN

Recently the antimicrobial and antibiofilm activities of h-BN NPs were reported by Merihet. al [62], against *Streptococcus mutans* 3.3, *Candida sp* M25, *Staphylococcus pasteuri* M3, and *S. mutans* ATTC 25175. The minimum inhibitory concentration (MIC) of h-BN NPs was determined and found higher for *Staphylococcus pasteuri* M3 and *Streptococcus mutans* ATTC 25175 and lower against *Candida sp* M25 and *Streptococcus mutans* 3.3. A high antibiofilm activity was shown by h-BN NPs, which inhibit biofilm growth of S. mutans ATTC 25175, S. mutans 3.3 and Candida sp. M25. The cells were exposed for 24 to 48 hours to 0.025-0.4 mg/mL concentration of h-BN nanoparticle suspension in cell viability tests. The results show no cytotoxic effect on MDCK and CRL-2120 cells in the concentration range from 0.025-0.1 mg/mL; however, h-BN caused mild cytotoxicity on CRL-2120 cells on both the first and second day when used in high concentration (0.2-0.4 mg/mL). According to this study, an appropriate concentration (0.1 mg/mL) of h-BN NPs can be considered a potentially safe oral care product.

Due to efficient dispersion in an aqueous environment and biodegradation behavior, hBN synthesized from boric acid (BA) can be used as a therapeutic option in wound healing. As it was suggested that hBN releases boron derivative(s), which enhance wound healing; therefore, in a recent study, the h-BNs for wound healing were performed in comparison with BA [63]. It was found that human dermal fibroblasts (HDFs) have low uptake capacity as compared to human umbilical vein endothelial cells (HUVECs), explaining the reason for the stimulation effects of hBNs. Considering the wound healing phases, the BA-treated cells showed little improvement compared to the hBN treated cultures because hBNs significantly increase the proliferation and migration of HUVECs and HDFs. Besides, the angiogenesis ability of HUVECs reacted with hBNs also proven encouraging results. Due to antioxidant capacity of hBNs similar to BA, it may also improve the wound healing process by lowering reactive oxygen species (ROS) [64]. Furthermore, the cells were rescued by hBNs from apoptosis; however, almost no effect was found on the cell death mechanism in the case of BA. These results demonstrate that both h-BNs and BA accelerate wound healing. However, hBNs offer slow degradation and acting as a controlled release source for BA, which overcomes the short half-life of BA. In conclusion, for wound healing the h-BNs might be a promising therapeutic option as shown in Fig. (**6a**).

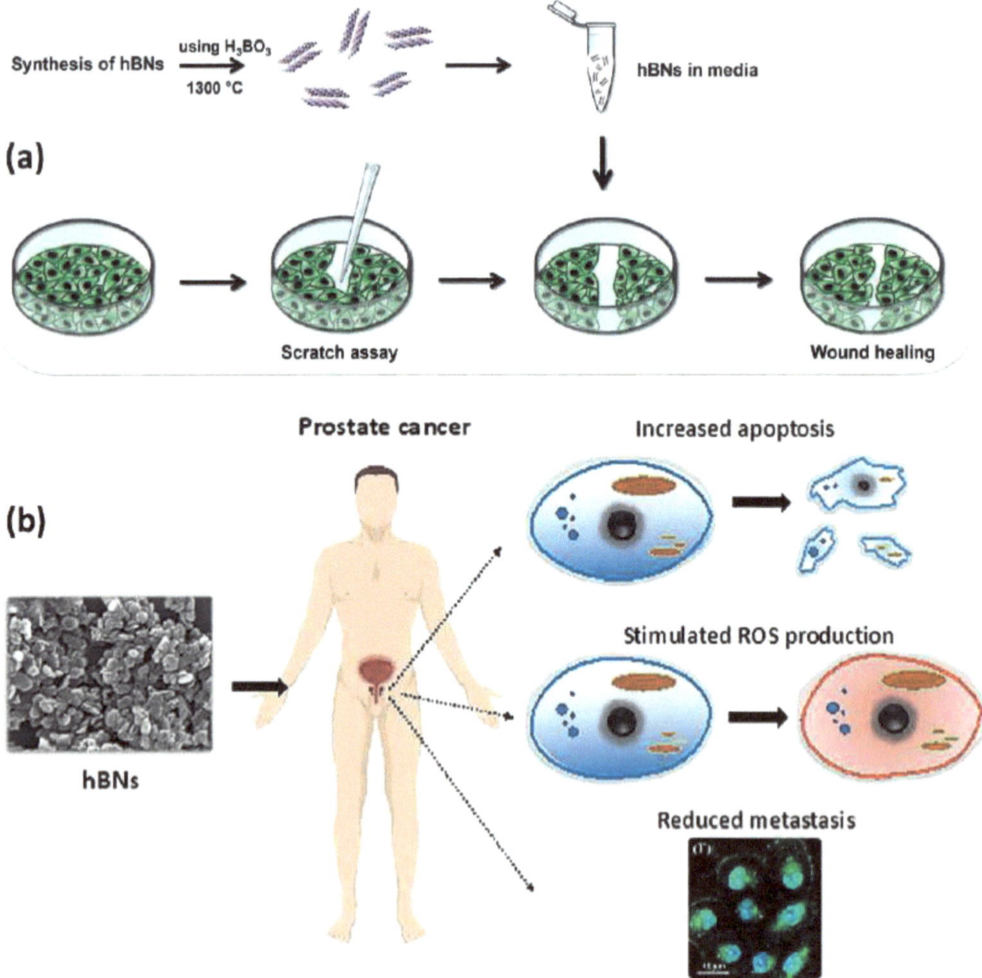

Fig. (6). Stimulatory effect of h-BNs in wound healing **(a)** (Reprint from Ref [63]), h-BN NPs for prostate cancer treatment **(b)**. (Reprint from Ref [65]).

2.3.2. h-BNs for Cancer Treatment

The hBN therapeutic efficiency against prostate cancer was recently examined as reported by Emanetet. al [65]. They reported that h-BN with an average size of 50 nm was suitable NMs for cellular internalization. Also, after efficient cellular uptake of hBN, their intracellular degradation studies *via* DU145 cells designate their slow degradation as compared to Boron atom (BA). A serious suppressive effect on cancer cells were indicated by the results, which was directly proportional to the h-BN concentration. These promising selective suppressive effects on cancer cells encouraged further investigation. Therefore, they also study the cell cycle analysis to support the sensitivity studies.The BA and hBN exposed DU145 cells in a comparative cell cycle analysis exhibited that at long incubation times the cells were arrested in the mitosis phase. The increased ROS production and mitochondrial response of DU145 cells deliver significant signs about their cellular response to h-BN. At long term incubation and highest concentration of hBN the seriously increased ROS generation and mitochondrial dysfunction was found, which significantly increased apoptosis rate (around 45%). However, a different effect on the cells by inducing decreased cell viability was demonstrated by BA, which is the possible degradation product of h-BN. The slow degradation of h-BN NPs in the long term may be responsible for differences in the effects of h-BN and BA. This long-term stay of hBN results in an efficient therapeutic effect on prostate cancer cells as shown in Fig. (**6b**).

2.4. Boron Nitride NPs for Cancer Treatment

In boron nitride NPs (BNNPs) the carbon atom is replaced by boron and nitrogen and are structural analogs of carbon materials [66]. As compare to its carbon counterparts, BNNPs are show low cytotoxicity and better biocompatibility because they are degradable [67]. Due to higher boron content in BNNPs, they are considered possible candidates for BNCT as boron delivery agents. Previously, it has been reported that BN nanotubes can be used as delivery agents for BNCT at the cellular level [56, 68]. BNNPs biodegradability is related to their crystalline structure. The treatment of prostate cancer can be ultimately achieved by using the hollow BN spheres with controlled crystallinity [57]. BNNPs need to be surface modified based on special physicochemical properties, to prevent decomposition to prolong the blood circulation. As shown in Fig. (**7a**) phase transitioned lysozyme (PTL) was used to coat BNNPs to prolong blood circulation because it could protect them from hydrolysis and could be detached when treated with vitamin C [69, 70], and thus on-demand delivery of boron for BNCT [71]. The PTL@BNNPs shown sufficient accumulation in tumor and maintain a good tumor-to-nontumor ratio. Also, in animal models the suppression of triple negative breast cancer was noteworthy and resulting a great promise for treating these cancers.

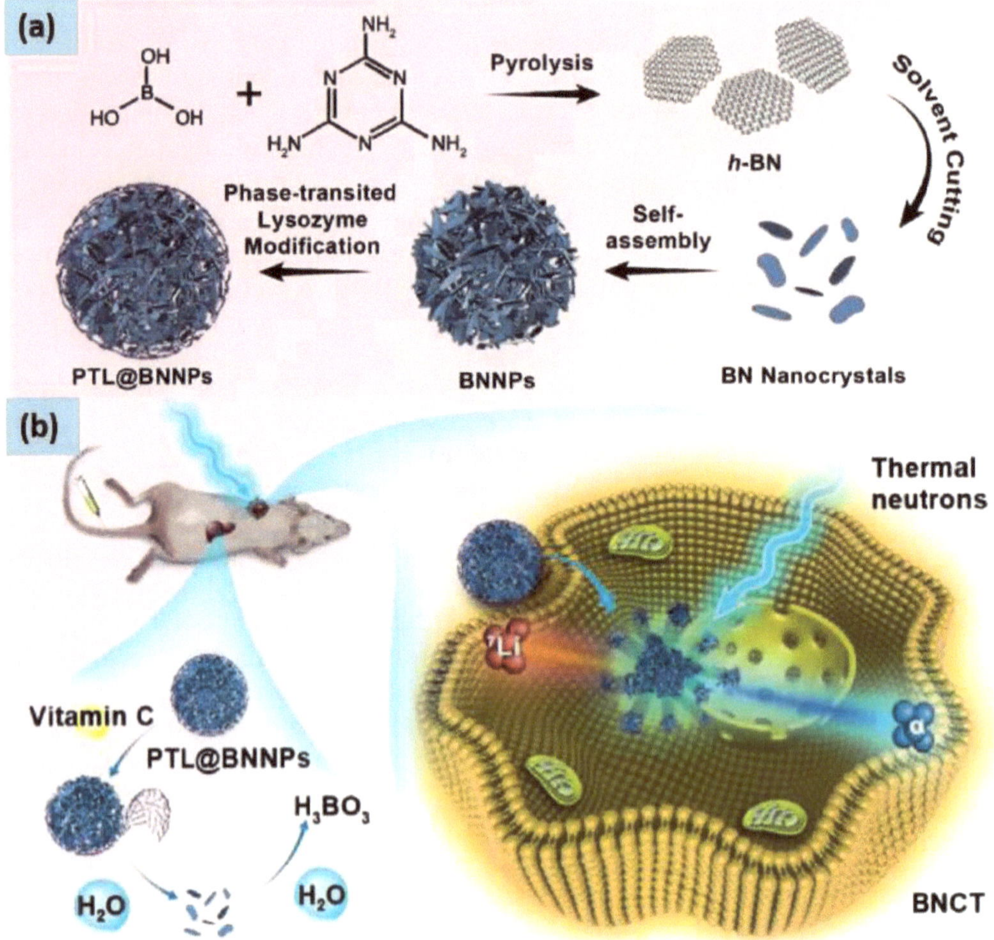

Fig. (7). Preparation of PTL@BNNPs **(a)**, Schematic Illustration of PTL@BNNPs BNCT and On-Demand Degradation **(b)**. (Reprint from Ref [71]).

2.5. Boron Nitride Nanotubes (BNNTs)

Boron nitride nanotubes (BNNTs) have substantial features such as high thermal stability, high resistance to oxidation, excellent thermal conductibility, piezoelectricity, high Young's modulus, and the ability to suppress thermal neutron radiation [72]. In addition to these properties, its surface has the ability to incorporate rare earth metals and various types of molecules, which gives it additional properties [73 - 75]. For instance, when BNNTs bound to a target molecule may be internalized by cancer cells and thus capable of promoting tumor death, it can be used as specific therapeutic agents in boron neutron capture therapy. This medical technique is helpful for cancer treatment, where the reaction occurs inside the destroying cells with the help of densely ionizing radiation. Therefore, BNNTs have been demonstrated as a useful drug delivery agent. Also, BNNTs have been shown to be non-toxic to HEK293 cells as a comparison to carbon nanotubes, and they can be functionalized to endorse water solubility [67]. A number of methods used for functionalizing BNNTs include coating with poly-l-lysine (PLL) or polyethyleneimine (PEI) [58], interacting with glycodendrimers [67], or reacting with substituted quinuclidine bases [76]. The correlation of different production methods of boron nitride, types of boron nitride, time of exposure, and concentration on different cells and their responses are summarized in Table **1**.

Table 1. Type of boron nitride and its preparation method, time of exposure and its concentration on different cells and their responses.

BN Form	Production Method	BNNT Geometry	Dispersion Agent	Cell type	Max Conc. of Exposure	Time of Exposure (Hours)	Results	Ref.
Boron nitrides	Solid reaction method	Branched nanoribbons, hydroxylated layered structure	None	Mouse embryonic fibroblast cells and human prostate cancerous cell	100 µg mL^{-1}	24	Non-cytotoxic	[77]
BNNPs	Ballmilling in argon	Spherical, amorphous-like, D 100–200 nm	None	Human osteosarcoma cells	1 mg mL^{-1}	168	Cytotoxic, the more the lower the D	[78]
BNNTs	Ball milling and annealing	----	Polyethyleneimine	Neuroblastoma cells	5 µg mL^{-1}	72	Non cytotoxic	[54]
BNNTs	Ball milling and annealing	L 200–300 nm	Poly-L-lysine	Myoblast cells	15 µg mL^{-1}	72	Non cytotoxic, optimal cell viability up to 10 µg mL−1	[79]
BNNTs	CVD + homogeneization + sonication	Multiwalled, L ˜1,5 µm, D 10–80 nm	Gum Arabica	Neuroblastoma cells and human umbilical vein epithelial cells	100 µg mL^{-1}	72	Non-cytotoxic up to 20 µg mL^{-1}	[58]
BNNTs	CVD	Multiwalled, L ˜10 µm, D < 80 nm	Tween 80	Human lung adenocarcinoma epithelial cells	20 µg mL^{-1}	120	Cytotoxic already at 2 µg mL−1	[80]
BNNTs	High-temperature synthesis	Both single and small aggregates of nanotubes, bamboo-like, L 200–600 nm, D ˜50 nm	Glycol-chitosan	Neuroblastoma human cells	100 µg mL^{-1}	48	Non-cytotoxic up to 20 µg mL^{-1}	[67]

(Table 1) contd.....

BN Form	Production Method	BNNT Geometry	Dispersion Agent	Cell type	Max Conc. of Exposure	Time of Exposure (Hours)	Results	Ref.
BNNTs	CVD	Multiwalled, straight, tubular, inner D ˜10, outer D ˜25 nm	Pluronic P123	Chang cells	1000 µg mL^{-1}	24	non-cytotoxic, IC50 125 µg mL^{-1} (still alive cells 50%)	[81]
BNNTs	CVD	Multiwalled, straight, tubular, inner D ˜10, outer D ˜25 nm	Pluronic P123	Vero cells	1000 µg mL^{-1}	24	Non-cytotoxic, IC50 125 µg mL^{-1}	[81]
BNNTs	CVD	Multiwalled, straight, tubular, inner D ˜10, outer D ˜25 nm	None	Vero and Chang cells	1000 µg mL^{-1}	24	Non cytotoxic,	[81]
BNNTs	Commercial	Cylindrical and bamboo-like structures, L 0.43–5.8 µm, D 32–145 nm	None	Osteoblasts and macrophages	1 µg mL^{-1}	60	Non-cytotoxic, normal cell growth	[82]
BNNTs film	Boron ink method	Bamboo-like and cylindrical NTs, 20–40 µm thick film	Plasma treated	Human mammary fibroblast, transformed breast tumor cells	35 mm diameter cell culture plate	48 (breast tumore cells) and 96 (fibroblasts)	Non-cytotoxic	[83]
BNNTs	Annealing method	Single and aggregate, bamboo-like structure, L 200–600 nm, D ˜50 nm	Glycol-chitosan	Nuronal-like cells (PC12)	100 µg mL^{-1}	216	Non-cytotoxic, no difference	[84]
BNNTs	Spark plasma sintering	L ˜0.43–5.8 µm, mean D 71 nm	2nd phase in HA	Human osteoblasts	4 wt%	120	Non-cytotoxic, normal cell growth	[85]
BNNTs	Milling and annealing	L < 500 nm, D 40–70 nm	Poly-L-lysine	Osteoblast cells	15 µg mL^{-1}	72	Non cytotoxic	[86]
BNNTs	Commercial	Bamboo-like structure, L 0.5–2.0 µm, D 30–100 nm	Glycol-chitosan	*In-vivo*	2 mL of a 1 mg mL^{-1}	72	Non-cytotoxic, higher platelet count	[87]
BNNTs layer	CVD + shortening + oxidation	L 1–2 µm	None	Mesenchymal stem cells	25 µg mL^{-1}	336	Non-cytotoxic, protein adsorption at 5 µg mL^{-1} after 14 days	[88]
BNNTs	Commercial	L ˜500 nm	Glycol-chitosan	*In-vivo*	10 mg kg^{-1}	168	Non-cytotoxic, no alteration	[43]
BNNTs	CVD + shortening	Crystalline, multiwalled, L 1.0–2.5 µm, D 10–80 nm	Gum arabica	*In-vivo*	Multiple injections	336	Non-cytotoxic	[89]

(Table 1) contd.....

BN Form	Production Method	BNNT Geometry	Dispersion Agent	Cell type	Max Conc. of Exposure	Time of Exposure (Hours)	Results	Ref.
BNNSs	Ballmilling in ammonia	100 nm D × 3 nm in thickness	None	Human osteosarcoma cells	1 mg mL^{-1}	168	Cytotoxic and non-cytotoxic	[78]

2.5.1. BNNTs for Cancer Treatment

Due to its relatively simple composition, the BNNT is also a potentially promising BNCT agent that can be functionalized for specific tumors [8, 90 - 92]. In addition, the synthesis of the ^{10}B-enriched BNNTs is experimentally feasible. Nakamura *et al.* [68], demonstrates for the first time the BNCT antitumor effects of BNNTs toward B16 melanoma cells. The BNNT–DSPEPEG2000 accumulated in B16 melanoma cells shows three times higher BNCT antitumor effect as compared to BSH, demonstrating that BNNT–DSPE-PEG2000 would be a probable applicant as a boron delivery vehicle [68]. Moreover, Fe-containing BNNTs have been prepared by Menichetti and coworkers by a convenient milling process with a Fe content of about 1.5 wt% [93]. Subsequently, in magnetic resonance imaging (MRI), the BNNT nanocomposite was used as contrast agents by encapsulating with poly(L-lysine). A good potential of the composite has been reported for negative MRI contrast agents, specifically as T(2) contrast-enhancement agents [93]. The potential application of BNNT for BNCT in cancer treatment have also been explored by Ferreira and coworkers [94]. They found that in the presence of a thermal neutron flux of around 6.6×108 n·cm^{-2}·s^{-1}, in the HeLa cell line, the BNNTs were selectively accumulated and demonstrated a high cell-killing effect, as shown in Fig. (**8**) [94]. Thus, evidence of the appropriateness of BNNTs for BNCT applications is provided by these results.

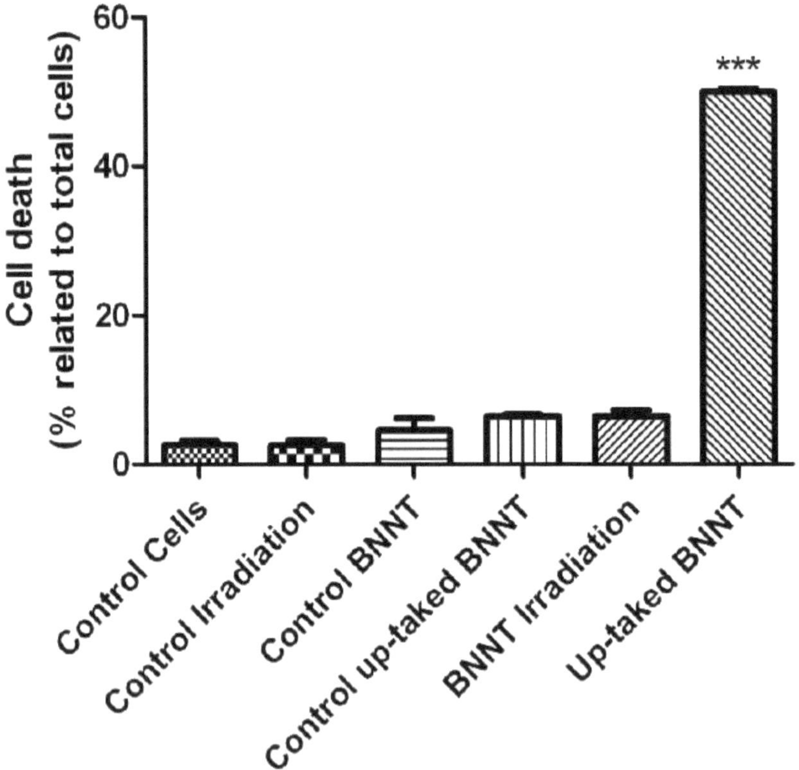

Fig. (8). Cytotoxic effects of BNNTs on HeLa cells with quantification of dead cells (% of total cells). (Reprint from Ref [94].)

2.6. Borophene

Since the two-dimensional boron sheet (borophene) was synthesized on Ag substrates in 2015, research on borophene has grown fast in the fields of condensed matter physics, chemistry, material science, and nanotechnology. Due to its unique physical and chemical properties, borophene has various potential applications. Borophene is composed purely of boron atoms and arranged in a hexagonal structure with conventional covalent bonds between each boron atom. Recently, researchers have shown an escalating research interest in borophene, not only regarding industrial applications but also in the field of biomedicine. An up-to-date summary of the recent advances in borophene-based nanomedicine is discussed here. Finally, we review the emerging use of borophenes as biosensors and therapeutics. We used strengths, weaknesses, opportunities, threats (SWOT) analysis to assess both the current and future marketing potential of 2D based NMs in cancer therapeutics.

2.6.1. Biomedical Applications of Borophene

In the field of biomedicine, borophene as a nanomaterial has been widely studied and paid attention to because of its good flexibility. This is because borophene has excellent molecular, physical, and mechanical properties in strip and tubular conformations.

In the biomedical applications of NMs, borophene is often used as a 2D nanomaterial combined with other metals and semiconductor materials to improve the performance of biological applications without any negative effects [95, 96]. DNA sequencing has been realized by different methods through the determination of base sequence, which has a great impact on the decoding of human biological code [97, 98]. However, the application of NMs in this technology will greatly accelerate the research of biology and medicine [99].

Due to the structural similarities of borophene and graphene, borophene may also be used in applications such as batteries. However, except for biosensors, biomedical applications have been rarely reported. However, 2D boron clusters, which interact with other elements, show great potential for tumor cell localization and therapy.

2.6.2. Biosensors

Borophene is effectively used for biosensors. By testing the energy and electron sensitivity of 2D borophene to the four bases (adenine (A), guanine (G), thymine (T), and cytosine (C)) on top of biological DNA, the scientists found that different bases attached to borophene produce different conductivities, resulting in different electrical signals. In addition, Das *et al.* also measured the sensitivity of borophene to different bases, $A > G > C > T$ [99]. Thus, borophenenanosheets could be used in biological DNA sequencing devices.

Borophene has been investigated as a gas sensor due to modification of its electronic structure. Omidavaret. a., [100] showed the sensitivity of B36 borophene to HCN concentration and pressure due to its altered electrical properties, various configurations providing a differential response to HCN. Besides HCN, other gases, such as CO, CO_2, NO, NO_2, and NH_3 [101 - 103] could also be detected by borophene following charge transfer after attachment of the gas onto borophene [102]. Gases have differential binding energy to borophene, higher binding energies representing stronger binding. Recently, the glucose sensing performance of Borophene and PANI: Borophene-based non-enzymatic electrochemical biosensors were investigated in comparison to the prepared

PANI-based biosensor [104]. PANI: Borophene-based biosensor detected 1–12 mM glucose with a sensitivity of 96.93 μAmM^{-1} cm^{-2} during 1 min cyclic voltammetry measurement. The results reveal that Borophene enhanced the glucose-sensing sensitivity of PANI. PANI: Borophene-based biosensor has higher sensitivity and better stability [104].

CONCLUSION AND FUTURE PERSPECTIVES

Boron-based compounds have the potential to be effective medications in the treatment of cancer and other disorders. Due to advances in nanotechnology and the creation of new neutron sources, boron-based NMs such as BNCT is expected to become a viable approach in the near future. After decades of research, the BNCT carriers were switched from tiny molecules to NCs. A high boron content is required for BNCT therapy, which can be achieved using NCs. Nanostructure boron compounds, on the other hand, have a very restricted excretion and metabolic potential. As a result, greater research into the pharmacokinetics of BNCT drugs is needed to better understand their possible harmful effects on human health. Preliminary exploration of NCs in BNCT use can lead to the development of "magic bullets" that selectively deliver various boron reagents intracellularly. Nonetheless, more *in vivo* investigations and clinical trials using all of the developed boron nano-carriers are required. The NCs are thought to be able to restore our hopes of finding a cure for cancer and other diseases by using a boron-based drug discovery pipeline.

CONSENT FOR PUBLICATION

Not applicable.

CONFLICT OF INTEREST

The author declares no conflict of interest, financial or otherwise.

ACKNOWLEDGMENT

The authors are grateful to the School of Pharmacy and State Key Laboratory of Quality Research in Chinese Medicine, Macau University of Science and Technology, Macau SAR, China, for providing research facilities.

REFERENCES

[1]   Capek I. Polymer decorated gold nanoparticles in nanomedicine conjugates. Adv Colloid Interface Sci 2017; 249: 386-99.
[http://dx.doi.org/10.1016/j.cis.2017.01.007] [PMID: 28259207]

[2]   Swierczewska M, Han HS, Kim K, Park JH, Lee S. Polysaccharide-based nanoparticles for theranostic

nanomedicine. Adv Drug Deliv Rev 2016; 99(Pt A): 70-84.
[http://dx.doi.org/10.1016/j.addr.2015.11.015] [PMID: 26639578]

[3]　Gao SM, Zhu YH, Hosmane N. Nanostructured boron compounds for boron neutron capture therapy (BNCT) in cancer treatment. Boron-based compounds: potential and emerging applications in medicine 2018; 371-88.

[4]　Barreto JA, O'Malley W, Kubeil M, Graham B, Stephan H, Spiccia L. Nanomaterials: applications in cancer imaging and therapy. Adv Mater 2011; 23(12): H18-40.
[http://dx.doi.org/10.1002/adma.201100140] [PMID: 21433100]

[5]　Jokerst JV, Gambhir SS. Molecular imaging with theranostic nanoparticles. Acc Chem Res 2011; 44(10): 1050-60.
[http://dx.doi.org/10.1021/ar200106e] [PMID: 21919457]

[6]　Ahmed N, Fessi H, Elaissari A. Theranostic applications of nanoparticles in cancer. Drug Discov Today 2012; 17(17-18): 928-34.
[http://dx.doi.org/10.1016/j.drudis.2012.03.010] [PMID: 22484464]

[7]　Grimm J, Scheinberg DA. Will nanotechnology influence targeted cancer therapy? Seminars in radiation oncology. Elsevier 2011; pp. 80-7.

[8]　Zhu Y, Hosmane NS. Nanostructured boron compounds for cancer therapy. Pure Appl Chem 2018; 90: 653-63.
[http://dx.doi.org/10.1515/pac-2017-0903]

[9]　Axtell JC, Saleh LM, Qian EA, Wixtrom AI, Spokoyny AM. Synthesis and applications of perfunctionalized boron clusters. ACS Publications 2018.
[http://dx.doi.org/10.1021/acs.inorgchem.7b02912]

[10]　Pitochelli AR, Hawthorne FM. The isolation of the icosahedral B12H12-2 Ion. J Am Chem Soc 1960; 82: 3228-9.
[http://dx.doi.org/10.1021/ja01497a069]

[11]　Emsley J. Nature's building blocks: an AZ guide to the elements. Oxford University Press 2011.

[12]　Goldbach HE, Wimmer MA. Boron in plants and animals: is there a role beyond cell-wall structure? J Plant Nutr Soil Sci 2007; 170: 39-48.
[http://dx.doi.org/10.1002/jpln.200625161]

[13]　Brokesh AM, Gaharwar AK. Inorganic biomaterials for regenerative medicine. ACS Appl Mater Interfaces 2020; 12(5): 5319-44.
[http://dx.doi.org/10.1021/acsami.9b17801] [PMID: 31989815]

[14]　Si PZ, Zhang M, You CY, Geng DY, Du JH, Zhao XG, *et al.* Amorphous boron nanoparticles and BN encapsulating boron nano-peanuts prepared by arc-decomposing diborane and nitriding. J Mater Sci 2003; 38: 689-92.
[http://dx.doi.org/10.1023/A:1021832209250]

[15]　Bellott BJ, Noh W, Nuzzo RG, Girolami GS. Nanoenergetic materials: boron nanoparticles from the pyrolysis of decaborane and their functionalisation. Chem Commun (Camb) 2009; (22): 3214-5.
[http://dx.doi.org/10.1039/b902371b] [PMID: 19587917]

[16]　He X, Joo S, Xiao H, Liang H. Boron-based nanoparticles for chemical-mechanical polishing of copper films. ECS J Solid State Sci Technol 2013; 2: 20-P5.
[http://dx.doi.org/10.1149/2.021301jss]

[17]　Icten O, Hosmane NS, Kose DA, Zumreoglu-Karan B. Production of magnetic nano-bioconjugates *via* ball milling of commercial boron powder with biomolecules. Z Anorg Allg Chem 2016; 642: 828-32.
[http://dx.doi.org/10.1002/zaac.201600181]

[18]　Icten O, Hosmane NS, Kose DA, Zumreoglu-Karan B. Magnetic nanocomposites of boron and vitamin C. New J Chem 2017; 41: 3646-52.

[http://dx.doi.org/10.1039/C6NJ03894H]

[19]   He X, Joo S, Xiao H, Liang H. Boron-based nanoparticles for chemical-mechanical polishing of copper films. ECS J Solid State Sci Technol 2012; 2: 20.
[http://dx.doi.org/10.1149/2.021301jss]

[20]   Exploring the structure of nitrogen-rich ionic liquids and their binding to the surface of oxide-free boron nanoparticles. J Phys Chem C 2013; 117: 5693-707.
[http://dx.doi.org/10.1021/jp3100409]

[21]   Wang JL, Gu YL, Li ZL, Wang WM, Fu ZY. Synthesis of nano-sized amorphous boron powders through active dilution self-propagating high-temperature synthesis method. Mater Res Bull 2013; 48: 2018-22.
[http://dx.doi.org/10.1016/j.materresbull.2013.01.053]

[22]   Seifolazadeh A, Mohammadi S. Synthesis and characterization of nanoboron powders prepared with mechanochemical reaction between B_2O_3 and Mg powders. Bull Mater Sci 2016; 39: 479-86.
[http://dx.doi.org/10.1007/s12034-016-1150-x]

[23]   Van Devener B, Perez JPL, Jankovich J, Anderson SL. Oxide-free, catalyst-coated, fuel-soluble, air-stable boron nanopowder as combined combustion catalyst and high energy density fuel. Energy Fuels 2009; 23: 6111-20.
[http://dx.doi.org/10.1021/ef900765h]

[24]   Perez JPL, McMahon BW, Anderson SL. Functionalization and Passivation of Boron Nanoparticles with a Hypergolic Ionic Liquid. J Propuls Power 2013; 29: 489-95.
[http://dx.doi.org/10.2514/1.B34724]

[25]   Shin WG, Calder S, Ugurlu O, Girshick SL. Production and characterization of boron nanoparticles synthesized with a thermal plasma system. J Nanopart Res 2011; 13: 7187-91.
[http://dx.doi.org/10.1007/s11051-011-0633-3]

[26]   Marzik JV, Suplinskas RJ, Wilke RHT, Canfield PC, Finnemore DK, Rindfleisch M, *et al.* Plasma synthesized doped B powders for MgB2 superconductors. Physica C 2005; 423: 83-8.
[http://dx.doi.org/10.1016/j.physc.2005.04.005]

[27]   Pickering AL, Mitterbauer C, Browning ND, Kauzlarich SM, Power PP. Room temperature synthesis of surface-functionalised boron nanoparticles. Chem Commun (Camb) 2007; (6): 580-2.
[http://dx.doi.org/10.1039/b614363f] [PMID: 17264897]

[28]   Xu TT, Zheng JG, Wu NQ, Nicholls AW, Roth JR, Dikin DA, *et al.* Crystalline boron nanoribbons: Synthesis and characterization. Nano Lett 2004; 4: 963-8.
[http://dx.doi.org/10.1021/nl0498785]

[29]   Kirihara K, Sasaki T, Koshizaki N, Kimura K. Seebeck coefficient and power factor of single-crystalline boron nanobelts. Appl Phys Express 2011; 4: 041201.
[http://dx.doi.org/10.1143/APEX.4.041201]

[30]   Wang XJ, Tian JF, Yang TZ, Bao LH, Hui C, Liu F, *et al.* Single crystalline boron nanocones: Electric transport and field emission properties. Adv Mater 2007; 19: 4480.
[http://dx.doi.org/10.1002/adma.200701336]

[31]   Guo L, Singh RN, Kleebe HJ. Nucleation and growth of boron nanowires on ZrB_2 particles. Chem Vap Depos 2006; 12: 448-52.
[http://dx.doi.org/10.1002/cvde.200606497]

[32]   Hieu ND, Chu NM, Tokoi Y, Do TMD, Nakayama T, Suematsu H, *et al.* Preparation of boron nanoparticles by pulsed discharge of compacted powder. Jap J App Phy 2020; 59 59:SCCC05.

[33]   El-Batal AI, El-Sayyad GS, Al-Hazmi NE, Gobara M. Antibiofilm and antimicrobial activities of silver boron nanoparticles synthesized by PVP polymer and gamma rays against urinary tract pathogens. J Cluster Sci 2019; 30: 947-64.
[http://dx.doi.org/10.1007/s10876-019-01553-4]

[34]   Uspenskii S, Khaptakhanova P, Zaboronok A, *et al.* Elemental boron nanoparticles: production by ultrasonication in aqueous medium and application in boron neutron capture therapy doklady chemistry. Springer 2020; pp. 45-8.

[35]   Bundy F, Wentorf R Jr. Direct transformation of hexagonal boron nitride to denser forms. J Chem Phys 1963; 38: 1144-9.
[http://dx.doi.org/10.1063/1.1733815]

[36]   Corrigan F, Bundy F. Direct transitions among the allotropic forms of boron nitride at high pressures and temperatures. J Chem Phys 1975; 63: 3812-20.
[http://dx.doi.org/10.1063/1.431874]

[37]   Vel L, Demazeau G, Etourneau J. Cubic boron-nitride - synthesis, physicochemical properties and applications. Mat Sci Eng B-Solid 1991; 10: 149-64.
[http://dx.doi.org/10.1016/0921-5107(91)90121-B]

[38]   Weng Q, Wang X, Wang X, Bando Y, Golberg D. Functionalized hexagonal boron nitride nanomaterials: emerging properties and applications. Chem Soc Rev 2016; 45(14): 3989-4012.
[http://dx.doi.org/10.1039/C5CS00869G] [PMID: 27173728]

[39]   Suryavanshi AP, Yu MF, Wen JG, Tang CC, Bando Y. Elastic modulus and resonance behavior of boron nitride nanotubes. Appl Phys Lett 2004; 84: 2527-9.
[http://dx.doi.org/10.1063/1.1691189]

[40]   Golberg D, Costa PMFJ, Lourie O, *et al.* Direct force measurements and kinking under elastic deformation of individual multiwalled boron nitride nanotubes. Nano Lett 2007; 7: 2146-51.
[http://dx.doi.org/10.1021/nl070863r]

[41]   Zettl A, Chang CW, Begtrup G. A new look at thermal properties of nanotubes. Phys Status Solidi, B Basic Res 2007; 244: 4181-3.
[http://dx.doi.org/10.1002/pssb.200776103]

[42]   Chen Y, Zou J, Campbell SJ, Le Caer G. Boron nitride nanotubes: Pronounced resistance to oxidation. Appl Phys Lett 2004; 84: 2430-2.
[http://dx.doi.org/10.1063/1.1667278]

[43]   Merlo A, Mokkapati VRSS, Pandit S, Mijakovic I. Boron nitride nanomaterials: biocompatibility and bio-applications. Biomater Sci 2018; 6(9): 2298-311.
[http://dx.doi.org/10.1039/C8BM00516H] [PMID: 30059084]

[44]   Habib T, Sundaravadivelu Devarajan D, Khabaz F, *et al.* Cosolvents as Liquid Surfactants for Boron Nitride Nanosheet (BNNS) Dispersions. Langmuir 2016; 32(44): 11591-9.
[http://dx.doi.org/10.1021/acs.langmuir.6b02611] [PMID: 27740775]

[45]   Li X, Li QF, Chen GX. Alkali metal surfactant-facilitated formation of thick boron nitride layers on carbon nanotubes by dip-coating. Mater Lett 2014; 134: 38-41.
[http://dx.doi.org/10.1016/j.matlet.2014.07.049]

[46]   Chae A, Park SJ, Min B, In I. Enhanced dispersion of boron nitride nanosheets in aqueous media by using bile acid-based surfactants. Mater Res Express 2018; 5: 015036.
[http://dx.doi.org/10.1088/2053-1591/aaa434]

[47]   Li LH, Xing T, Chen Y, Jones R. Boron nitride nanosheets for metal protection. Adv Mater Interfaces 2014; 1: 1300132.
[http://dx.doi.org/10.1002/admi.201300132]

[48]   Li LH, Chen Y. Atomically thin boron nitride: unique properties and applications. Adv Funct Mater 2016; 26: 2594-608.
[http://dx.doi.org/10.1002/adfm.201504606]

[49]   Deepika , Li LH, Glushenkov AM, Hait SK, Hodgson P, Chen Y. High-efficient production of boron nitride nanosheets *via* an optimized ball milling process for lubrication in oil. Sci Rep 2014; 4: 7288.

[http://dx.doi.org/10.1038/srep07288] [PMID: 25470295]

[50] Zhang H, Tong CJ, Zhang YS, Zhang YN, Liu LM. Porous BN for hydrogen generation and storage. J Mater Chem A Mater Energy Sustain 2015; 3: 9632-7.
[http://dx.doi.org/10.1039/C5TA01052G]

[51] Ma R, Bando Y, Zhu H, Sato T, Xu C, Wu D. Hydrogen uptake in boron nitride nanotubes at room temperature. J Am Chem Soc 2002; 124(26): 7672-3.
[http://dx.doi.org/10.1021/ja026030e] [PMID: 12083917]

[52] Butts M, Sinha M, Genovese SE, Yamada M. Cosmetic compositions comprising sub-micron boron nitride particles. Google Patents 2007.

[53] Falin A, Cai Q, Santos EJG, et al. Mechanical properties of atomically thin boron nitride and the role of interlayer interactions. Nat Commun 2017; 8: 15815.
[http://dx.doi.org/10.1038/ncomms15815] [PMID: 28639613]

[54] Jiang XF, Weng QH, Wang XB, et al. Recent progress on fabrications and applications of boron nitride nanomaterials: A review. J Mater Sci Technol 2015; 31: 589-98.
[http://dx.doi.org/10.1016/j.jmst.2014.12.008]

[55] Ali F, S Hosmane N, Zhu Y. Boron chemistry for medical applications. Molecules 2020; 25(4): 828.
[http://dx.doi.org/10.3390/molecules25040828] [PMID: 32070043]

[56] Singh B, Kaur G, Singh P, et al. Nanostructured boron nitride with high water dispersibility for boron neutron capture therapy. Sci Rep 2016; 6: 35535.
[http://dx.doi.org/10.1038/srep35535] [PMID: 27759052]

[57] Li X, Wang X, Zhang J, et al. Hollow boron nitride nanospheres as boron reservoir for prostate cancer treatment. Nat Commun 2017; 8: 13936.
[http://dx.doi.org/10.1038/ncomms13936] [PMID: 28059072]

[58] Ciofani G, Raffa V, Menciassi A, Cuschieri A. Cytocompatibility, interactions, and uptake of polyethyleneimine-coated boron nitride nanotubes by living cells: confirmation of their potential for biomedical applications. Biotechnol Bioeng 2008; 101(4): 850-8.
[http://dx.doi.org/10.1002/bit.21952] [PMID: 18512259]

[59] Su CY, Wang JC, Chen CY, Chu K, Lin CK. Spherical composite powder by coupling polymethyl methacrylate and boron nitride *via* spray drying for cosmetic application. Materials (Basel) 2019; 12(5): 706.
[http://dx.doi.org/10.3390/ma12050706] [PMID: 30823370]

[60] Jedrzejczak-Silicka M, Trukawka M, Piotrowska K, Mijowska E. Few-layered hexagonal boron nitride: functionalization, nanocomposites, and physicochemical and biological properties. Biochemical Toxicology-Heavy Metals and Nanomaterials: IntechOpen; 2020.

[61] Wu H, Kessler MR. Multifunctional cyanate ester nanocomposites reinforced by hexagonal boron nitride after noncovalent biomimetic functionalization. ACS Appl Mater Interfaces 2015; 7(10): 5915-26.
[http://dx.doi.org/10.1021/acsami.5b00147] [PMID: 25726956]

[62] Kıvanç M, Barutca B, Koparal AT, Göncü Y, Bostancı SH, Ay N. Effects of hexagonal boron nitride nanoparticles on antimicrobial and antibiofilm activities, cell viability. Mater Sci Eng C 2018; 91: 115-24.
[http://dx.doi.org/10.1016/j.msec.2018.05.028] [PMID: 30033238]

[63] Şen Oz, Emanet M, Çulha M. Stimulatory effect of hexagonal boron nitrides in wound healing. ACS Appl Bio Mater 2019; 2: 5582-96.
[http://dx.doi.org/10.1021/acsabm.9b00669]

[64] O'Toole EA, Goel M, Woodley DT. Hydrogen peroxide inhibits human keratinocyte migration. Dermatol Surg 1996; 22(6): 525-9.
[http://dx.doi.org/10.1111/j.1524-4725.1996.tb00368.x] [PMID: 8646466]

[65]   Emanet Ciofani M. Şen Oz, Çulha M. Hexagonal boron nitride nanoparticles for prostate cancer treatment. ACS Appl Nano Mater 2020; 3: 2364-72.
[http://dx.doi.org/10.1021/acsanm.9b02486]

[66]   Suenaga K, Colliex C, Demoncy N, Loiseau A, Pascard H, Willaime F. Synthesis of nanoparticles and nanotubes with well-separated layers of boron nitride and carbon. Science 1997; 278: 653-5.
[http://dx.doi.org/10.1126/science.278.5338.653]

[67]   Chen X, Wu P, Rousseas M, *et al.* Boron nitride nanotubes are noncytotoxic and can be functionalized for interaction with proteins and cells. J Am Chem Soc 2009; 131(3): 890-1.
[http://dx.doi.org/10.1021/ja807334b] [PMID: 19119844]

[68]   Nakamura H, Koganei H, Miyoshi T, Sakurai Y, Ono K, Suzuki M. Antitumor effect of boron nitride nanotubes in combination with thermal neutron irradiation on BNCT. Bioorg Med Chem Lett 2015; 25(2): 172-4.
[http://dx.doi.org/10.1016/j.bmcl.2014.12.005] [PMID: 25522821]

[69]   Ha Y, Yang J, Tao F, Wu Q, Song Y, Wang H, *et al.* Phase-transited Lysozyme as a universal route to bioactive hydroxyapatite crystalline film. Adv Funct Mater 2018; 28: 1704476.
[http://dx.doi.org/10.1002/adfm.201704476]

[70]   Gao A, Wu Q, Wang D, Ha Y, Chen Z, Yang P. A superhydrophobic surface templated by protein self-assembly and emerging application toward protein crystallization. Adv Mater 2016; 28(3): 579-87.
[http://dx.doi.org/10.1002/adma.201504769] [PMID: 26607764]

[71]   Li L, Li J, Shi Y, *et al.* On-demand biodegradable boron nitride nanoparticles for treating triple negative breast cancer with boron neutron capture therapy. ACS Nano 2019; 13(12): 13843-52.
[http://dx.doi.org/10.1021/acsnano.9b04303] [PMID: 31697475]

[72]   da Silva WM, de Andrade Alves E Silva RH, Cipreste MF, *et al.* Boron nitride nanotubes radiolabeled with ^{153}Sm and ^{159}Gd: Potential application in nanomedicine. Appl Radiat Isot 2020; 157: 109032.
[http://dx.doi.org/10.1016/j.apradiso.2019.109032] [PMID: 32063327]

[73]   da Silva WM, Hilário Ferreira T, de Morais CA, Soares Leal A, Barros Sousa EM. Samarium doped boron nitride nanotubes. Appl Radiat Isot 2018; 131: 30-5.
[http://dx.doi.org/10.1016/j.apradiso.2017.10.045] [PMID: 29100156]

[74]   da Silva WM, Monteiro GAA, Gastelois PL, de Sousa RG, de Almeida Macedo WA, Sousa EMB. Efficient sensitive polymer-grafted boron nitride nanotubes by microwave-assisted process. Nano-Structures & Nano-Objects 2018; 15: 186-96.
[http://dx.doi.org/10.1016/j.nanoso.2017.09.014]

[75]   da Silva WM, de Andrade Alves E Silva RH, Cipreste MF, *et al.* Boron nitride nanotubes radiolabeled with ^{153}Sm and ^{159}Gd: Potential application in nanomedicine. Appl Radiat Isot 2020; 157: 109032.
[http://dx.doi.org/10.1016/j.apradiso.2019.109032] [PMID: 32063327]

[76]   Maguer A, Leroy E, Bresson L, Doris E, Loiseau A, Mioskowski C. A versatile strategy for the functionalization of boron nitride nanotubes. J Mater Chem 2009; 19: 1271-5.
[http://dx.doi.org/10.1039/b815954h]

[77]   Mateti S, Wong CS, Liu Z, *et al.* Biocompatibility of boron nitride nanosheets. Nano Res 2018; 11: 334-42.
[http://dx.doi.org/10.1007/s12274-017-1635-y]

[78]   Wu P, Chen X, Hu N, *et al.* Biocompatible carbon nanotubes generated by functionalization with glycodendrimers. Angew Chem Int Ed Engl 2008; 47(27): 5022-5.
[http://dx.doi.org/10.1002/anie.200705363] [PMID: 18509843]

[79]   Pinto AM, Gonçalves IC, Magalhães FD. Graphene-based materials biocompatibility: a review. Colloids Surf B Biointerfaces 2013; 111: 188-202.
[http://dx.doi.org/10.1016/j.colsurfb.2013.05.022] [PMID: 23810824]

[80]   Gurunathan S, Kim JH. Synthesis, toxicity, biocompatibility, and biomedical applications of graphene and graphene-related materials. Int J Nanomedicine 2016; 11: 1927-45.
[http://dx.doi.org/10.2147/IJN.S105264] [PMID: 27226713]

[81]   Kang S, Herzberg M, Rodrigues DF, Elimelech M. Antibacterial effects of carbon nanotubes: size does matter! Langmuir 2008; 24(13): 6409-13.
[http://dx.doi.org/10.1021/la800951v] [PMID: 18512881]

[82]   Motskin M, Wright DM, Muller K, *et al.* Hydroxyapatite nano and microparticles: correlation of particle properties with cytotoxicity and biostability. Biomaterials 2009; 30(19): 3307-17.
[http://dx.doi.org/10.1016/j.biomaterials.2009.02.044] [PMID: 19304317]

[83]   Ciofani G, Danti S, D'Alessandro D, Moscato S, Menciassi A. Assessing cytotoxicity of boron nitride nanotubes: Interference with the MTT assay. Biochem Biophys Res Commun 2010; 394(2): 405-11.
[http://dx.doi.org/10.1016/j.bbrc.2010.03.035] [PMID: 20226164]

[84]   Nithya JSM, Pandurangan A. Aqueous dispersion of polymer coated boron nitride nanotubes and their antibacterial and cytotoxicity studies. RSC Advances 2014; 4: 32031-46.
[http://dx.doi.org/10.1039/C4RA04846F]

[85]   Li X, Zhi C, Hanagata N, Yamaguchi M, Bando Y, Golberg D. Boron nitride nanotubes functionalized with mesoporous silica for intracellular delivery of chemotherapy drugs. Chem Commun (Camb) 2013; 49(66): 7337-9.
[http://dx.doi.org/10.1039/c3cc42743a] [PMID: 23851619]

[86]   Li LH, Chen Y, Glushenkov AM. Boron nitride nanotube films grown from boron ink painting. J Mater Chem 2010; 20: 9679-83.
[http://dx.doi.org/10.1039/c0jm01414a]

[87]   Ciofani G, Danti S, D'Alessandro D, *et al.* Enhancement of neurite outgrowth in neuronal-like cells following boron nitride nanotube-mediated stimulation. ACS Nano 2010; 4(10): 6267-77.
[http://dx.doi.org/10.1021/nn101985a] [PMID: 20925390]

[88]   Meng WJ, Huang Y, Fu YQ, Wang ZF, Zhi CY. Polymer composites of boron nitride nanotubes and nanosheets. J Mater Chem C Mater Opt Electron Devices 2014; 2: 10049-61.
[http://dx.doi.org/10.1039/C4TC01998A]

[89]   Danti S, Ciofani G, Moscato S, *et al.* Boron nitride nanotubes and primary human osteoblasts: *in vitrol* compatibility and biological interactions under low frequency ultrasound stimulation. Nanotechnology 2013; 24(46): 465102.
[http://dx.doi.org/10.1088/0957-4484/24/46/465102] [PMID: 24150892]

[90]   Lee CH, Bhandari S, Tiwari B, Yapici N, Zhang D, Yap YK. Boron nitride nanotubes: recent advances in their synthesis, functionalization, and applications. Molecules 2016; 21(7): 922.
[http://dx.doi.org/10.3390/molecules21070922] [PMID: 27428947]

[91]   Ciofani G, Raffa V, Menciassi A, Cuschieri A. Folate functionalized boron nitride nanotubes and their selective uptake by glioblastoma multiforme cells: implications for their use as boron carriers in clinical boron neutron capture therapy. Nanoscale Res Lett 2008; 4(2): 113-21.
[http://dx.doi.org/10.1007/s11671-008-9210-9] [PMID: 20596476]

[92]   Buzatu DA, Wilkes JG, Miller D, Darsey JA, Heinze T, Birls A, *et al.* Nanotubes for cancer therapy and diagnostics. Google Patents 2011.

[93]   Menichetti L, De Marchi D, Calucci L, Ciofani G, Menciassi A, Forte C. Boron nitride nanotubes for boron neutron capture therapy as contrast agents in magnetic resonance imaging at 3 T. Appl Radiat Isot 2011; 69(12): 1725-7.
[http://dx.doi.org/10.1016/j.apradiso.2011.02.032] [PMID: 21398132]

[94]   Ferreira TH, Miranda MC, Rocha Z, Leal AS, Gomes DA, Sousa EMB. An assessment of the potential use of BNNTs for boron neutron capture therapy. Nanomaterials (Basel) 2017; 7(4): 82.
[http://dx.doi.org/10.3390/nano7040082] [PMID: 28417903]

[95]　Piazza ZA, Hu H-S, Li W-L, Zhao Y-F, Li J, Wang L-S. Planar hexagonal B(36) as a potential basis for extended single-atom layer boron sheets. Nat Commun 2014; 5: 3113.
[http://dx.doi.org/10.1038/ncomms4113] [PMID: 24445427]

[96]　Duo Y, Xie Z, Wang L, Abbasi NM, Yang T, Li Z, *et al.* Borophene-based biomedical applications: Status and future challenges. Coord Chem Rev 2021; 427: 213549.
[http://dx.doi.org/10.1016/j.ccr.2020.213549]

[97]　Kim HS, Kim Y-H. Recent progress in atomistic simulation of electrical current DNA sequencing. Biosens Bioelectron 2015; 69: 186-98.
[http://dx.doi.org/10.1016/j.bios.2015.02.020] [PMID: 25744599]

[98]　Raoof M, Jans K, Bryce G, Ebrahim S, Lagae L, Witvrouw A. Improving the selectivity by using different blocking agents in DNA hybridization assays for SiGe bio-molecular sensors. Microelectron Eng 2013; 111: 421-4.
[http://dx.doi.org/10.1016/j.mee.2013.04.035]

[99]　Xie Z, Meng X, Li X, *et al.* Two-dimensional borophene: Properties, fabrication, and promising applications. Research 2020.

[100]　Omidvar A. Borophene: A novel boron sheet with a hexagonal vacancy offering high sensitivity for hydrogen cyanide detection. Comput Theor Chem 2017; 1115: 179-84.
[http://dx.doi.org/10.1016/j.comptc.2017.06.018]

[101]　Beheshtian J, Soleymanabadi H, Peyghan AA, Bagheri Z. A DFT study on the functionalization of a BN nanosheet with PCX,(PC= phenyl carbamate, X= OCH_3, CH_3, NH_2, NO_2 and CN). Appl Surf Sci 2013; 268: 436-41.
[http://dx.doi.org/10.1016/j.apsusc.2012.12.119]

[102]　Rezaei-Sameti M, Hemmati NN. 2 O interaction with the pristine and 1Ca-and 2Ca-doped beryllium oxide nanotube: a computational study. J Nanostructure Chem 2016; 6: 343-55.
[http://dx.doi.org/10.1007/s40097-016-0206-1]

[103]　Taşaltın N, Taşaltın C, Baytemir G, Karakuş S. S. β12 Phase Borophene Enhanced PANI Gas Sensor for CO and NH_3 Detection. 2021.

[104]　Taşaltın C, Türkmen TA, Taşaltın N, Karakuş S. Highly sensitive non-enzymatic electrochemical glucose biosensor based on PANI: β12 Borophene. J Mater Sci Mater Electron 2021; 32: 1-11.

CHAPTER 9

Metal Nanoparticle Synthesis Through Biological Entities

Robaica Khan[1], Muhammad Bilal[1], Fahad Hassan Shah[2], Song Ja Kim[2,*], Junaid Dar[1], Ayesha Sajjad[1], Kashif Iqbal[1] and Saad Salman[1,*]

[1] *The University of Lahore, Islamabad Campus, Islamabad-44000, Pakistan*

[2] *Department of Biological Sciences, College of Natural Sciences, Kongju National University, Gongju, 32588, Republic of Korea*

Abstract: During recent years, the development of suitable green chemistry methods for the synthesis of metallic nanoparticles has become the main focus of researchers. The investigations are under process for the creation of standardized nanoparticles (NPs). One of the most frequent ways for NPs synthesis is using plants that are ideally suited for nanoparticle production. The nanoparticles created from various organisms vary in physical appearance, and the plant-based NPs enable the researchers to explore the plant mechanisms for the uptake and creation of metallic NPs. Nanotechnology is emerging as a crucial discipline of science and technology that examines the cell-level interaction between synthetic and biological materials. The use of this technology is rising worldwide due of its advantages and simplicity. Organisms from primitive prokaryotes to complex eukaryotes and angiosperm plants are used for the production of NPs. Further investigation and study are required in this field to enhance the biological synthesis of nanoparticles. This book chapter discussed the plants employed in NPs synthesis. It also represents the many biological systems that create the art of fabrication of NPs and the development of this advanced technology.

Keywords: Applications, Biological based nanoparticles, Characterization, Metallic Nanoparticles, Nanotechnology, Physiochemical Properties, Toxicity.

1. INTRODUCTION

The newly created field of nanobiotechnology in recent years is focused on using nanotechnologies for the creation of nanometer-size particles *via* biological resources. Nanoparticles (NPs) are of immense importance because of their

* Corresponding author Saad Salman and Song Ja Kim: The University of Lahore, Islamabad Campus, Islamabad-44000, Pakistan. and Department of Biological Sciences, College of Natural Sciences, Kongju National University, Gongju, 32588, Republic of Korea; E-mail: ksj85@kongju.ac.kr; E-mail: saad.salman@pharm.uol.edu.pk

magnetic, electro-optic, and physicochemical properties which are determined by their morphology [1 - 3]. Due to the large surface area to volume ratio and extremely small size, the differences in their properties is very significant *i.e.* catalytic activity, biological activity, optical immersion, heat and electrical conduction, mechanical properties, melting point, as compared to the substances that are present in bulk or at large scales [4 - 7]. Due to the uniquely extensive range of physicochemical characteristics, NPs play a part in various techniques, including medical diagnosis and imaging, medical treatment protocols, pharmaceutical products, chemical sensors, *etc.* For example, inert metals like gold (Au), silver (Ag), palladium (Pd), and platinum (Pt) are being widely used in medical and pharmaceutical products. As Ag NPs are used in anti-inflammatory and antibacterial activities, along with that, they are also used in dressing wounds and medical implant coating [8, 9]. Similarly, the gold NPs are also used in biomedical applications such as disease diagnosis and pharmaceutics [10, 11]. The palladium NPs are used in chemical sensors, catalysis, and electrocatalysis applications [12, 13]. The platinum is either used as a pure form or its alloy is made with other NPs and universally used in NPs applications. In addition to those, the non-metallic NPs comprising Cu, ZnO, Se, and iron are involved in medical treatment, cosmetics, and pharmaceuticals. These NPs are synthesized and stabilized by various techniques, including lithography, laser ablation, and high-energy irradiation, *etc* [14]. Studies have shown that many variables (such as concentration, temperature, *etc*) affect the production of NPs [15]. So, consequently, during the synthesis of the NPs, the physicochemical properties, stability, and morphology of NPs are to be effectively monitored. With the wide range of applications of NPs, there comes a slight drawback as the conventional synthesis of NPs often uses toxic materials that have potential hazards for instance, carcinogenicity, cytotoxicity and environmental toxicity. But luckily these hazards can be controlled by the biological monitored production of the NPs. And therefore the outcome will be an ecofriendly process *i.e.*, the biotic production of NPs [16, 17]. This method is now highly efficient, reliable, and biologically compatible with the traditional method for the synthesis of the NPs. The biological synthesis eventually resulted in the use of green chemistry comprising of unicellular and multicellular biological organizations including actinomycetes, bacteria, viruses, algae, bryophytes, *etc.* The biosynthesis of NPs may result in the creation of a wide variety of NPs based on their shape, size, stability, compositions, and physicochemical properties. The production of NPs through biological objects such as plants is an advantageous approach as compared to micro-organisms or other entities as it does not require difficult steps and stages for its production. It is a faster method and especially cost-effective and also used in the synthesis of NPs at a large scale.

2. CHARACTERIZATION TECHNIQUES

The production of NPs is initiated by many methods. But all those methods and techniques fall under two major approaches, including the bottom-up approach and the top-down approach [18, 19]. In either of these approaches, the NPs produced are used in various techniques and their characterized properties are determined such as their shape, size, *etc.* In a bottom-up approach [20], the NPs are simply made from their monomers, while in the top-down approach [21], the material of interest is selected and it undergoes the side reduction by various physical or chemical methods to produce NPs. Due to their significantly high dependency on their size, shape, and surface structures, there is a possible risk of producing surface imperfections by these techniques [22 - 25]. For a particular application, the NPs need to be homogeneous. During the biological synthesis of the NPs, the appearance of the color changes in the action combination is the primary positive indication that NPs are present afterward, the Tyndall effect is used for detection of the NPs in the solution in which a colloidal solution is present. A laser beam is passed through it [26]. After this, a high-speed centrifugation process is applied in which the NPs separate from the colloidal solution and then various characterization techniques are applied for their examination. Some of the commonly used characterization techniques, including spectroscopy and microscopy are, Transmission Electron Microscopy (TEM), Scanning Electron Microscopy (SEM), Atomic Force Microscopy (AFM), Powder X-Ray Diffraction (XRD), UV-visible spectroscopy (UV-vis), Dynamic Light Scattering (DLS), Fourier Transform Infrared Spectroscopy (FT-IR), Energy Dispersive Spectroscopy (EDS), *etc.* The techniques based on microscopy including SEM, AFM, and TEM are the direct method to obtain the images of NPs, which are then applied to find the size and structural features of NPs. In comparison to that, the techniques based on spectroscopy are the indirect methods such as UV-vis, DLS, EDS, FT-IR that are used to find out the composition, period, and characteristics of the NPs. UV-vis uses a wide range to determine the interaction of radiation with matter and also used to determine the electronic transitions of the particles from the low to high energy states. The XRD technique uses special diffraction patterns to conclude the structural information of the constituent part while the DLS method is used to plot the size spreading and evaluate the surface charge on NPs in a liquid suspension.

3. SYNTHESIS OF NPS

3.1. Biological Synthesis of NPs

In recent times, various researches have reported that the NPs produced by microorganisms and plants are economical and ecological [17, 27, 28]. These NPs as a result of both of these biological entities have shown less toxic effects and are less hazardous to the environment. These distinct properties of the NPs have led to the use of the inherent biochemical processes that apply the manufacture of MNPs by transforming the inorganic metallic ions, thus leading to an un-researched field of science. New methods for biological processes such as bioremediation and bioleaching are been introduced due to the microorganism's improbable ability of interaction, extraction, and accumulation of the metallic materials from the ground and surroundings. Due to biochemical conversions occurring by the microorganisms, it has been seen that both unicellular and multicellular organisms make micro and nano-sized materials that aids in oxidation-reduction phenomena [29].

It's a laborious job to synthesize NPs from micro-organisms. The advantage of using plants in NPs synthesis is diverse. These advantages are such that the plant-based NPs are eco-friendly and less hazardous to the environment, these do not involve the use of the specific techniques that are costly. In other words, the production of NPs from the plants is safe, has a very short production time, is cost-effective in the case of cultivation, and also can be used for massive production as compared to other biological entities. For the production of NPs, various biological entities can be used including, bacteria, viruses, algae, plants, *etc.* Firstly, the selection of the entities is done for the synthesis purpose to produce NPs of correct size and morphology, as all the entities are not appropriate for the biological synthesis and have different biochemical processing capabilities. For micro-organisms, culturing techniques are of great importance. It has been observed that those biological entities that have the potential to accumulate heavy metals give the best results for the synthesis of NPs. So, pH, buffer, light, temperature, and nutrients are most effective and can remarkably increase enzyme activity. The utilization of plants for the production of NPs is an alternative and the most effective method for NPs production. The general biological syntheses of metallic NPs are summarized in the Fig. (**1**).

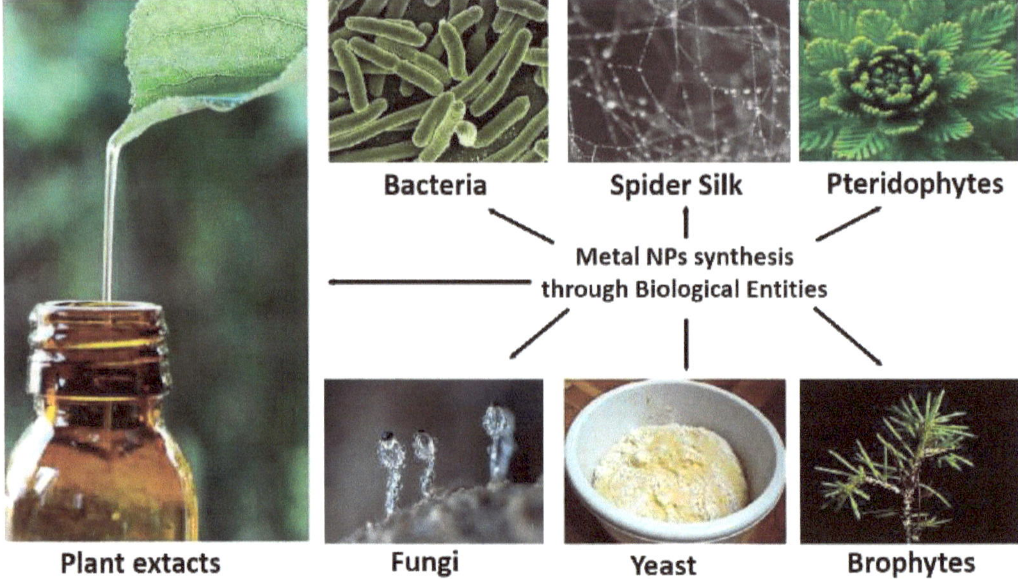

Fig. (1). General synthesis of metallic NPs with the help of biological entities.

3.2. Microorganisms for Nanoparticle Synthesis

As discussed earlier, the production of NPs occurs because of the oxidation-reduction reactions of metal ions by different molecules *e.g.*, enzymes, proteins that are secreted by the micro-organisms. This is because every micro-organism behaves and acts differently to the metal ion. These interactions of the NPs and the effect of ecological features like temperature, pH play role in determining the morphology of NPs. The NPs can either be synthesized extracellular or intracellular based on the kind of micro-organism. Similarly, the techniques for plants are also different in each case. The following sections contain some microbial routes for the production of NPs from plants and micro-organisms.

3.2.1. Actinomycetes

Actinomycetes have been used for the synthesis of NPs intracellularly and extracellularly [30 - 32]. Gold ions reduction intracellularly by Rhodococcus sp. has disclosed that reduction of Au particles took place in the cell wall and cell membrane whereas no reduction took place in the cytosol [33]. The interacting enzymes that were excreted from the cell wall and cell membrane were liable for the lessening of Au ions. Mono-dispersed AuNPs were produced by the biosynthetic process which was nontoxic to the cell. Many studies proved that Au and Ag's NPs undergo intracellular reduction to produce metallic monomers that start the NPs growth. To analyze these conditions which favored the extracellular synthesis of NPs, Karthik *et al.* took Streptomyces sp. LK-3 for the reduction of Ag ions, and it led to the development of AgNPs [34]. This study indicated that (NADH) dependent nitrate reductase enzyme was liable for the lessening of Ag ion, which led to the production of stabilized NPs. For the lessening of Au ions from aqueous solutions comprising gold chloride ($AuCl_4$) ions a similar nitrate reductase enzyme mechanism was. During the electron transfer, the Au ion gains an electron and is reduced to $Au°$, and stable NPs are formed. Proper stabilization is important to prevent clumping and for the protection of NPs. NPs produced *via* biologic methods have been observed to show higher antimicrobial activity in contrast to those that are produced *via* ancient methods. Synergetic proteins produce stable NPs, which are also the cause of antimicrobial activity.

3.2.2. Bacteria

In nature, bacteria have to deal with extremely harsh environments. To survive such situations, they have a natural defense system to combat these stressful situations like the poisonousness from high metallic ion concentration. Some techniques for dealing with high metallic ion concentration include the accumulation of metals, intracellular precipitation, redox state changes *via* efflux systems, and extracellular formation of complexes [35]. *Actinobacteria* sp., *Corynebacterium* sp., *Bacillus cereus*, *Lactobacillus* spp., *Klebsiella pneumonia*, *Escherichia coli*, and *Pseudomonas* sp. are some of the most commonly used bacteria for the production of MNPs [36]. Bacteria may either use intracellular or extracellular mechanisms for the production of NPs. For example, *Pseudomonas stutzeri* AG259 bacterium has been used for the production of AgNPs by NADH-dependent reductase enzyme mechanism in which it donates an electron and then oxidizes to NAD [37]. This donation causes the production of Ag NPs from Ag ions. Likewise in a similar study, Husseiny *et al.* used Pseudomonas aeruginosa to reduce Au ions and it resulted in the extracellular production of AuNPs [38]. However, the non-involvement of biological enzymes has been suggested by some other researchers. For example, Au NPs were produced by Liu *et al.* from dried cells of Bacillus megaterium [39]. Likewise, Sneha *et al.* also used a non-enzymatic reduction mechanism in NPs production using a *Corynebacterium* sp [40]. A lot of factors are considered to be the cause of the reduction of NPs, like organic functional groups on the cell wall which is the rudimentary factor while other factors like pH and temperature are also considered. For example, AgNPs can be produced by the *Lactobacillus* sp. A09 dried biomass and *Bacillus Megaterium* D01 through the collaboration of functional groups existent on the cell wall and can reduce the Ag ions [41]. NPs shape and size are affected by the pH and temperature. Determination of particle size is important as the distinct physical and chemical characteristics are more noticeable at reduced sizes. The foundation of the NPs production and its yield depends upon a suitable culture medium and the salt concentration. Experiments by He *et al.* using bacterium Rhodopseudomonas Capsulata have shown that both metallic salt concentration and medium pH affected the morphology and particle size [42]. Spherical AuNPs were produced at pH 6, with dilute concentrations of $AuCl_4$. On increasing salt concentration Au nanowires were produced at the same pH. Also, when pH was reduced to 4 then both the spheres and triangular nanometer-scale plates were produced. Therefore, it is revealed by the studies that the NPs morphology is changed by altering the medium pH directly.

3.2.3. Fungi

The production of NPs *via* fungi is spreading at a global level and this covers both the intracellular and extracellular processes. For example, the production of gold and AgNPs is possible by the biosynthetic activity of *Fusarium* sp, *aspergillus* sp, and *penicillin* sp [43]. In addition to this, the studies have revealed that fungi can produce mono-dispersed NPs with a large range of particle sizes. Fungi can produce metallic NPs because of their additional applications as compared to bacteria. For example, fungi secrete proteins and enzymes in large numbers which leads to the production of MNPs. Studies revealed that due to the high intracellular uptake volume of some fungi, the synthesized particle size is smaller. On the other hand, the culture conditions can affect NPs synthesis. For example, the extracellular NPs were produced by Au ions reduction by using Trichothecium sp, but the agitation of this mixture produced intracellular NPs [44]. This result leads to the conclusion that the release of enzymes was due to the non-agitation while the agitation prevented the release of enzymes. Fluorescence spectrum analysis showed that the act of bio-reactive reducing agents present in the cell wall caused extracellular NPs synthesis. The study was also helpful in suggesting that the proteins that were released by fungal biomass. Those proteins were also a part of the solution and were attached to the surfaces of the NPs [28]. Using fungi, both the extracellular and intracellular synthesis has been investigated and it was found that the intracellular synthesis suffers low yield, while in extracellular synthesis recovery is fast as the NPs are produced at the surface or periphery of the cell. A distinct feature of fungi is that they can produce NPs having dissimilar organic configurations. For example, *Fusarium oxysporum* can be used to produce Si and Ti NPs *via* aqueous solutions of Si62′ and TiF62′ respectively [45]. Along with that, the synthesis of nanometer-scale material like magnetite, zirconia, CdS quantum dots, and oxide NPs has also been reported [43, 46, 47].

3.2.4. Viruses

The delivery of inorganic materials like silicon dioxide, cadmium oxide, iron oxide, and zinc sulfide has become possible due to viruses [48 - 50]. Thus the viruses can be used for NPs synthesis. Electronic industries show special interest in methods that are used for the synthesis of semiconductor materials like CdS and ZnS. The research on the synthesis of quantum dots by viruses has been expedited in recent years. A special structural feature about viruses is that they possess capsid proteins on their outer surface which can interact with the metal ions. TMV a plant virus can have as many as 2130 capsid proteins which may serve as sites for the settling of materials or may be used for the production of the 3-D vessel for pharmaceuticals. In recent researches, when low concentrations of TMV were used and added before the plant extracts, it was observed that the viruses diminished the size of NPs by increasing their production amount [51, 52]. It was also revealed that the high concentration of TMV can produce fewer free NPs and can also lead to the formation of nanowires and nanotubes because the viruses have a special tendency to do so.

3.2.5. Yeasts

Like many other microorganisms, yeasts can enthrall and collect a large number of toxic metals from their surroundings. This adaptation has led to the development of many mechanisms like bio-sorption, chelation, bio-precipitation, and, extracellular sequestration in yeasts. The size and shape variations of NPs occur because yeasts use different mechanisms during NPs synthesis. Experiments showed that CdS quantum dots were produced when yeast *Candida Glabrata* was exposed to the salts of cadmium [53, 54]. Similar studies showed that there was an association between the period of growth of yeast and the generation of CdS quantum dots [55, 56]. In addition to this PbS quantum dots were synthesized when a yeast *Torulopsis* sp. was exposed to the Pb^{+2} ions [57]. *Pichia Jadinii* has been used for the production of gold NPs [58]. It was observed by managing the growth and the cellular activities of *P.Jadinii* the morphology of NPs could be regulated during NPs synthesis. A marine yeast *Yarrowia lipolytica* was used to check the impact of Au salt concentration and biomass which exposed that both the gold salt concentration and the biomass affected the particle size and shape of the NPs [59, 60]. For example, by increasing the Au salt concentration the nanometer-scale spheres were produced along with nanometer-scale plates, and Ag tolerant yeast strain of MKY3 also produced Ag sphere-shaped NPs whose size range was observed in between 2 to 5 nm [61].

4. METALLIC NPS BIOSYNTHESIS THROUGH MICROBES

In recent years, chemical and physical techniques are being applied for NPs synthesis, but these methods are seemed to be costly with the production of toxic chemicals. But although due to their disadvantages the methods are still applied as the production of toxic chemicals is an area of concern in recent times. For this purpose, the biosynthesis of NPs is the main focus to reduce the cause. NPs can be synthesized in two ways; physical synthesis but is very costly, requires a large amount of energy while chemical synthesis is less costly but produces toxic chemicals as a by-product. Thus, the biological synthesis by organisms like yeast, bacteria can lead to the environment-friendly synthesis of NPs. This method includes techniques like simple under cellular, molecular biochemical and, microbial cultivation mechanisms which can lead to an improved rate of synthesis of NPs. Biotechnological processes like biomineralization, bleaching and, bioremediation are common for the metals and microbes inter-linkage. The properties of NPs synthesized from microbes are similar to chemically synthesized NPs. Many extracellular inorganic materials are produced by unicellular and multicellular organisms. These materials' sizes and shapes can be changed by monitoring the culture variables or parameters. Different microorganisms use different methods for the production of NPs inside and outside the cell. For example, in the intracellular nanoparticle synthesis, the negative ion interaction is used for the transport of ions bearing positive charges inside the wall of the cell. After that, the enzymes present inside the wall of the cell reduce the metal ion and thus causing the production of NPs which are afterward diffused across the bacterial cell wall. Similarly in fungi, the nitrate reductase enzyme which causes the bioreduction of metal ions is responsible for the production of NPs.

4.1. Bacteria Mediated

In bacteria, the cell wall is of great importance as the metal atoms have to cross and shifted back through the mesh of fibers in the cell wall. The peptidoglycan present in the wall contains poly-anions that are responsible for metal and chemical interactions. The groups like amines and carboxyl can be used to react with the cell wall metal-binding sites, thus changing the charge from positive to negative. By the change in the chemical composition of peptidoglycan present, Bacillus Subtilis;s cell wall has developed in the alteration of the carboxyl group present in the glutamic acid, causing the penetration electron easily through the metal [62]. Fe_3O_4 crystal mechanism occurs when hydrates iron oxide are present as a precursor during the crystal growth [63]. The cadmium (Cd) was used for the production of NPs from *Klebsiella pneumonia.* The CdS particles were produced on the cell surface in the existence of Cd ions [64]. The CdS quantum dots deposited on the cell wall of the bacteria were shown to have a characteristic for the protection of the biological membrane against corrosion so to be called bio CdS. It can be used for bio semiconductors applications as it has photophysical and photochemical characteristics which prevent the hazardous effects of Cd species. *Pseudomonas stuzeri*, a remote strain obtained from an Ag mine, was used to synthesize cermet NPs [37]. Crystalline AgNPs that were derived by biosynthesis were assumed to have an organic carbon matrix of various shapes and sizes. The optical properties could be combined after providing the requirement of heat, suitable medium, and change in metal volume for production. Biologically synthesized NPs have useful technological applications they have properties that are similar to conventional thin film coating technologies. The Ag resistance of *P.stutzeri* allows the production and gathering of the metal residue by metal flux and binding of metal [65]. The bacterial tolerance is affected by physical and chemical growth factors towards metal ions and NPs formation [35]. The NPs produced from bacteria can be collected and they have shown to have great applications in metal ion recovery, the medical field during rheumatology, analytical chemistry, and drug delivery [28]. The biological processed Pd has the properties of a chemical catalyst and can be used for industrial wastewater processes of metal recovery [66]. The metal recovery process from the environment by bio-sorption process causes the production of NPs by the bioreduction of metals. Thus, bio-sorption combined with bio-reduction is a compelling procedure for the production of NPs by heavy metals waste at an industrial scale. By using living and non-living organisms the synthesis of spherical platinum NPs suggests the industries a great substitute as compared to chemicals. Surgical instruments made of titanium are hazardous as it reacts with the serum of humans and cancer-causing agents are produced, but this problem can be solved by bacteria, the instruments made of nano-titanium can lead to better prospects.

4.2. Fungal Mediated

The production of NPs *via* fungi is more beneficial than bacteria [43]. Fungal mediated NPs are manufactured by more advanced techniques and are monodisperse. Also, the NPs produced by fungi are profitable [47, 67, 68]. AuNPs are produced by *Fusarium* oxysporum that resulted in the excretion of reducing agents in the solution when treated with aq $AuCl_4$ ions [69 - 72]. The resulted NPs were far more stable because of the linkages of cysteine and lysine leftovers. Restriction of motion on the film surfaces for various applications became possible because of this ability. Lack of colliding with metallic particles and hydrolyzing ability of *F. Oxysporum* resulted in the manufacture of zirconia

NPs when treated with K2ZrF6 solution. *F.Oxysporum* is unique in this ability as compared to bacteria [73 - 75]. Fungi have a reproductive property that is very beneficial for the massive production of NPs, when the aqueous solutions are available, fungi can produce the respective NPs. For instance, Au and AgNPs can be produced when $AuCl_4$ and $AgNO_3$ solutions are available [76], Pt NPs can be produced when H_2PtCl_6 solution is present [77]. The change in pH and temperature affected the morphology and structure of the NPs produced *via* bacteria and yeasts [36, 43, 47]. Verticillium luteoalbum produced various NPs after the changes in morphology and were isolated. AgNPs, which were monodispersive were formulated by *aspergillus* flavus, with a size of 8.92 nm, they also possessed a unique "sil" gene which leads to the massive production of AgNPs [58, 78]. Even in the unavailability of surfactants and other excipients, C.versicolor produced AgNPs [79]. Using glucose as an agent for the stabilization of AgNPs by fungi created stabilized NPs. These NPs had vast applications, such as being a water-soluble metallic catalyst for living cells.

4.3. Virus Mediated

Synthesis of inorganic NPs with required arrays is difficult for bacteria and fungi, therefore the techniques like DNA recognizing linkers, protein cages and surfactant assembled pathways are used but they have limitations. For the problem of the limitations, the engineered viruses having the ability to self-support the semi-conductors surface and having great quantum dots arrangements with monodispersed size and shape are produced [80]. By the genetic selection and molecular cloning techniques, NPs of specific lengths engineered phage-based tobacco mosaic virus (TMV), which could arrange in a line and adjust inert nano-crystals in 3D arrangements [81]. The manufacture of pathological films can be preserved for up to seven months without causing any bacterial infection. It can also be used to store high-density engineered DNA, which has a wide range of applications in medicine [82].

5. ANIMAL WORLD AND SYNTHESIS OF METALLIC NPS

There are various applications of metallic NPs, like their antimicrobial activity by cooperating with proteins, enzymes, and DNA for the purpose of hindering cell division. Along with their advantage, metallic NPs show a wide range of toxicity. Metallic NPs are also used in some biomedical types of equipment such as dental equipment and materials, catheters, medical devices, and implants. Different methods are recently being used for the infusion of metallic NPs in tissues. Bio and nanomedicines offer great applications in medical diagnosis and therapy as they generate no toxicity in host tissues. Metallic NPs can affect tumors;

therefore, they are used in cancer treatment. Thus, the animal models are used for experimenting and positive results were obtained with improved tissue development. There are fewer reports about animal-mediated MNPs. Silk fibroin is the most extensively studied case that is synthesized by arachnids and worms, which have catalytic activity and molecular recognition thus, they can be used as seam materials.

5.1. Animal-Derived Materials

Novel materials are produced by nano-fibers due to their exclusive properties such as their expanse, small pore diameter, and their activity as a microbial barricade. In the host, the cell reactions for growth characteristics and physiology can be evaluated by the NPs. Organisms can be a primary source to obtain inorganic material, which causes the production of NPs. For example, bones, shellac, and spicules are inorganic composite materials produced by multicellular organisms, while unicellular organisms produce magnetic NPs to build different structures.

5.2. Silk Proteins (Fibroin and Sericin) and Spider Silk

Silk fibroin is a natural semi-crystalline biopolymer. It is fabricated by several insects and spiders. Components of fibroin mostly include amino acids, such as serine, glycine, and alanine. The proliferation and attachment properties of silk fibroin make it a valuable item to be used in the textiles industries. Along with it allows easy manufacturing of textile products such as gels, films, and mats. Because of its non-immunogenic and non-toxic properties, it is used in the engineering of skin, bone, blood vessels, ligaments, and nerves. It has been reported by a few research articles that silk fibroin is recyclable [83, 84], but the extent of the degradation rate is not yet very clear. Some spiders and fossil species naturally produce silk. The silk produced by the spider can be of many natures like non-sticky or dry for making spider webs and capturing prey. Bombyx mori, a silkworm, produces silk that is used for commercial purposes due to its catalytic activity and molecular identification [85]. Some species can produce silk in the early metamorphosis stage, while other produce silk at adult age. The Trichoptera larvae can produce silk from sand grains or fragments of the plant. Fibroin is a component such as fibroin TiO_2 or nano-hydroxyapatite (silk fibroin), can also be used in the manufacturing of nanocomposites [86, 87]. In addition to this, sericin can also produce NPs that are released in the wastewater from silk industries. The sericin is recovered from wastewater can be utilized to produce nano sericin by reducing it by rotation techniques. A concentrated solution is obtained which is then converted to powdered form by ultrasonication to decrease particle size. These fibers exhibit remarkable properties as they resist oxidation and have antibacterial activity. With those properties, they also show biocompatibility and are resistant to UV rays [88, 89]. The spider nets have a sticky glycoprotein by which they trap insects, also produce adhesive nano-filaments.

5.3. Invertebrate Mediated

The materials derived from various sources of invertebrates are of significant importance in the medicinal field. Such as the sponges and starfishes have mineralized biological material, which has structural and compositional similarity to the mammalian tooth. The formation of microstructure by the conversion of biomaterials such as hydroxyapatite and bio-silica is an important part of the research. Hydroxyapatite is obtained from fishbone and is present in the natural mineralized form of calcium apatite. It has nano-sized collagenous and non-collagenous proteins present in it. It is used to provide osteoconductivity, safety, and biocompatibility to the bone graft. In sponges, the enzyme silicatein causes the formation of bio or biologic silica. It has a shiny appearance and an amorphous silica structure. It is also made by other aquatic organisms, including sponges, diatoms, choano-flagellates, and radiolarians. The procedure includes the layering of lamellae that have silica NPs. NPs of hydroxyapatite (HA) have been reported to be beneficial for clinical procedures, such as osteogenesis. Gunduz by thermo-gravimetry induced a technique to acquire nano-hydroxyapatite from corals, which was then further studied and with chitosan [90, 91]. The production of NPs from a variety of classes of earthworms has been reported. For instance, nano-red gold was obtained from the earthworm [92 - 94], when reacted to $AuCl_4$. AgNPs were produced from marine worms [94]. These solutions act as a reducer and a preservative for nanoparticle production from $AgNO_3$.

5.4. Chitosan

Chitosan is a peptide obtained from invertebrates. Chitosan contains nanofibers that can be used as coloring agents. Chitosan is also used in the field of medicine as nanocapsules for cancer treatment. Chitosans can be used as a carrier of other compounds as Mahmoodian *et al.* researched the activity of a poly HEMA chitosan MWCNT nanocomposite that may be beneficial for pharmaceutical industries [95]. Nanochitosan can remove pollutants from the environment. For this purpose, ZnS/chitosan nano-photocatalysts with a size less than 4 nm were reported by Mansur *et al.* reported for decomposition by the light of some hazardous biological pollutants that were present in the used water [96]. In addition to this, another environment-friendly application that was done by Sahab *et al.* concluded the anti-fungal activity by prepared chitosan polyacrylic acid (PAA) NPs [97]. The compound exhibited antifungal activity for 3 species

(*Aspergillus terreus*, *Fusarium oxysporum*, and *F. Solani*) and also hindered the egg deposition of different insect classes as *Callosobruchus maculatus* and *Aphis gossypii* that were usually found to damage the soybean crops. Salah *et al.* used nanosized hydroxyapatite chitosan composite sorbents and reported the cadmium removal from wastewater [98]. For the removal of organic dyes magnetic graphene (chitosan) was found beneficial because the hydroxyl and amino groups together with Fe_3O_4 showed adsorption properties [99]. Bentonite chitosan nanocomposites were found helpful in removing synthetic dyes [100]. Recently, a TiO_2 composite and chitosan were proved beneficial for the elimination of biological contaminants from the used water [101], it also retains its photocatalytic activity after 10 cycles. Under UV radiations, nano ZnS quantum dots have similar applications.

6. BIOLOGICAL SYNTHESIS OF METAL NPS *VIA* PLANTS

Plants have the natural ability to accumulate and decrease the number of metal ions from their surroundings. Due to these characteristics, plants are assumed to be a great source for the synthesis of MNPs [28]. Plant extracts are assumed to have an essential role in reducing and stabilizing the metal ions that contain phenolic acids, sugars, proteins, polyphenols, terpenoids, and bioactive alkaloids. The difference between the active constituent's concentration and composition among different plants is the cause of varying size and shapes of the NPs and also forms the basis for the interaction of metal ions. The NPs are synthesized at room temperature initially by mixing the plant extract in the metal salt solution. After the mixing, the biological reduction of the metal salt occurs in the mixture which is indicated by the color change. In the process, firstly the activation period is present in which the mono and divalent metal ions are transformed to the zero-valent metal ion. After which a growth period is accompanied, the reduction of metal ions occurs by the neighboring atoms that join with the NPs to form larger NPs. As the growth process advances, the NPs build up to form different types of structures such as pentagons, hexagons, spheres, cubes, triangles, wires, and rods. In the last stage, the nanoparticle formed is stabilized and represented in its most suitable forms. The NPs synthesis by this method can vary in their size and shape as the plant extract properties such as pH, temperature, concentration, and reaction time play a significant role [102].

6.1. Angiosperms

Angiosperms are favorably oppressed for GS of MNPs. This group of plants is extremely common among the masses. They are an attractive source for scientific research due to their edible nature. These plants are advantageous for the GS of

NPs and the Asian countries are contributing a lot in this regard due to the extensive availability of these plant species. But all the plants of this species cannot be used for GS, and this is the basic drawback of this methodology. Because of this reason, the search for suitable plants is undergoing. The updating and tracing of all the angiosperms are not possible. An effort has been made to create a brief view of the demonstrative species of angiosperm plants. This is an indication that plants having high reducing potential phytochemicals can neutralize uni- or multivalent metallic cations into neutral atoms (Mo) for MNPs synthesis. The plants having lower ionization potentials lessen the metallic cations with larger and smaller standard reduction potentials. Maximum data was based on the GS of AU or AgNPs, and there is not enough data available on other MNPs.

It may be due to the disability of the plant molecules to reduce metal cations with lower reduction potentials. The GS of MNPs can be enhanced by using the plants that have the high electron-donating capability; for this purpose, the biological features and the edibility of plants are kept under check. The Arbitrary collection of plants may lead to the synthesis of NPs but it may not produce standardized NPs. *Azadirachta indica, Camellia sinensis, Aloe vera*, and *Centella Asiatica* are examples of plant species that have been discovered for their medicinal values and clinical relevancy. It has been confirmed from the cytotoxicity assay that the Capping behavior of the phytochemical molecules makes MNPs biocompatible, but the size and shape of MNPs serve as a hurdle in the biocompatibility determination. Therefore, to solve this issue, the particle size is suggested to be 100nm. In addition to the size and shape, the atom economy also serves as a challenge for the researchers. The temperature for the GS of MNPs has been tested from as low as 25°C to as high as 80-150°C because the time for the completion of a reaction is determined by the reaction kinetics, which is greatly influenced by the temperature.

GS methodologies that are based on temperature variations result in the change of shape and structure. The process of GS has been made profitable by the photosynthesis of Pd NPs with Asparagus racemosus by the use of sunlight [103]. This method of GS can be made common by using other species of angiosperms. In addition to their synthesis, the creation of nontoxic MNPs is also an indication that must be considered, and for this purpose, water has been the solvent of choice and is used on a large scale. The mechanism of NP synthesis is not much discovered in GS methodologies; therefore, some plant species like Camellia sinensis (tea) serve as a perfect example for the study of the mechanism of NP synthesis. Separation and purification of tea biomolecules like catechins, the aflavins, and the origins and their trialing with Au3 cations ensured they were involved in the GS of AuNPs [104, 105]. Likewise, tetra-nortriterpenoid azadirachtin separation and clearance have depicted the reducing and capping activity of *Azadirachta indica* for the green synthesis of Au and AgNPs [106]. The Pt NPs have been produced by the use of pure tea polyphenol (from Sigma). All this knowledge paves the way for the production of MNPs on a massive scale. The use of compounds whose pure formulations are commercially available is beneficial like quercetin-glucuronide and epicatechin for the production of MNPs (*e.g.,* Fe_2O_3). The plant *Jatropha curcas L* diminishes the metal cations through recurring peptide molecules, curcacycline B, and curcacycline A that is present in its sap. Essential clarification of peptide molecules provides a greater sense of the activity of these molecules. Researches on *in situ* syntheses (live plant) of MNPs are not much. An important example is the *in situ* synthesis of AgNPs by Alfa sprouts [107]. Furthermore, the researchers are looking for a general method for the production of MNPs *via* GS it has been found that phenols, alkaloids, terpenoids, and some pigments are involved in this method. Now, it's time to clarify the reduction potentials of all these constituents so that the metal ion reduction becomes convenient. Analysis techniques like energy-dispersive X-ray spectroscopy (EDAX) and Fourier transform infrared spectroscopy (FTIR) confirm the capping nature of the molecules of the plant throughout the GS of MNPs, although these tools are not very much trustworthy. The downstream processing of MNPs produced *via* GS may differ from the findings of FTIR and EDAX. In addition to this, cytotoxic analysis is also lacking in the GS techniques. The main purpose of the GS technique was to create MNPs that are non-toxic, and through various experiments, it has been confirmed that nature can fulfill this purpose. But the lack of cytotoxic study in the GS techniques crushes the true goal. The developments made in this field are remarkable and attractive to the researchers; however, certain parameters must be brought under consideration, like the plant collection methods, biocompatibility check of MNPs, and preferred features for clinical applications. Besides, proper guidelines for the manufacture of GS on a largescale must also be taken under consideration.

6.2. Gymnosperms

The gymnosperms are the first seed plants and are present everywhere on the Earth. Each plant species has unique and special features that make them distinguishable among others. These metabolites reduce metal ions to NPs. Biological reduction in prokaryotes has been studied for many years and recently, eukaryotes have also been found to reduce metal ions. Different plummeting and alleviating agents resulted in the formation and bioaccumulation of MNPs, and new research about eukaryotes provided information about their genetic code and their function. Sharma *et al.* and Curtis *et al.* presented that these compact and steadied MNPs in plant cells were used as a reagent in purifying pollutants [108,

109]. Plants need copper Cu as a micronutrient, and plants detoxify their higher concentration by reducing Cu ions to neutral atoms and then to Cu NPs. There isn't much material on the biosynthesis of MNPs using gymnosperms, maybe because these species have not been investigated much. Thus, the research about metallic nanoparticle synthesis using gymnosperms is yet to be done. It was supposed that the morphology of NPs depends on the plant type and its part, along with the pH and availability of materials. Research has been done on angiosperm species for nanoparticle synthesis along with metal reduction and stabilization techniques. Gymnosperms have common phytochemical families as compared to angiosperms so they may be useful for extrapolation of NPs formation mechanism. Jha and Prasad demonstrated that AgNPs are produced by the stimulation of the antioxidative system in the Cycas plant by the metallic stress (AgNO$_3$) [110]. Gymnosperm plants are unique to some of the organic groups like phenols, carbonyls, and thiols, where phenols are present in the Cycas plants' leaves. The comparison of Ag nanoparticle synthesis with the angiosperms shows that they are similar in phytochemicals and functional groups, but this affects the biochemical and physical characteristics of the resulting NPs. Noruzi *et al.* stated that the production of gold NPs is possible by reduction ability of cypress (Thuja orientalis) leaves, which was accomplished within 10 min with 90% progress [111]. The formed Au NPs were spherical, with sizes ranging from 5 to 94 nm. Their FTIR and X-ray showed that they are crystalline and bind capping molecules to the particle surface. Cu NPs of 15-20 nm were produced by the leaf extricate of Ginkgo biloba Linn by Nasrollahzadeh and Sajadi [112]. It was an environment-friendly synthesis since no toxic chemicals were used. The leaf extricates of Torreya Nucifera were used by Kalpana *et al.* for the production of AgNPs [113]. It was found that the morphology of NPs was exaggerated by the temperature and concentration of extract. The formed NPs were spherical and 10 to 125 nm in size. A parallel study, by Prabu and Johnson, detected the lessening capability of Cycas circinalis leaves extracts for Ag ions which caused the production of crystal-like AgNPs, which were spherical with 13-15 nm diameter [114]. In the pine family of gymnosperms, phenolic compounds were found. Velmurugan *et al.* proposed that carboxyl, hydroxyl, and phenolic groups were included in the production of MNPs in Pinus thunbergia [115, 116], although the bioprocess mechanism was not well understood in pine plants. Researches proved that the properties of NPs are controlled positively by higher concentrations of pH, temperature, and duration. Thus, the synthesis of NPs by gymnosperm plant species is a better way as compared to the traditional techniques.

6.3. Pteridophytes

The antibacterial activity of Pteridophytes has made them widely useful over the centuries. The extracts from these plants are collected and used as antibacterial agents. De Britto *et al.* used three dissimilar species of Pteridophyte plants of Petri's kind for the production of (Ag) NPs [117]. In the NPs produced, it was detected that AgNPs from the plant *Pteris Laurita* had shown the greatest antibacterial activity. Some plants of the Pteridophytes are also used in the production of metallic NPs. Along with these, some of the NPs that are derived from the ferns like *Nephrolepis exaltata* also show antiseptic action alongside many microbes. Certain pteridophytes such as *Adiantum philippense. L* has a structural similarity with the angiosperms, makes the extract of the plant oxidant and is involved in the synthesis of Ag and gold NPs [118]. The metallic NPs that are derived have shown enhanced antioxidant and antibacterial activity due to the plant's natural medicinal values. Many types of research have shown different results for the production of NPs. For example, Azolla pinnata whole plant was used for the production of sphere-shaped AgNPs; similarly, the aqueous extract of Azolla pinnata was used as a stabilizer and reducer for the production of rod-shaped NPs [119] Likewise, the pigments existing in Azolla microphylla assisted as a plummeting and stabilizing agent for the synthesis of gold NPs [120].

6.4. Bryophytes

Being second in the largest group of land plants, which are ancient terrestrial plants that do not have a vascular system and have an important part in the discovery of the land plant's evolution. These plants, just like pteridophytes, produce active compounds to protect themselves. These plants produce phytochemicals that help to produce many active compounds that are helpful in many ways. Along with that, the bryophytes also help in the production of MNPs [121 - 124]. Sarkar and Acharya synthesized AuNPs by using the extract of *Taxithelium Nepalese* gametophyte and these NPs were observed to be triangular, hexagonal, and sphere shapes varying in size ranges [125].

6.5. Algae

There are three basic requirements for the production of green MNPs, a suitable solvent, a reducing and agent, and a capping agent. One of them is Algae-mediated biological synthesis. Algae are eukaryotic autotrophs and are used for the production of MNPs like Ag, platinum, gold, zinc oxide, and palladium. The bioreduction of algae causes the production of these MNPs [28, 48, 50, 121, 126, 127]. Several different algae can synthesize different NPs. There is not much understanding of the involved principles and size and shape control. Thus, many researchers have shown keen interest in the production of NPs interceded from algae. Algae have the ability the production of complex inorganic structures but the thorough process of synthesis of Au NPs is still not known. The static attraction between the ions and the carboxylate ions on the surface of the cell is the factor that traps the metal ion. Subsequently, the nuclei are formed due to the reduction of enzymes by cellular enzymes and the nuclei grow with the reduction of metal ions. *Sesbania drummondii*, accepts a high amount of Au (III) ions which are converted to Au (0) ions through reduction [108]. For the algae like *Spirulina subsalsa* and *Lyngbya majuscula*, the gold NPs are present either inside or outside the medium at the same time [128]. Amongst the metallic NPs, Au and AgNPs are of supreme importance. The attachment of the single-cell green algae is strong with tetrachloroaurate ions and Ag nitrate. This allows the formation of bound Ag or gold algal which is then reduced to null forms of Au and Ag [129]. 88% of metallic gold is reduced by *Chlorella Vulgaris*, dried algae, and then it was amassed in cell parts with a variety of different structures [130]. Various species of dried algae like *Spirulina Platensis* have been used in the synthesis of bimetallic nano particles [131]. Lately, an algae *Tetraselmis kochinensis* was used for the intracellular production of gold NPs [132]. Similarly, *Fucus vesiculosus,* a brown alga, was reported for the reduction of Au3 to Au0. The synthesis of MNPs is also associate with cyanobacteria [133]. A study showed that the protein present inside the cell of algae named *Oscillatoria willei,* aided in the reduction of Ag ions and the formation of metallic Ag, which was further secreted out of the dead cell [134]. Many functional groups, including the amine and hydroxyl groups, were reported robust for reducing Ag ions and the production of AgNPs. Hypnea musciformis algae extricate used for reducing and stabilizing the NPs that were produced by single-step synthesis [135]. The resulted NPs were mostly spherical. Other NPs, including CdS, MgO, microorganisms, PbS, and ZnS, seem to be found from algae. Algae collect heavy metals and are used in NP synthesis. *C. Vulgaris* has been used for the production of tetra-chloroaurate ions, as mentioned above [126, 130]. Similarly, it was also found that Ag nanometer-scale plates were also produced by *C. Vulgaris* at room temperature [136, 137]. Recent studies showed that the proteins obtained from the extracts have shown reducing and stabilizing properties for the NPs, and they also act as shape-controlling modifiers. Recently, Singaravelu *et al.* proposed that Au NPs can be produced by *S. wightii* [138]. Rajasulochana *et al.* proposed that Au NPs can be produced from *Kappaphycus alvarezii* [139], and Mata *et al.* explained that Fucus vesiculosus brown algae, its biomass can be used for the bioreduction of Au NPs [133]. In addition to this, intracellular synthesis of gold NPs was presented by Senapati *et al.* using *Tetraselmis kochinensis* [132].

7. MAJOR NPS SYNTHESIZED FROM PLANT EXTRACTS

7.1. Au and AgNPs

AuNPs have unique properties concerning their morphology and particle size. They have been examined for their applications in various fields like bio sensing and hyperthermia therapy, which provide a way for the development of antibacterial drugs. The employment of plants as the biological factories for the free production of AuNPs. For instance, Das *et al.* used Nyctanthes arborists (night jasmine) flower extract and produced gold NPs circular in shape [140]. Also, Narayanan and Sakthivel used *Coriandrum sativum* (coriander) leaf extricate for the synthesis of Au NPs in a large amount of 7 to 58nm [141]. The formed NPs varied had distinct shapes. A study by Armendarizet *et al.* proposed that Avenasativa produced gold NPs in the range of 5 to 85nm based on pH [142]. A careful look demonstrated that various shapes could be produced based on pH. In the recent research by Poinern *et al.*, it was proposed that AuNPs can be produced from *Eucalyptus macrocarpa* [143]. A general distillation apparatus for the synthesis of NPs through plant extracts is shown in Fig. (**2**). As a result of this deeper look, it was found that the main focus particles were those ranging from 20 to 80nm; furthermore, alongside the spheres, several other shapes were found and every shape ranged from 50 to 100nm, as mentioned in personage 2. From the historical point of view, Ag showed antimicrobial properties and was widely used and since then, the synthesis of AgNPs has always been the primary goal. The synthesis was Ag NPs by plants was then brought forward. For instance, Edison and Sethuraman produced AgNPs from the fruit of Terminalia chebula (Harad) [144]. Similarly, Poinern *et al.* used *Eucalyptus macrocarpa* to form cube-shaped AgNPs ranging from 50 to 200nm [145]. Geetha *et al.* also proposed the antibacterial properties of AgNPs using Cymbopogancitratus (lemongrass) sheet extract [146]. Those Ag NPs that were cube-shaped or rectangular structures were effective against many bacterias such as *Escherichia coli* and *Klebsiellapneumonia*. Many reports by authors suggested that the alloy of gold and Ag NPs for the production of bi-metallic NPs should be more focused than plants. The production of the bimetallic NPs can be done by competitive fall using an aqueous solution containing the ions that are held with the extracts. As a result, a core shell-like structure will be formed due to the more cutting-edge ability of Au. After this, the falling of Ag particles increases the size of the shell structure. Some ancient plants that were used for the production of Au & Ag bimetallic NPs include cruciferous vegetable extracts, *Azadirachta indica* (neem) extracts, and *Anacardium occidentale* (cashew nut) extracts.

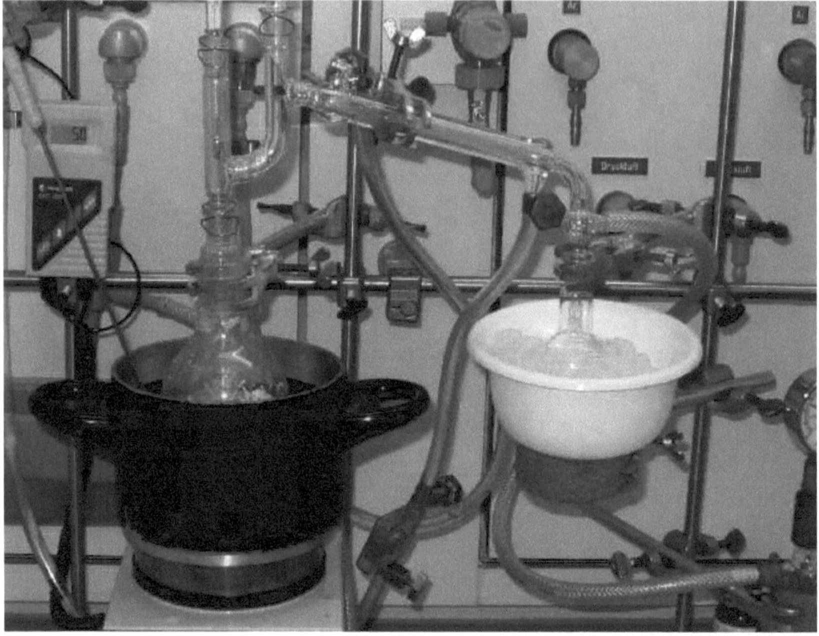

Fig. (2). Synthesis of plant derived metallic NPs through plant extracts in a distillation apparatus.

7.2. Copper and Copper Oxide NPs

NPs synthesized by different forms of plant extracts also include copper and copper oxide NPs. *Magnolia kobus* extract, which is produced physically, is used to produce even NPs of Cu in abundance ranging from 40 to 100 nm [147]. The Cu NPs were observed to show antibacterial resistance against some bacteria's such as *Escherichia coli*. Cu NPs produced by *Syzygium aromaticum* (Clove) extract had a particle size of about 40nm [148]. Similarly, *Euphoria nivulia* (common milk hedge) stem latex can also be used for the synthesis of Cu NPs [149]. The latex contains terpenoids and peptides that help in the stabilization of NPs and may be lethal to the adenocarcinomas present on the basal surface of alveolar epithelial cells (A549 cells). In addition to this, *Sterculia urens* (Karaya gum was used to make round Cuprous Oxide NPs having a center magnitude of 4.8nm of the particles [150]. Antimicrobial properties along with antioxidant and antibacterial activities of these NPs were also observed.

7.3. Palladium and Platinum NPs

C. zeylanicum bark extricate was utilized for the production of Pd NPs by Satishkumar *et al.* in 2009 [151].]. Modifying the bark pull-out focus, result from pH, and fever during combination was made for non-influencing the molecule mass (15 to 20 nm) and shape and structure. Pd NPs ranging from 75 to 85 nm arrange moreover been synthesized using *Annona squamosa* (Custard apple) rind wheedle out, whereas the folio extorts of soybean (Glycine max) state been bright to produce NPs with a shameful mass of 15 nm [152]. Also still, normal business-related foodstuffs like *Camellia sinensis* (tea) extracts and *Coffea arabica* (Coffee) are being used for the production of palladium NPs with a face-centered cubic arrangement [153]. Furthermore, Moreover, palladium NPs could not be synthesized from *Gardenia jasminoides* (Cape jasmine) antioxidants such as crocetin, chlorogenic acid, Geniposide, and crocins served as plummeting and stabilizing agents [154]. The production of platinum NPs was reported for the first time by Song *et al.* in 2010 by a folio wheedle out full from *Diospyros kaki* (Persimmon) [155]. Significant NPs were 2 to 12 nm in size and presented that 90% of the Pt ions were transformed through a 10% quantity of leaf biomass at 95°C. A leaf extricates taken from Ocimum sanctum (Holy basil) also had a size of 23 nm from aqueous chloroplatinic acid at a hotness of 100 ″C [156]. Likewise, the biologic production of Pt NPs with particle magnitude and form check has as well been reported *via* place timber nanometer climb equipment. For example, Coccia *et al.* proposed the production of Pd and Pt NPs by lignin from burgundy pout *(Pinus resinosa)* [157].

7.4. Titanium Dioxide and Zinc Oxide NPs

ZnO and TiO$_2$ NPs have been synthesized by using various plant species like Roopan *et al.*, proposed that TiO$_2$ particles can be produced by Annona squamosa [158], on the other hand, round NPs of about 100 to 150 nm have been produced by leaf extricates of *Nyctanthes arbor-tristis* [159] and *Eclipta prostrata* are considered to produce particles of about 36 to 68 nm in size [160]. Velayutham *et al.* produced amorphous TiO$_2$ particles of about 25 to 110 nm size, and [161] and it was discovered that they are adulticidal and parricidal against *Bovicola Ovis* (sheep louse) and *Hippobosca maculate* (hematophagous fly). TiO$_2$ particles produced from *Psidium guajava* were examined for antibacterial and antioxidant properties against different microbes and pathogens [162]. The resulting NPs were excellent against *Escherichia coli* and *Staphylococcus aureus* and also, these properties were lethal for many bacterial strains. ZnO NPs are an important component of the cosmetic and biomedical industry. The *Calotropis procera* extract has been used to produce round ZnO NPs [163] Although, steady and sphere-shaped Nps have already been produced by using extract of *Aloe vera* [164]. Furthermore, crystalline ZnO NPs have been produced by *Physalis alkekengi* extract of 72.5nm size, and NPs produced from Sedum alfredii were almost sphere-shaped with a size of 53.7nm [165]. The latest research by Vimala *et al.* proposed that ZnO NPs produced as a result of GS can serve as a base of drug delivery system for doxorubicin, which demonstrates the significance of GS methodologies for the production of NPs [166].

7.5. Indium Oxide, Iron Oxide, Lead, and Selenium NPs

Metal oxide and metal NPs have been produced *via* plant extracts. For instance, indium oxide NPs have been produced from *Aloe vera* leaf extract. After initial treatment, the particles were heated at 400 to 600 °C and as a result, the resulted particles ranged from 5 to 50 nm. FeNPs are extremely important,which is why all the focus has been shifted towards the GS of FeNPs. For instance, Fe NPs were biologically produced *via* sorghum bran extracts [168]. Lately, Pattanayak *et al.* produced sphere-shaped Fe NPs from *Azadirachta indica* (Neem) leaf extracts which were almost 100nm in size [169]. Also, Shah *et al.* synthesized Fe NPs from *Tridax procumbens, Euphorbia milii*, Datura innoxia, Tinospora cordifolia, Calotropisprocera, and *Cymbopogoncitratus* (lemongrass tea) [170]. The slightest sphere-shaped NPs were produced from *Euphorbia milii* of almost 13 to 21 nm and the largest NPs were produced from *Cymbopogon citratus* of almost 43 to 342 nm. Some other NPs produced *via* biological methods include selenium (Se) and lead (Pb). For the production of sphere-shaped Pb NPs, Joglekar *et al.* used latex from Jatropha curcas, which resulted in the particle size of 10 to 12.5nm [171]. Lately, sphere-shaped Se NPs were produced *via* the extracts of Citrus reticulate, which produced a particle size of almost 70 nm [172].

8. FACTORS AFFECTING BIOLOGICAL SYNTHESIS OF METAL NPS

The biotic production of MNPs involves many factors like temperature, reaction time, concentration, and pH. These factors have discoursed in the upcoming lines.

8.1. Influence of pH

In the production of NPs, pH plays a primary role [27, 50]. Change in the pH can cause a change in the morphology of the NPs, and the magnitude of NP was found to be greater at high pH as compared to the low pH [2, 27, 28]. For instance, Au NPs were larger at the pH of 2 and were smaller at pH 3 and 4 [142]. It has been revealed that more accessible, functional groups were available between the pH of 3 and 4. Likewise, at pH 2 few functional groups were existing and lead to the formation of rod-shaped Au NPs. Cinnamon zeylancium bark extricate used to manufacture AgNPs. It was found that with the rise in the quantity of bark and raising the pH value, the resulting particles also increased and at the higher pH value, the particles became spherical [173]. Cinnamon bark also increased the Palladium NPs size when pH was greater than 5 and *vice versa* [151].

8.2. Influence of Reactant Concentration

The synthesis of NPs is altered by the quantities of biological molecules found in plant extracts. A study by Huang *et al.* found that the morphology of the synthesized Au and AgNPs can be affected by changing the concentrations of leaf extricates of *Cinnamomum camphora* (camphor) in the resulting solution [174]. For instance, the morphology of the resulting NPs changed by introducing chloroauric acid in the plant extract, which resulted in increased concentration. Using this observation, Chandran *et al.* changed the shape of AuNPs [175]. Ti was also found that particle shape was also affected by carbonyl compounds and the concentration change produced the particle size variation between 50 and 350 nm. Also, the change in concentration of leaf extract of *Plectranthus amboinicus* resulted in the production of different shaped NPs [176].

8.3. Influence of Reaction Time

The latest research of Ahmad *et al.* demonstrated that the production of AgNPs by extricating of *Ananas comosus* (Pineapple) is an essential requirement as like here the color change occurred in just 2 mins [177, 178]. Aqueous $Ag(NO)_3$ within the reply standard was speedily low-price and NPs became visible in 2 min. The result remained continuous utes, but thenfor five minutes, barely a fragile deviation in color is often detected. The NPs created were round and had a proposed extent of 12 nm. Likewise, research by Gopal and Dwivedi suggested that the Ag and AuNPs produced from the album leaf extract became visible after 15 mins, although the process continued for 2 hours [179]. Furthermore, Prathna *et al.* proposed that the interaction of $AgNO_3$ and leaf extract of *Azadirachta indica* produced enlarged NPs which were 10 to 35nm, after the increase in concentration [180].

8.4. Influence of Reaction Temperature

Temperature is an essential requirement when it comes to the determination of particle morphology and structure [181, 182]. For instance, a change in the size of AgNPs was observed when Citrus sinensis, also known as sweet orange peel extract, having a size of 35nm, was used at 25°C, but its size decreased with the temperature was raised to 60°C [183]. Similarly, Song *et al.* produced AgNPs at 25 to 95°C using leaf extract of *Diospyros kaki* (persimmon) [181]. Another research by Armendariz *et al.* showed that the gold NPs morphology was affected by the changes in the temperature of *Avena sativa* (oat) biomass [142]. In addition to this, Gericke and Pinches proposed the production of gold NPs increased with the increase in temperature and decreased when the temperature was decreased, which suggested that temperature was directly related to the number of NPs produced [58].

9. OPPORTUNITIES AND OBSTACLES RELATED TO BIOLOGICAL SYNTHESIS OF MNP'S

9.1. Biological Methods in Variance with Chemical Methods for Synthesis of NPs

The long-established methods for the production of NPs were based on the evaporation phenomenon, milling techniques, vapourization processes, and lithographic techniques. The chemical process that was present was based on the chemical reactions that occurred in the solutions, electrolysis processes, sol-gel conversions, radiation effects, and shift transmutations. Previous researches on the physicochemical techniques showed that the change in the conditions required for the reaction affected the morphology, structure, and stability of NPs. Therefore, the synthesis of NPs by chemical and physical methods is maintained according to the particle morphology and stability [27, 29, 36, 49]. The main biotic methods are the production of NPs from plant extracts and microbial agents. The production of MNPs is the result of enzymatic activity that occurs both within and outside of the cell by which the metal ions are converted to their elements [48]. The methods of production of NPs have been discussed already, although the chemical methods are in great use but are strictly prohibited in clinical settings because of the involvement of toxic compounds. There is another flaw with the use of chemical methods as they are not economical and are energy-yielding; furthermore, they have negative effects on the environment. The purpose of GS is to generate environment-friendly methods for the production of MNPs; therefore, the clinical methods are not very much preferred. The NPs produced from plants, and natural sources are safe as compared to those synthesized from chemicals and therefore are applied in clinical and biomedical settings. The production of stabilized NPs can be enhanced by considering factors like organism type, growth of the cell, catalysts and reaction conditions. The secretion of enzymes by the microbial organisms and the proteins serve as important factors for the production of MNPs. Furthermore, the NPs produced from chemical methods are poly dispersed in comparison to the biologically produced NPs. The morphology of the NPs controls the crucial catalytic, optical, magnetic and electronic properties of that particle. However, a major drawback related to the manufacture of NPs by biological methods is that the microbes require specific conditions to flourish, which may be the point of concern for later researches.

9.2. Toxicity Issue Related to Biological Synthesis of NP's

The harmful effects of chemical synthesis are minimized in biological synthesis. The NPs produced by biological methods have a variety of applications like tumor destruction, targeted delivery of drugs, MRI scan (magnetic resonance imaging), and gene therapies. This wide range of applications is impossible to achieve by chemical methods because of the toxic solvents, the biological methods are safe from these types of solvents. However, in certain cases, the use of toxic chemicals becomes a necessity; therefore, the use of environment-friendly solvents like water must be preferred.

9.3. Environmental Issues

Environmental problems are closely related to the synthesis of NPs. Over the recent years, the synthesis of NPs has increased due to the spread of industries, resulting in anthropogenic NPs. Many organisms are affected by these as their vital organs are always in close contact with their living habitat. For instance, in humans, the skin, lungs, and GI tract are in constant contact with the environment. As the NPs are very small in size, they can easily penetrate the respiratory and lymphatic systems and ultimately damage the body organs. In some cases the damage becomes irreversible. Varying reasons of NPs based on their size, surface area, structure, shape, concentration, and other features like their screen proportion, function, and chemistry of the particles can be the reason for the produced toxicity in the metallic NPs [184]. But along with that, it should be understood that all NPs are not toxic, some of them don't exhibit any toxic effect at all and some do have beneficial health effects. In addition to this, along with the study of the physical behavior of NPs, their toxicology must also be monitored along with particle aging so that this information can be used in future processes and the betterment of the NP production processes.

10. FUTURE PERSPECTIVE(S)

The production of NPs *via* biological methods is a new scheme and is also facing initial starting issues related to the morphology, stability, and growth of crystals for the produced NPs. [214]. These problems are mostly related to the production of NPs, but more attention is diverted towards the synthesis of NPs by biological techniques as they are assumed to be more sustainable, safe, and environmentally friendly. Some important points in this regard are as follows:

1. The mechanism of the produced NPs is not very much understood; therefore, this point must be given attention in the future. The NP properties must be considered keenly along with other chemical properties.
2. Another unmapped point is the downstream process of MNPs. It involves the separation of NPs from impure substances. It must be kept under consideration that the NPs must remain nontoxic to investigate physical processes like ultrasound, centrifugation, *etc.*
3. Until now, this process is limited to labs; for mass production, this process must be taken to the industrial level where stabilized and nontoxic MNPs could be produced.
4. The process must also be economical and less costly; therefore, the analysis must be performed with the chemical methods. It has already been mentioned that this process has yet to be transferred to the industrial scale. For instance, different solvents are used for chemical methods while salts and microbes will play that part in the biological methods. It can serve as a valuable approach to recycling the products.
5. In the future, the fast production of NPs must be a target, and some research is already on the way.
6. Current research has proved that the GS can serve as a profitable way to produce NPs, which will serve as a direction towards the enhancement of green synthesis.

11. BIOLOGICALLY IMPORTANT NPS APPLICATIONS

Green nanotechnology is an emerging and continuously growing branch of science. It is expected that operational and working NPs will be a necessity of this field. As the applications of NPs are unceasing so they are being applied in various medical techniques. The biologically produced NPs are a part of a few applications like Ag NPs antimicrobial activities and are being used in medical and other products. AgNPs are also effective against plant pathogens, cancer cells, and plasmodial pathogens [185]. Au has successfully gained interest and is now being used in the treatment of tumors [186]. Au NPs have also been used in the targeted drug delivery of anticancerous drugs with eliminating the side effects caused by it. AuNPs are also active against various bacterial strains. AuNPs can also be used for the targeted delivery of anticancer drugs by reducing the hurdles and side effects. AuNPs are also active against various bacterial strains. The antimicrobial properties of Cu and CuO NPs can be used for the coating of hospital equipment. For several applications like water electrolysis and decomposition, Pt NPs have been used. The TiO_2 NPs are being used in wastewater treatment and process like sterilization and antibacterial coatings. While ZnO NPs are being used in the foodstuff packaging and sewage treatment works. Furthermore, template-supported the manufacture of complex structures using biological entities occurs at both micro and nano metric levels. Microbes such as bacteria are favored for the creation of one dimensional structure. For instance, Ag, gold, and platinum NPs have been assembled by TMV, and silica fibers have been produced *via* filamentous bacteriophages. For the creation of 1D assemblies, the nanometer scales are very efficient, while sericin has been used for the production of nano-fibrous particles 3D arrays produced from iron oxide NPs support the growth of stem cells. Thus, MNPs are involved in the production of beneficial products. NPs synthesized *via* biological methods are ecofriendly and are involved in various applications. The synthesis of NPs depends upon the morphology and stability and these factors are affected by changes in the pH, reactant concentration, and temperature. This variation can result in different results of the same experiment by the laboratories. Although the plant extracts are being used for the production of stabilized NPs following all the limitations the chances of a major failure are still there. For instance, Shankar *et al.*, reduced a large amount of AgNPs using *Cymbopogon flexuosus* (Lemongrass) extract. Many NPs reduced from aqueous chloroaurate were composed of gold nano triangles similar to the Ag nano triangles. Also, continuous centrifugation leads to the improvement of the nano triangles. It is quite interesting that despite all the advancements in physical and chemical methodologies, certain physical methods still require improvements. The chemical methods applied for the synthesis of NPs from toxic chemicals are of significant importance as they are much safer and environmentally friendly.

CONCLUSION

Due to advancements in science and technology, NPs, especially metallic NPs are becoming the field of interest. The use of metallic NPs in the pharmaceutical, medicinal, agricultural, and electronic industries is helping in various new developments due to their vast range of applications. The article has explained how metallic NPs can be synthesized by various biological practices. The synthesis of NPs using biological methods results in the creation of stable and non-toxic products. This method of green synthesis is completely different from physical and chemical methods that were used in the past. The production of NPs *via* biological methods provides a way of creating particles that do not require any special conditions. This method is economical and environmentally friendly. The NPs have also shown their worth in medical procedures such as the targeted drug delivery, cancer cell destruction, detection of antigen, and antibodies by fluorescent labeling methods. Also, the NPs produced *via* biological methods are being used in agricultural methods. Furthermore, the residue of agricultural plants and crops serves as a fuel for the biological production of MNPs. Although the process of GS is economical and beneficial, it also has some failures like morphology, stability, and consistency issues. When it comes to the NPs production *via* plants the methods are different therefore, their mechanisms must be studied keenly to get maximum benefits from the process of GS.

CONSENT FOR PUBLICATION

Not applicable.

CONFLICT OF INTEREST

The author declares no conflict of interest, financial or otherwise.

ACKNOWLEDGEMENTS

This work was supported by the National Research Foundation of Korea (NRF) funded by the Korean Government (MEST) (2020R1I1A3069699).

REFERENCES

[1]   Hasan S. A review on nanoparticles: their synthesis and types. Res J Recent Sci 2015; 2277: 2502.

[2]   Priyadarsini S, Mukherjee S, Mishra M. Nanoparticles used in dentistry: A review. J Oral Biol Craniofac Res 2018; 8(1): 58-67.
[http://dx.doi.org/10.1016/j.jobcr.2017.12.004] [PMID: 29556466]

[3]   Ramos AP, Cruz MAE, Tovani CB, Ciancaglini P. Biomedical applications of nanotechnology. Biophys Rev 2017; 9(2): 79-89.
[http://dx.doi.org/10.1007/s12551-016-0246-2] [PMID: 28510082]

[4]   Leon L, Chung EJ, Rinaldi C. 2020.

[5]   He X, Hwang H-M. Nanotechnology in food science: Functionality, applicability, and safety assessment. J Food Drug Anal 2016; 24(4): 671-81.
[http://dx.doi.org/10.1016/j.jfda.2016.06.001] [PMID: 28911604]

[6]   Kumar P, Mahajan P, Kaur R, Gautam S. Nanotechnology and its challenges in the food sector: a review. Mater Today Chem 2020; 17100332
[http://dx.doi.org/10.1016/j.mtchem.2020.100332] [PMID: 32835156]

[7]   Krishna VD, Wu K, Su D, Cheeran MCJ, Wang J-P, Perez A. Nanotechnology: Review of concepts and potential application of sensing platforms in food safety. Food Microbiol 2018; 75: 47-54.
[http://dx.doi.org/10.1016/j.fm.2018.01.025] [PMID: 30056962]

[8]   Burduşel A-C, Gherasim O, Grumezescu AM, Mogoantă L, Ficai A, Andronescu E. Biomedical applications of silver nanoparticles: An up-to-date overview. Nanomaterials (Basel) 2018; 8(9): 681.
[http://dx.doi.org/10.3390/nano8090681] [PMID: 30200373]

[9]   Shanmuganathan R, Karuppusamy I, Saravanan M, *et al.* Synthesis of Silver nanoparticles and their biomedical applications-A comprehensive review. Curr Pharm Des 2019; 25(24): 2650-60.
[http://dx.doi.org/10.2174/1381612825666190708185506] [PMID: 31298154]

[10]   Elahi N, Kamali M, Baghersad MH. Recent biomedical applications of gold nanoparticles: A review. Talanta 2018; 184: 537-56.

[http://dx.doi.org/10.1016/j.talanta.2018.02.088] [PMID: 29674080]

[11]   Jeong H-H, Choi E, Ellis E, Lee T-C. Recent advances in gold nanoparticles for biomedical applications: from hybrid structures to multi-functionality. J Mater Chem B Mater Biol Med 2019; 7(22): 3480-96.
[http://dx.doi.org/10.1039/C9TB00557A]

[12]   Yaqoob SB, Adnan R, Rameez Khan RM, Rashid M. Gold, silver, and palladium nanoparticles: a chemical tool for biomedical applications. Front Chem 2020; 8: 376.
[http://dx.doi.org/10.3389/fchem.2020.00376] [PMID: 32582621]

[13]   Phan TTV, Huynh T-C, Manivasagan P, Mondal S, Oh J. An up-to-date review on biomedical applications of palladium nanoparticles. Nanomaterials (Basel) 2019; 10(1): 66.
[http://dx.doi.org/10.3390/nano10010066] [PMID: 31892149]

[14]   Nagarajan R, Hatton TA. Nanoparticles: synthesis, stabilization, passivation, and functionalization. ACS Publications 2008.
[http://dx.doi.org/10.1021/bk-2008-0996]

[15]   Rao BG, Mukherjee D, Reddy BM. Novel approaches for preparation of nanoparticles.Nanostructures for novel therapy. Elsevier 2017; pp. 1-36.
[http://dx.doi.org/10.1016/B978-0-323-46142-9.00001-3]

[16]   Razavi M, Salahinejad E, Fahmy M, Yazdimamaghani M, Vashaee D, Tayebi L. Green chemical and biological synthesis of nanoparticles and their biomedical applications. Green Process Nanotechnol 2015; pp. 207-35.
[http://dx.doi.org/10.1007/978-3-319-15461-9_7]

[17]   Singh P, Kim Y-J, Zhang D, Yang D-C. Biological synthesis of nanoparticles from plants and microorganisms. Trends Biotechnol 2016; 34(7): 588-99.
[http://dx.doi.org/10.1016/j.tibtech.2016.02.006] [PMID: 26944794]

[18]   Singh AV, Mehta KK. K Mehta K. Top-down versus bottom-up nanoengineering routes to design advanced oropharmacological products. Curr Pharm Des 2016; 22(11): 1534-45.
[http://dx.doi.org/10.2174/1381612822666151210124001] [PMID: 26675228]

[19]   Gregorczyk K, Knez M. Hybrid nanomaterials through molecular and atomic layer deposition: Top down, bottom up, and in-between approaches to new materials. Prog Mater Sci 2016; 75: 1-37.
[http://dx.doi.org/10.1016/j.pmatsci.2015.06.004]

[20]   Kumar S, Bhushan P, Bhattacharya S. Fabrication of Nanostructures with Bottom-up Approach and Their Utility in Diagnostics, Therapeutics, and Others BT - Environmental, Chemical and Medical Sensors.Singapore: Springer Singapore 2018; pp. 167-98.

[21]   Iqbal P, Preece JA, Mendes PM. Nanotechnology: The "Top-Down" and "Bottom-Up" Approaches. Supramolecular Chemistry 2012.

[22]   Titus D, James Jebaseelan Samuel E, Roopan SM. Nanoparticle characterization techniques. In: Shukla AK, Iravani Characterization and Applications of Nanoparticles SBT-GS, editors. Micro and Nano Technologies Elsevier;. 2019; pp. 303-19.

[23]   Mourdikoudis S, Pallares RM, Thanh NTK. Characterization techniques for nanoparticles: comparison and complementarity upon studying nanoparticle properties. Nanoscale 2018; 10(27): 12871-934.
[http://dx.doi.org/10.1039/C8NR02278J] [PMID: 29926865]

[24]   Srivastava R. Synthesis and characterization techniques of nanomaterials. Int J Green Nanotechnol 2012; 4(1): 17-27.
[http://dx.doi.org/10.1080/19430892.2012.654738]

[25]   Mahmood S, Mandal UK, Chatterjee B, Taher M. Advanced characterizations of nanoparticles for drug delivery: investigating their properties through the techniques used in their evaluations. Nanotechnol Rev 2017; 6(4): 355-72.
[http://dx.doi.org/10.1515/ntrev-2016-0050]

[26]   Carvalho PM, Felício MR, Santos NC, Gonçalves S, Domingues MM. Application of light scattering techniques to nanoparticle characterization and development. Front Chem 2018; 6: 237.
[http://dx.doi.org/10.3389/fchem.2018.00237] [PMID: 29988578]

[27]   Li X, Xu H, Chen Z-S, Chen G. Biosynthesis of Nanoparticles by Microorganisms and Their Applications. 2011.
[http://dx.doi.org/10.1155/2011/270974]

[28]   Das RK, Pachapur VL, Lonappan L, Naghdi M, Pulicharla R, Maiti S, *et al.* Biological synthesis of metallic nanoparticles: plants, animals and microbial aspects. Nanotechnol Environ Eng 2017; 2(1): 18.
[http://dx.doi.org/10.1007/s41204-017-0029-4]

[29]   Khan I, Saeed K, Khan I. Nanoparticles: Properties, applications and toxicities. Arab J Chem 2019; 12(7): 908-31.
[http://dx.doi.org/10.1016/j.arabjc.2017.05.011]

[30]   Rasool U, Hemalatha S. Marine endophytic actinomycetes assisted synthesis of copper nanoparticles (CuNPs): Characterization and antibacterial efficacy against human pathogens. Mater Lett 2017; 194: 176-80.
[http://dx.doi.org/10.1016/j.matlet.2017.02.055]

[31]   Hassan SE-D, Salem SS, Fouda A, Awad MA, El-Gamal MS, Abdo AM. New approach for antimicrobial activity and bio-control of various pathogens by biosynthesized copper nanoparticles using endophytic actinomycetes. J Radiat Res Appl Sci 2018; 11(3): 262-70.
[http://dx.doi.org/10.1016/j.jrras.2018.05.003]

[32]   Manimaran M, Kannabiran K. Actinomycetes-mediated biogenic synthesis of metal and metal oxide nanoparticles: progress and challenges. Lett Appl Microbiol 2017; 64(6): 401-8.
[http://dx.doi.org/10.1111/lam.12730] [PMID: 28267874]

[33]   Ahmad A, Senapati S, Khan M, Kumar R, Ramani R, Srinivas V, *et al.* Intracellular synthesis of gold nanoparticles by a novel alkotolerant actinomycetes, Rhodococcus species. Nanotechnology 2003; 14: 824.
[http://dx.doi.org/10.1088/0957-4484/14/7/323]

[34]   Karthik L, Kumar G, Kirthi AV, Rahuman AA, Bhaskara Rao KV. Streptomyces sp. LK3 mediated synthesis of silver nanoparticles and its biomedical application. Bioprocess Biosyst Eng 2014; 37(2): 261-7.
[http://dx.doi.org/10.1007/s00449-013-0994-3] [PMID: 23771163]

[35]   Chandrangsu P, Rensing C, Helmann JD. Metal homeostasis and resistance in bacteria. Nat Rev Microbiol 2017; 15(6): 338-50.
[http://dx.doi.org/10.1038/nrmicro.2017.15]

[36]   Iravani S. Bacteria in Nanoparticle Synthesis: Current Status and Future Prospects. Labrenz M, editor Int Sch Res Not. 2014.

[37]   Klaus T, Joerger R, Olsson E, Granqvist C-G. Silver-based crystalline nanoparticles, microbially fabricated. Proc Natl Acad Sci USA 1999; 96(24): 13611-4.
[http://dx.doi.org/10.1073/pnas.96.24.13611] [PMID: 10570120]

[38]   Husseiny MI, El-Aziz MA, Badr Y, Mahmoud MA. Biosynthesis of gold nanoparticles using Pseudomonas aeruginosa. Spectrochim Acta A Mol Biomol Spectrosc 2007; 67(3-4): 1003-6.
[http://dx.doi.org/10.1016/j.saa.2006.09.028] [PMID: 17084659]

[39]   Wen L, Lin Z, Gu P, Zhou J, Yao B, Chen G, *et al.* Extracellular biosynthesis of monodispersed gold nanoparticles by a SAM capping route. J Nanopart Res 2009; 11(2): 279-88.
[http://dx.doi.org/10.1007/s11051-008-9378-z]

[40]   Sneha K. M. S, Mao J, Kwak I, Yun Y-S. Corynebacterium glutamicum-mediated crystallization of silver ions through sorption and reduction processes. Chem Eng J 2010; 162: 989-96.

[http://dx.doi.org/10.1016/j.cej.2010.07.006]

[41] Fu JK, Liu YY, Gu PY, Tang D, Lin ZY, Yao BX, *et al.* Spectroscopic Charcterization on the Biosorption and Bioreduction of Ag(I) by Lactobacillus sp.A09*. Wuli Huaxue Xuebao 2000; 16: 781-2.

[42] He S, Zhang Y, Guo Z, Gu N. Biological synthesis of gold nanowires using extract of Rhodopseudomonas capsulata. Biotechnol Prog 2008; 24(2): 476-80.
[http://dx.doi.org/10.1021/bp0703174] [PMID: 18293997]

[43] Boroumand Moghaddam A, Namvar F, Moniri M. Md. Tahir P, Azizi S, Mohamad R. Nanoparticles Biosynthesized by Fungi and Yeast: A Review of Their Preparation, Properties, and Medical Applications. Vol. 20. Molecules 2015.
[http://dx.doi.org/10.3390/molecules200916540]

[44] Ahmad A, Senapati S, Khan M, Kumar R, Sastry M. Extra-/Intracellular biosynthesis of gold nanoparticles by an alkalotolerant fungus, *trichothecium* sp. J Biomed Nanotechnol 2005; 1: 47-53.
[http://dx.doi.org/10.1166/jbn.2005.012]

[45] Bansal V, Rautaray D, Bharde A, Ahire K, Sanyal A, Ahmad A, *et al.* Fungus-mediated biosynthesis of silica and titania particles. J Mater Chem 2005; 15(26): 2583-9.
[http://dx.doi.org/10.1039/b503008k]

[46] Silva LP, Bonatto CC, Polez VLP. Green Synthesis of Metal Nanoparticles by Fungi: Current Trends and Challenges BT - Advances and Applications Through Fungal Nanobiotechnology.Cham: Springer International Publishing 2016; pp. 71-89.

[47] Siddiqi KS, Husen A. Fabrication of Metal Nanoparticles from Fungi and Metal Salts: Scope and Application. Nanoscale Res Lett 2016; 11(1): 98.

[48] Salem SS, Fouda A. Green Synthesis of Metallic Nanoparticles and Their Prospective Biotechnological Applications: an Overview. Biol Trace Elem Res 2021; 199(1): 344-70.
[http://dx.doi.org/10.1007/s12011-020-02138-3] [PMID: 32377944]

[49] Yaqoob AA, Ahmad H, Parveen T, *et al.* Recent advances in metal decorated nanomaterials and their various biological applications: a review. Front Chem 2020; 8: 341.
[http://dx.doi.org/10.3389/fchem.2020.00341] [PMID: 32509720]

[50] Zhang D, Ma X-L, Gu Y, Huang H, Zhang G-W. Green synthesis of metallic nanoparticles and their potential applications to treat cancer. Front Chem 2020; 8: 799.
[http://dx.doi.org/10.3389/fchem.2020.00799] [PMID: 33195027]

[51] Love AJ, Makarov VV, Sinitsyna OV, *et al.* A genetically modified tobacco mosaic virus that can produce gold nanoparticles from a metal salt precursor. Vol. 6. Front Plant Sci 2015; 6: 984.
[http://dx.doi.org/10.3389/fpls.2015.00984] [PMID: 26617624]

[52] Bruckman MA, Czapar AE, VanMeter A, Randolph LN, Steinmetz NF. Tobacco mosaic virus-based protein nanoparticles and nanorods for chemotherapy delivery targeting breast cancer. J Control Release 2016; 231: 103-3.

[53] Krumov N, Oder S, Perner-Nochta I, Angelov A, Posten C. Accumulation of CdS nanoparticles by yeasts in a fed-batch bioprocess. J Biotechnol 2007; 132(4): 481-6.
[http://dx.doi.org/10.1016/j.jbiotec.2007.08.016] [PMID: 17900736]

[54] Dameron CT, Smith BR, Winge DR. Glutathione-coated cadmium-sulfide crystallites in Candida glabrata. J Biol Chem 1989; 264(29): 17355-60.
[http://dx.doi.org/10.1016/S0021-9258(18)71500-7] [PMID: 2793859]

[55] Mei J, Yang L-Y, Lai L, *et al.* The interactions between CdSe quantum dots and yeast Saccharomyces cerevisiae: adhesion of quantum dots to the cell surface and the protection effect of ZnS shell. Chemosphere 2014; 112: 92-9.
[http://dx.doi.org/10.1016/j.chemosphere.2014.03.071] [PMID: 25048893]

[56] Cui R, Liu H-H, Xie H-Y, Zhang Z-L, Yang Y-R, Pang D-W, *et al.* Living yeast cells as a controllable biosynthesizer for fluorescent quantum dots. Adv Funct Mater 2009; 19: 2359-64.
[http://dx.doi.org/10.1002/adfm.200801492]

[57] Kowshik M, Vogel W, Urban J, Kulkarni S, Paknikar K. Microbial Synthesis of Semiconductor PbS Nanocrystallites. Adv Mater 2002; 14: 815-8.
[http://dx.doi.org/10.1002/1521-4095(20020605)14:11<815::AID-ADMA815>3.0.CO;2-K]

[58] Gericke M, Pinches A. Microbial production of gold nanoparticles. Gold Bull 2006; 39(1): 22-8.
[http://dx.doi.org/10.1007/BF03215529]

[59] Agnihotri M, Joshi S, Kumar AR, Zinjarde S, Kulkarni S. Biosynthesis of gold nanoparticles by the tropical marine yeast Yarrowia lipolytica NCIM 3589. Mater Lett 2009; 63(15): 1231-4.
[http://dx.doi.org/10.1016/j.matlet.2009.02.042]

[60] Apte M, Girme G, Nair R, Bankar A, Ravi Kumar A, Zinjarde S. Melanin mediated synthesis of gold nanoparticles by Yarrowia lipolytica. Mater Lett 2013; 95: 149-52.
[http://dx.doi.org/10.1016/j.matlet.2012.12.087]

[61] Kowshik M, Ashtaputre S, Kharrazi S, Vogel W, Urban J, Kulkarni S, *et al.* Extracellular synthesis of silver nanoparticles by a silver-tolerant yeast strain MKY3. Nanotechnology 2003; 14: 95-100.
[http://dx.doi.org/10.1088/0957-4484/14/1/321]

[62] Beveridge TJ, Murray RG. Sites of metal deposition in the cell wall of Bacillus subtilis. J Bacteriol 1980; 141(2): 876-87.
[http://dx.doi.org/10.1128/jb.141.2.876-887.1980] [PMID: 6767692]

[63] Mann S. Structure, morphology, and crystal growth of bacterial magnetite.Magnetite biomineralization and magnetoreception in organisms. Springer 1985; pp. 311-32.
[http://dx.doi.org/10.1007/978-1-4613-0313-8_15]

[64] Malarkodi C, Rajeshkumar S, Paulkumar K, Vanaja M, Gnanajobitha G, Annadurai G. Biosynthesis and Antimicrobial Activity of Semiconductor Nanoparticles against Oral Pathogens 2014.
[http://dx.doi.org/10.1155/2014/347167]

[65] Slawson RM, Lohmeier-Vogel EM, Lee H, Trevors JT. Silver resistance in *Pseudomonas stutzeri.* Biometals 1994; 7(1): 30-40.
[http://dx.doi.org/10.1007/BF00205191] [PMID: 8118170]

[66] Yong P, Rowson NA, Farr JP, Harris IR, Macaskie LE. Bioreduction and biocrystallization of palladium by Desulfovibrio desulfuricans NCIMB 8307. Biotechnol Bioeng 2002; 80(4): 369-79.
[http://dx.doi.org/10.1002/bit.10369] [PMID: 12325145]

[67] Khandel P, Shahi SK. Mycogenic nanoparticles and their bio-prospective applications: current status and future challenges. J Nanostructure Chem 2018; 8(4): 369-91.
[http://dx.doi.org/10.1007/s40097-018-0285-2]

[68] Alghuthaymi MA, Almoammar H, Rai M, Said-Galiev E, Abd-Elsalam KA. Myconanoparticles: synthesis and their role in phytopathogens management 2015.
[http://dx.doi.org/10.1080/13102818.2015.1008194]

[69] Thakker JN, Dalwadi P, Dhandhukia PC. Biosynthesis of gold nanoparticles using *fusarium oxysporum* f. sp. cubense JT1, a plant pathogenic fungus Int Scholarly Res Notices,. 2013.

[70] Pourali P, Yahyaei B, Afsharnezhad S. Bio-synthesis of gold nanoparticles by fusarium oxysporum and assessment of their conjugation possibility with two types of β-lactam antibiotics without any additional linkers. Microbiology 2018; 87(2): 229-37.
[http://dx.doi.org/10.1134/S0026261718020108]

[71] Naimi-Shamel N, Pourali P, Dolatabadi S. Green synthesis of gold nanoparticles using Fusarium *oxysporum* and antibacterial activity of its tetracycline conjugant. J Mycol Med 2019; 29(1): 7-13.
[http://dx.doi.org/10.1016/j.mycmed.2019.01.005] [PMID: 30709721]

[72]   Mukherjee P, Senapati S, Mandal D, *et al.* Extracellular synthesis of gold nanoparticles by the fungus *Fusarium oxysporum.* ChemBioChem 2002; 3(5): 461-3.
[http://dx.doi.org/10.1002/1439-7633(20020503)3:5<461::AID-CBIC461>3.0.CO;2-X]   [PMID: 12007181]

[73]   Bansal V, Rautaray D, Ahmad A, Sastry M. Biosynthesis of zirconia nanoparticles using the fungus Fusarium oxysporum. J Mater Chem 2004; 14(22): 3303-5.
[http://dx.doi.org/10.1039/b407904c]

[74]   Bahrulolum H, Nooraei S, Javanshir N, *et al.* Green synthesis of metal nanoparticles using microorganisms and their application in the agrifood sector. J Nanobiotechnology 2021; 19(1): 86.
[http://dx.doi.org/10.1186/s12951-021-00834-3] [PMID: 33771172]

[75]   Dhanasekaran D, Latha S, Saha S, Thajuddin N, Panneerselvam A. Biosynthesis and antimicrobial potential of metal nanoparticles. Int J Green Nanotechnol 2011; 3(1): 72-82.
[http://dx.doi.org/10.1080/19430892.2011.574545]

[76]   Senapati S, Ahmad A, Khan MI, Sastry M, Kumar R. Extracellular biosynthesis of bimetallic Au-Ag alloy nanoparticles. Small 2005; 1(5): 517-20.
[http://dx.doi.org/10.1002/smll.200400053] [PMID: 17193479]

[77]   Syed A, Ahmad A. Extracellular biosynthesis of platinum nanoparticles using the fungus Fusarium oxysporum. Colloids Surf B Biointerfaces 2012; 97: 27-31.
[http://dx.doi.org/10.1016/j.colsurfb.2012.03.026] [PMID: 22580481]

[78]   Gericke M, Pinches A. Biological synthesis of metal nanoparticles. Hydrometallurgy 2006; 83(1–4): 132-40.
[http://dx.doi.org/10.1016/j.hydromet.2006.03.019]

[79]   Deniz F, Adigüzel AO, Mazmanci MA. The biosynthesis of silver nanoparticles with coriolus versicolor. Turkish J Eng 2019; 3(2): 92-6.
[http://dx.doi.org/10.31127/tuje.429072]

[80]   Lee S-W, Mao C, Flynn CE, Belcher AM. Ordering of quantum dots using genetically engineered viruses. Sci 2002; 296(5569): 892-5.
[http://dx.doi.org/10.1126/science.1068054]

[81]   Bruckman MA, VanMeter A, Steinmetz NF. Nanomanufacturing of tobacco mosaic virus-based spherical biomaterials using a continuous flow method. ACS Biomater Sci Eng 2015; 1(1): 13-8.
[http://dx.doi.org/10.1021/ab500059s] [PMID: 25984569]

[82]   Love AJ, Makarov V, Yaminsky I, Kalinina NO, Taliansky ME. The use of tobacco mosaic virus and cowpea mosaic virus for the production of novel metal nanomaterials. Virology 2014; 449: 133-9.
[http://dx.doi.org/10.1016/j.virol.2013.11.002] [PMID: 24418546]

[83]   Fan S, Zhang Y, Huang X, Geng L, Shao H, Hu X, *et al.* Silk materials for medical, electronic and optical applications. Sci China Technol Sci 2019; 62(6): 903-18.
[http://dx.doi.org/10.1007/s11431-018-9403-8]

[84]   Mathur AB, Gupta V. Silk fibroin-derived nanoparticles for biomedical applications. Nanomedicine (Lond) 2010; 5(5): 807-20.
[http://dx.doi.org/10.2217/nnm.10.51] [PMID: 20662650]

[85]   Gholipourmalekabadi M, Sapru S, Samadikuchaksaraei A, Reis RL, Kaplan DL, Kundu SC. Silk fibroin for skin injury repair: Where do things stand? Adv Drug Deliv Rev 2020; 153: 28-53.
[http://dx.doi.org/10.1016/j.addr.2019.09.003] [PMID: 31678360]

[86]   Kim J-H, Kim D-K, Lee OJ, *et al.* Osteoinductive silk fibroin/titanium dioxide/hydroxyapatite hybrid scaffold for bone tissue engineering. Int J Biol Macromol 2016; 82: 160-7.
[http://dx.doi.org/10.1016/j.ijbiomac.2015.08.001] [PMID: 26257379]

[87]   Kim MH, Kim BS, Lee J, Cho D, Kwon OH, Park WH. Silk fibroin/hydroxyapatite composite

hydrogel induced by gamma-ray irradiation for bone tissue engineering. Biomater Res 2017; 21(1): 12.
[http://dx.doi.org/10.1186/s40824-017-0098-2] [PMID: 28652926]

[88]   Elahi M, Ali S, Tahir HM, Mushtaq R, Bhatti MF. Sericin and fibroin nanoparticles—natural product for cancer therapy: a comprehensive review. Int J Polym Mater Polym Biomater 2021; 70(4): 256-69.
[http://dx.doi.org/10.1080/00914037.2019.1706515]

[89]   Huang L, Tao K, Liu J, *et al.* Design and fabrication of multifunctional sericin nanoparticles for tumor targeting and pH-responsive subcellular delivery of cancer chemotherapy drugs. ACS Appl Mater Interfaces 2016; 8(10): 6577-85.
[http://dx.doi.org/10.1021/acsami.5b11617] [PMID: 26855027]

[90]   Gunduz O, Sahin YM, Agathopoulos S, Ben-Nissan B, Oktar FN. A New Method for Fabrication of Nanohydroxyapatite and TCP from the Sea Snail *Cerithium vulgatum.* J Nanomater . 2014; 382861.

[91]   Gunduz O. A simple method of producing hydroxyapatite and tri calcium phosphate from coral *(Pocillopora verrucosa).* J Aust Ceram Soc 2014; 50: 52-8.

[92]   Kim HK, Choi M-J, Cha S-H, *et al.* Earthworm extracts utilized in the green synthesis of gold nanoparticles capable of reinforcing the anticoagulant activities of heparin. Nanoscale Res Lett 2013; 8(1): 542.
[http://dx.doi.org/10.1186/1556-276X-8-542] [PMID: 24369090]

[93]   Unrine JM, Hunyadi SE, Tsyusko OV, Rao W, Shoults-Wilson WA, Bertsch PM. Evidence for bioavailability of Au nanoparticles from soil and biodistribution within earthworms (Eisenia fetida). Environ Sci Technol 2010; 44(21): 8308-13.
[http://dx.doi.org/10.1021/es101885w] [PMID: 20879765]

[94]   Bourdineaud J-P, Štambuk A, Šrut M, *et al.* Gold and silver nanoparticles effects to the earthworm *Eisenia fetida* - the importance of tissue over soil concentrations. Drug Chem Toxicol 2021; 44(1): 12-29.
[http://dx.doi.org/10.1080/01480545.2019.1567757] [PMID: 30945571]

[95]   Mahmoodian H, Moradi O, Shariatzadeha B, Salehf TA, Tyagi I, Maity A, *et al.* Enhanced removal of methyl orange from aqueous solutions by poly HEMA–chitosan-MWCNT nano-composite. J Mol Liq 2015; 202: 189-98.
[http://dx.doi.org/10.1016/j.molliq.2014.10.040]

[96]   Mansur HS, Mansur AAP. Nano-photocatalysts based on ZnS quantum dots/chitosan for the photodegradation of dye pollutants. IOP conference series: materials science and engineering. IOP Publishing 2015; p. 12003.
[http://dx.doi.org/10.1088/1757-899X/76/1/012003]

[97]   Sahab A, Waly AI, Sabbour M, Nawar LS. Synthesis, antifungal and insecticidal potential of chitosan (CS)-g-poly (acrylic acid) (PAA) nanoparticles against some seed borne fungi and insects of soybean. Int J Chemtech Res 2015; 8: 589-98.

[98]   Salah TA, Mohammad AM, Hassan MA, El-Anadouli BE. Development of nano-hydroxyapatite/chitosan composite for cadmium ions removal in wastewater treatment. J Taiwan Inst Chem Eng 2014; 45(4): 1571-7.
[http://dx.doi.org/10.1016/j.jtice.2013.10.008]

[99]   Wu X-L, Xiao P, Zhong S, Fang K, Lin H, Chen J. Magnetic $ZnFe_2O_4$@chitosan encapsulated in graphene oxide for adsorptive removal of organic dye. RSC Advances 2017; 7(45): 28145-51.
[http://dx.doi.org/10.1039/C7RA04100D]

[100] Bhattacharyya R, Ray S. Micro- and nano-sized bentonite filled composite superabsorbents of chitosan and acrylic copolymer for removal of synthetic dyes from water. Appl Clay Sci 2014; (Nov): 101.
[http://dx.doi.org/10.1016/j.clay.2014.09.015]

[101] Ali F, Khan SB, Kamal T, Alamry KA, Asiri AM. Chitosan-titanium oxide fibers supported zero-valent nanoparticles: Highly efficient and easily retrievable catalyst for the removal of organic

pollutants. Sci Rep 2018; 8(1): 6260.
[http://dx.doi.org/10.1038/s41598-018-24311-4] [PMID: 29674721]

[102] Chatterjee A, Kwatra N, Abraham J. Nanoparticles fabrication by plant extracts.Micro and Nano Technologies. Elsevier 2020; pp. 143-57.

[103] Raut R, Sana A, Malghe Y, Nikam B, Sahebrao K. Rapid biosynthesis of platinum and palladium metal nanoparticles using root extract of asparagus racemosus linn. Adv Mater Lett 2013; 4: 650-4.
[http://dx.doi.org/10.5185/amlett.2012.11470]

[104] Boruah S, Boruah P, Sarma P, Medhi C, Kumar O. Green synthesis of gold nanoparticles using camellia sinensis and kinetics of the reaction. Adv Mater Lett 2012; 3.

[105] Jia J-L, Xu H-H, Li D-Q, Ye W-H, Liu W-J. Biosynthesis of silver and gold nanoparticles using huangdan *(camellia sinensis)* leaf sxtract. synth react inorganic. Met Nano-Metal Chem 2015; 45(7): 941-6.
[http://dx.doi.org/10.1080/15533174.2013.862817]

[106] Shankar SS, Rai A, Ahmad A, Sastry M. Rapid synthesis of Au, Ag, and bimetallic Au core-Ag shell nanoparticles using Neem *(Azadirachta indica)* leaf broth. J Colloid Interface Sci 2004; 275(2): 496-502.
[http://dx.doi.org/10.1016/j.jcis.2004.03.003] [PMID: 15178278]

[107] Gardea-Torresdey J. Alfalfa sprouts: A Natural source for the synthesis of silver nanoparticles. Langmuir 2003; 19.
[http://dx.doi.org/10.1021/la020835i]

[108] Sharma NC, Sahi SV, Nath S, Parsons JG, Gardea-Torresdey JL, Pal T. Synthesis of plant-mediated gold nanoparticles and catalytic role of biomatrix-embedded nanomaterials. Environ Sci Technol 2007; 41(14): 5137-42.
[http://dx.doi.org/10.1021/es062929a] [PMID: 17711235]

[109] Cirtiu CM, Dunlop-Brière AF, Moores A. Cellulose nanocrystallites as an efficient support for nanoparticles of palladium: application for catalytic hydrogenation and Heck coupling under mild conditions. Green Chem 2011; 13(2): 288-91.
[http://dx.doi.org/10.1039/C0GC00326C]

[110] Jha AK, Prasad K. Green synthesis of silver nanoparticles using cycas leaf. Int J Green Nanotechnol Phys Chem 2010; 1(2): 110-7.
[http://dx.doi.org/10.1080/19430871003684572]

[111] Noruzi M, Zare D, Davoodi D. A rapid biosynthesis route for the preparation of gold nanoparticles by aqueous extract of cypress leaves at room temperature. Spectrochim Acta A Mol Biomol Spectrosc 2012; 94: 84-8.
[http://dx.doi.org/10.1016/j.saa.2012.03.041] [PMID: 22522293]

[112] Nasrollahzadeh M, Sajadi SM. Green synthesis of copper nanoparticles using Ginkgo biloba L. leaf extract and their catalytic activity for the Huisgen [3+2] cycloaddition of azides and alkynes at room temperature. J Colloid Interface Sci 2015; 457: 141-7.
[http://dx.doi.org/10.1016/j.jcis.2015.07.004] [PMID: 26164245]

[113] Kalpana D, Han J, Park W, Lee S, Lee Y, Wahab R. Green Biosynthesis of Silver Nanoparticles Using *Torreya nucifera* and their Antibacterial Activity. Arab J Chem 2014; (Sep): 8.

[114] Johnson I, Prabu HJ. Green synthesis and characterization of silver nanoparticles by leaf extracts of Cycas circinalis, Ficus amplissima, Commelina benghalensis and Lippia nodiflora. Int Nano Lett 2015; 5(1): 43-51.
[http://dx.doi.org/10.1007/s40089-014-0136-1]

[115] Velmurugan P, Lee S-M, Iydroose M, Lee K-J, Oh B-T. Pine cone-mediated green synthesis of silver nanoparticles and their antibacterial activity against agricultural pathogens. Appl Microbiol Biotechnol 2012; (Jan): 97.

[PMID: 22290649]

[116]   Velmurugan P, Park J-H, Lee S-M, *et al.* Synthesis and characterization of nanosilver with antibacterial properties using Pinus densiflora young cone extract. J Photochem Photobiol B 2015; 147: 63-8.
[http://dx.doi.org/10.1016/j.jphotobiol.2015.03.008] [PMID: 25846578]

[117]   Britto AJ, Gracelin DHS, Jeya PB, Kumar R, Nadu T. Biogenic silver nanoparticles by Adiantum caudatum and their antibacterial activity. Int J Univers Pharm Life Sci 2012; 2: 92-8.

[118]   Sant DG, Gujarathi TR, Harne SR, Ghosh S, Kitture R, Kale S, *et al.* Adiantum philippense L. Frond Assisted Rapid Green Synthesis of Gold and Silver Nanoparticles. Agarwal G, editor. J Nanoparticles. 2013; 182320.

[119]   Chumpol J, Siri S. In vivo formation of spherical and rod lead nanoparticles in root cells of water velvet *(Azolla pinnata)*. Biotechnol Appl Biochem 2020; 67(6): 991-9.
[http://dx.doi.org/10.1002/bab.1871] [PMID: 31821601]

[120]   Kunjiappan S, Chowdhury R, Bhattacharjee C. A green chemistry approach for the synthesis and characterization of bioactive gold nanoparticles using Azolla microphylla methanol extract. Front Mater Sci 2014; 8: 123-35.
[http://dx.doi.org/10.1007/s11706-014-0246-8]

[121]   Smitha PS, Sheeja TT, Manju M. Green nanoparticles from different plant groups.Micro and Nano Technologies. Elsevier 2020; pp. 51-70.

[122]   Canivet L, Dubot P, Garçon G, Denayer F-O. Effects of engineered iron nanoparticles on the bryophyte, Physcomitrella patens (Hedw.) Bruch & Schimp, after foliar exposure. Ecotoxicol Environ Saf 2015; 113: 499-505.
[http://dx.doi.org/10.1016/j.ecoenv.2014.12.035] [PMID: 25576736]

[123]   Ghosh I, Sadhu A, Moriyasu Y, Bandyopadhyay M, Mukherjee A. Manganese oxide nanoparticles induce genotoxicity and DNA hypomethylation in the moss Physcomitrella patens. Mutat Res Toxicol Environ Mutagen 2019; 842: 146-57.
[http://dx.doi.org/10.1016/j.mrgentox.2018.12.006] [PMID: 31471003]

[124]   Ovais M, Khalil AT, Islam NU, *et al.* Role of plant phytochemicals and microbial enzymes in biosynthesis of metallic nanoparticles. Appl Microbiol Biotechnol 2018; 102(16): 6799-814.
[http://dx.doi.org/10.1007/s00253-018-9146-7] [PMID: 29882162]

[125]   Acharya K, Sarkar J. Bryo-synthesis of gold nanoparticles. Int J Pharm Sci Rev Res 2014; 29(1): 82-6.

[126]   Khanna P, Kaur A, Goyal D. Algae-based metallic nanoparticles: Synthesis, characterization and applications. J Microbiol Methods 2019; 163105656
[http://dx.doi.org/10.1016/j.mimet.2019.105656] [PMID: 31220512]

[127]   Chundawat* AA and TS. Metal Nanoparticles from Algae: A Green Approach for the Synthesis, Characterization and their Biological Activity. Vol. 10. Nanosci Nanotechnol Asia 2020; 185-202.

[128]   Parial D, Pal R. Green Synthesis of Gold Nanoparticles Using Cyanobacteria and their Characterization. Indian J Appl Res 2011; 4: 69-72.
[http://dx.doi.org/10.15373/2249555X/JAN2014/22]

[129]   Castro L, Blázquez ML, Muñoz JA, González F, Ballester A. Biological synthesis of metallic nanoparticles using algae. IET Nanobiotechnol 2013; 7(3): 109-16.
[http://dx.doi.org/10.1049/iet-nbt.2012.0041] [PMID: 24028809]

[130]   Annamalai J, Nallamuthu T. Characterization of biosynthesized gold nanoparticles from aqueous extract of *Chlorella vulgaris* and their anti-pathogenic properties. Appl Nanosci 2015; 5(5): 603-7.
[http://dx.doi.org/10.1007/s13204-014-0353-y]

[131]   Govindaraju K, Basha SK, Kumar VG, Singaravelu G. Silver, gold and bimetallic nanoparticles production using single-cell protein *(Spirulina platensis)* Geitler. J Mater Sci 2008; 43(15): 5115-22.

[http://dx.doi.org/10.1007/s10853-008-2745-4]

[132]   Senapati S, Syed A, Moeez S, Kumar A, Ahmad A. Intracellular synthesis of gold nanoparticles using alga Tetraselmis kochinensis. Mater Lett 2012; 79: 116-8.
[http://dx.doi.org/10.1016/j.matlet.2012.04.009]

[133]   Mata YN, Torres E, Blázquez ML, Ballester A, González F, Muñoz JA. Gold(III) biosorption and bioreduction with the brown alga Fucus vesiculosus. J Hazard Mater 2009; 166(2-3): 612-8.
[http://dx.doi.org/10.1016/j.jhazmat.2008.11.064] [PMID: 19124199]

[134]   Sasikala M, Gunasekaran M, Thajuddin N. Biosynthesis and characterization of silver nanoparticles using marine cyanobacterium, Oscillatoria willei NTDM01. Dig J Nanomater Biostruct 2011; 6: 385-90.

[135]   Roni M, Murugan K, Panneerselvam C, *et al.* Characterization and biotoxicity of Hypnea musciformis-synthesized silver nanoparticles as potential eco-friendly control tool against *Aedes aegypti* and *Plutella xylostella.* Ecotoxicol Environ Saf 2015; 121: 31-8.
[http://dx.doi.org/10.1016/j.ecoenv.2015.07.005] [PMID: 26184431]

[136]   Torabfam M, Yüce M. Microwave-assisted green synthesis of silver nanoparticles using dried extracts of *Chlorella vulgaris* and antibacterial activity studies. Green Process Synth 2020; 9(1): 283-93.
[http://dx.doi.org/10.1515/gps-2020-0024]

[137]   Soleimani M, Habibi-Pirkoohi M. Biosynthesis of Silver Nanoparticles using *Chlorella vulgaris* and Evaluation of the Antibacterial Efficacy Against *Staphylococcus aureus.* Avicenna J Med Biotechnol 2017; 9(3): 120-5.
[PMID: 28706606]

[138]   Singaravelu G, Arockiamary JS, Kumar VG, Govindaraju K. A novel extracellular synthesis of monodisperse gold nanoparticles using marine alga, Sargassum wightii Greville. Colloids Surf B Biointerfaces 2007; 57(1): 97-101.
[http://dx.doi.org/10.1016/j.colsurfb.2007.01.010] [PMID: 17350236]

[139]   Rajasulochana P, Dhamotharan R, Murugakoothan P, Subbiah M, Krishnamoorthy P. Biosynthesis and characterization of gold nanoparticles using the alga Kappaphycus alvarezii. Int J Nanosci 2010; 9(05): 511-6.

[140]   Das RK, Gogoi N, Bora U. Green synthesis of gold nanoparticles using *Nyctanthes arbortristis* flower extract. Bioprocess Biosyst Eng 2011; 34(5): 615-9.
[http://dx.doi.org/10.1007/s00449-010-0510-y] [PMID: 21229266]

[141]   Narayanan K, Sakthivel N. Coriander leaf mediated biosynthesis of gold nanoparticles. Mater Lett 2008; 62: 4588-90.
[http://dx.doi.org/10.1016/j.matlet.2008.08.044]

[142]   Armendariz V, Herrera I. Size controlled gold nanoparticle formation by Avena sativa biomass: use of plants in nanobiotechnology. J Nanopart Res 2004; 6(4): 377-82.
[http://dx.doi.org/10.1007/s11051-004-0741-4]

[143]   Poinern GEJ, Chapman P, Le X, Fawcett D. Green biosynthesis of gold nanometre scale plates using the leaf extracts from an indigenous Australian plant Eucalyptus macrocarpa. Gold Bull 2013; 46(3): 165-73.
[http://dx.doi.org/10.1007/s13404-013-0096-7]

[144]   Edison TJI, Sethuraman MG. Instant green synthesis of silver nanoparticles using Terminalia chebula fruit extract and evaluation of their catalytic activity on reduction of methylene blue. Process Biochem 2012; 47(9): 1351-7.
[http://dx.doi.org/10.1016/j.procbio.2012.04.025]

[145]   Poinern GEJ, Chapman P, Shah M, Fawcett D. Green biosynthesis of silver nanocubes using the leaf extracts from *Eucalyptus macrocarpa.* Nano Bull 2013; 2(1)

[146]   Geetha N, Geetha TS, Manonmani P, Thiyagarajan M. Green synthesis of silver nanoparticles using

Cymbopogan Citratus (Dc) Stapf. Extract and its antibacterial activity. Aust J Basic Appl Sci 2014; 8(3): 324-31.

[147]   Lee H-J, Song JY, Kim BS. Biological synthesis of copper nanoparticles using Magnolia kobus leaf extract and their antibacterial activity. J Chem Technol Biotechnol 2013; 88(11): 1971-7.

[148]   Rajesh KM, Ajitha B, Reddy YAK, Suneetha Y, Reddy PS. Assisted green synthesis of copper nanoparticles using *Syzygium aromaticum* bud extract: Physical, optical and antimicrobial properties. Optik (Stuttg) 2018; 154: 593-600.
[http://dx.doi.org/10.1016/j.ijleo.2017.10.074]

[149]   Valodkar M, Nagar PS, Jadeja RN, Thounaojam MC, Devkar RV, Thakore S. Euphorbiaceae latex induced green synthesis of non-cytotoxic metallic nanoparticle solutions: A rational approach to antimicrobial applications. Colloids Surf A Physicochem Eng Asp 2011; 384(1): 337-44.
[http://dx.doi.org/10.1016/j.colsurfa.2011.04.015]

[150]   Thekkae Padil VV, Černík M. Green synthesis of copper oxide nanoparticles using gum karaya as a biotemplate and their antibacterial application. Int J Nanomedicine 2013; 8(8): 889-98.
[PMID: 23467397]

[151]   Sathishkumar M, Sneha K, Kwak IS, Mao J, Tripathy SJ, Yun YS. Phyto-crystallization of palladium through reduction process using Cinnamom zeylanicum bark extract. J Hazard Mater 2009; 171(1-3): 400-4.
[http://dx.doi.org/10.1016/j.jhazmat.2009.06.014] [PMID: 19576689]

[152]   Petla RK, Vivekanandhan S, Misra M, Mohanty A, Satyanarayana N. Soybean (Glycine max) leaf extract based green synthesis of palladium nanoparticles. J Biomater Nanobiotechnol 2012; 03

[153]   Bogireddy N, Martinez Gomez L, Osorio Roman I, Agarwal V. Synthesis of gold nanoparticles using Coffea Arabica fruit extract 2017.

[154]   Jia L, Zhang Q, Li Q, Song H. The biosynthesis of palladium nanoparticles by antioxidants in Gardenia jasminoides Ellis: long lifetime nanocatalysts for p-nitrotoluene hydrogenation. Nanotechnology 2009; 20(38)385601
[http://dx.doi.org/10.1088/0957-4484/20/38/385601] [PMID: 19713585]

[155]   Song JY, Kwon E-Y, Kim BS. Biological synthesis of platinum nanoparticles using Diopyros kaki leaf extract. Bioprocess Biosyst Eng 2010; 33(1): 159-64.
[http://dx.doi.org/10.1007/s00449-009-0373-2] [PMID: 19701776]

[156]   Soundarrajan C, Sankari A, Dhandapani P, *et al.* Rapid biological synthesis of platinum nanoparticles using Ocimum sanctum for water electrolysis applications. Bioprocess Biosyst Eng 2012; 35(5): 827-33.
[http://dx.doi.org/10.1007/s00449-011-0666-0] [PMID: 22167464]

[157]   Coccia F, Tonucci L, Bosco D, Bressan M, d'Alessandro N. One-pot synthesis of lignin-stabilised platinum and palladium nanoparticles and their catalytic behaviour in oxidation and reduction reactions. Green Chem 2012; 14(4): 1073-8.
[http://dx.doi.org/10.1039/c2gc16524d]

[158]   Roopan SM, Bharathi A, Prabhakarn A, *et al.* Efficient phyto-synthesis and structural characterization of rutile TiO_2 nanoparticles using Annona squamosa peel extract. Spectrochim Acta A Mol Biomol Spectrosc 2012; 98: 86-90.
[http://dx.doi.org/10.1016/j.saa.2012.08.055] [PMID: 22983203]

[159]   Sundrarajan M, Gowri S. Green synthesis of titanium dioxide nanoparticles by nyctanthes arbor-tristis leaves extract. Chalcogenide Lett 2011; (Aug): 8.

[160]   Rajakumar G, Rahuman AA, Priyamvada B, Khanna VG, Kumar DK, Sujin PJ. Eclipta prostrata leaf aqueous extract mediated synthesis of titanium dioxide nanoparticles. Mater Lett 2012; 68: 115-7.
[http://dx.doi.org/10.1016/j.matlet.2011.10.038]

[161]   Velayutham K, Rahuman AA, Rajakumar G, *et al.* Evaluation of Catharanthus roseus leaf extract-

mediated biosynthesis of titanium dioxide nanoparticles against Hippobosca maculata and Bovicola ovis. Parasitol Res 2012; 111(6): 2329-37.
[http://dx.doi.org/10.1007/s00436-011-2676-x] [PMID: 21987105]

[162]   Santhoshkumar T, Rahuman AA, Jayaseelan C, *et al.* Green synthesis of titanium dioxide nanoparticles using Psidium guajava extract and its antibacterial and antioxidant properties. Asian Pac J Trop Med 2014; 7(12): 968-76.
[http://dx.doi.org/10.1016/S1995-7645(14)60171-1] [PMID: 25479626]

[163]   Chaudhuri SK, Malodia L. Biosynthesis of zinc oxide nanoparticles using leaf extract of Calotropis gigantea: characterization and its evaluation on tree seedling growth in nursery stage. Appl Nanosci 2017; 7(8): 501-12.
[http://dx.doi.org/10.1007/s13204-017-0586-7]

[164]   Ali K, Dwivedi S, Azam A, *et al.* Aloe vera extract functionalized zinc oxide nanoparticles as nanoantibiotics against multi-drug resistant clinical bacterial isolates. J Colloid Interface Sci 2016; 472: 145-56.
[http://dx.doi.org/10.1016/j.jcis.2016.03.021] [PMID: 27031596]

[165]   Qu J, Luo C, Hou J. Synthesis of ZnO nanoparticles from Zn-hyperaccumulator (Sedum alfredii Hance) plants. Micro Nano Lett IET 2011; 6: 174-6.
[http://dx.doi.org/10.1049/mnl.2011.0004]

[166]   Vimala K, Sundarraj S, Paulpandi M, Vengatesan S, Kannan S. Green synthesized doxorubicin loaded zinc oxide nanoparticles regulates the Bax and Bcl-2 expression in breast and colon carcinoma. Process Biochem 2014; 49(1): 160-72.
[http://dx.doi.org/10.1016/j.procbio.2013.10.007]

[167]   Ebrahiminezhad A, Zare-Hoseinabadi A, Sarmah AK, Taghizadeh S, Ghasemi Y, Berenjian A. Plant-mediated synthesis and applications of iron nanoparticles. Mol Biotechnol 2018; 60(2): 154-68.
[http://dx.doi.org/10.1007/s12033-017-0053-4] [PMID: 29256163]

[168]   Pattanayak M, Nayak PL. Green synthesis and characterization of zero valent iron nanoparticles from the leaf extract of Azadirachta indica (Neem). World J Nano Sci Technol 2013; 2(1): 6-9.

[169]   Shah S, Dasgupta S, Chakraborty M, Vadakkekara R, Hajoori M. Green synthesis of iron nanoparticles using plant extracts. Int J Biol Pharm Res 2014; 05: 549-52.

[170]   Joglekar S, Kodam K, Dhaygude M, Hudlikar M. Novel route for rapid biosynthesis of lead nanoparticles using aqueous extract of Jatropha curcas L. latex. Mater Lett 2011; 65(19): 3170-2.
[http://dx.doi.org/10.1016/j.matlet.2011.06.075]

[171]   Sasidharan S, Sowmiya R, Balakrishnaraja R. Biosynthesis of selenium nanoparticles using citrus reticulata peel extract. World J Pharm Res 2015; 4: 1322-30.

[172]   Sathishkumar M, Sneha K, Won SW, Cho C-W, Kim S, Yun Y-S. Cinnamon zeylanicum bark extract and powder mediated green synthesis of nano-crystalline silver particles and its bactericidal activity. Colloids Surf B Biointerfaces 2009; 73(2): 332-8.
[http://dx.doi.org/10.1016/j.colsurfb.2009.06.005] [PMID: 19576733]

[173]   Huang J, Li Q, Sun D, Lu Y, Su Y, Yang X, *et al.* Biosynthesis of silver and gold nanoparticles by novel sundried Cinnamomum camphora leaf. Nanotechnology 2007; 18(10)105104
[http://dx.doi.org/10.1088/0957-4484/18/10/105104]

[174]   Chandran SP, Chaudhary M, Pasricha R, Ahmad A, Sastry M. Synthesis of gold nanotriangles and silver nanoparticles using Aloe vera plant extract. Biotechnol Prog 2006; 22(2): 577-83.
[http://dx.doi.org/10.1021/bp0501423] [PMID: 16599579]

[175]   Narayanan KB, Sakthivel N. Phytosynthesis of gold nanoparticles using leaf extract of Coleus amboinicus Lour. Mater Charact 2010; 61(11): 1232-8.
[http://dx.doi.org/10.1016/j.matchar.2010.08.003]

[176]   Razali Z, Masdar NW, Nasir NAHA, Rahim NS, Kawi RM. Green synthesis of silver nanoparticles

from ananas comosus core extract and their antibacterial activity BT - charting the sustainable future of ASEAN in science and technology.Singapore: Springer Singapore 2020; pp. 455-63.

[177]   Ahmad N. Green synthesis of silver nanoparticles using extracts of ananas comosus. Green Sustain Chem 2012; 02: 141-7.
[http://dx.doi.org/10.4236/gsc.2012.24020]

[178]   Dwivedi AD, Gopal K. Biosynthesis of silver and gold nanoparticles using Chenopodium album leaf extract. Colloids Surf A Physicochem Eng Asp 2010; 369(1): 27-33.
[http://dx.doi.org/10.1016/j.colsurfa.2010.07.020]

[179]   Prathna TC, Chandrasekaran N, Raichur AM, Mukherjee A. Kinetic evolution studies of silver nanoparticles in a bio-based green synthesis process. Colloids Surf A Physicochem Eng Asp 2011; 377(1): 212-6.
[http://dx.doi.org/10.1016/j.colsurfa.2010.12.047]

[180]   Song JY, Jang H-K, Kim BS. Biological synthesis of gold nanoparticles using Magnolia kobus and Diopyros kaki leaf extracts. Process Biochem 2009; 44(10): 1133-8.
[http://dx.doi.org/10.1016/j.procbio.2009.06.005]

[181]   Sathishkumar M, Sneha K, Yun Y-S. Immobilization of silver nanoparticles synthesized using Curcuma longa tuber powder and extract on cotton cloth for bactericidal activity. Bioresour Technol 2010; 101(20): 7958-65.
[http://dx.doi.org/10.1016/j.biortech.2010.05.051] [PMID: 20541399]

[182]   Kaviya S, Santhanalakshmi J, Viswanathan B, Muthumary J, Srinivasan K. Biosynthesis of silver nanoparticles using citrus sinensis peel extract and its antibacterial activity. Spectrochim Acta A Mol Biomol Spectrosc 2011; 79(3): 594-8.
[http://dx.doi.org/10.1016/j.saa.2011.03.040] [PMID: 21536485]

[183]   Singh J, Dutta T, Kim K-H, Rawat M, Samddar P, Kumar P. 'Green' synthesis of metals and their oxide nanoparticles: applications for environmental remediation. J Nanobiotechnology 2018; 16(1): 84.
[http://dx.doi.org/10.1186/s12951-018-0408-4] [PMID: 30373622]

[184]   Vivek M, Kumar PS, Steffi S, Sudha S. Biogenic silver nanoparticles by *gelidiella acerosa* extract and their antifungal effects. Avicenna J Med Biotechnol 2011; 3(3): 143-8.
[PMID: 23408653]

[185]   Yue S, Luo M, Liu H, Wei S. Recent Advances of Gold Compounds in Anticancer Immunity. Front Chem 2020; 8: 543.
[http://dx.doi.org/10.3389/fchem.2020.00543] [PMID: 32695747]

[186]   Murugan K, Benelli G, Panneerselvam C, *et al.* Cymbopogon citratus-synthesized gold nanoparticles boost the predation efficiency of copepod Mesocyclops aspericornis against malaria and dengue mosquitoes. Exp Parasitol 2015; 153: 129-38.
[http://dx.doi.org/10.1016/j.exppara.2015.03.017] [PMID: 25819295]

SUBJECT INDEX

A

Acid(s) 29, 35, 36, 44, 64, 75, 76, 77, 108,
109, 110, 115, 116, 117, 118, 119, 124,
143, 148, 149, 152, 153, 157, 161, 165,
166, 167, 190, 195, 203
  boric (BA) 161, 165, 166, 167
  carboxylic 149
  chlorogenic 148, 203
  deoxyribonucleic 143, 152
  fatty 109
  folic 64, 76, 77, 116, 117
  glutamic 190
  hyaluronic 36, 110, 118, 124
  lactic 29, 44, 119
  lactic-co-glycolic 29, 108
  nucleic 75, 76, 115, 116, 153, 157
  phenolic 195
  polyglutamic 110
  polyglycolic 110
  polylactic 35, 110
  zoledronic 115
Activation 24, 43, 74, 77, 78, 150
  cytoplast 24
  metabolic 150
Acute lymphoblastic lymphoma 91
Adenocarcinomas 202
Algae 199, 200
    mediated biological synthesis 199
    tetraselmis kochinensis 200
Alzheimer's disease 23
Amphiphilic copolymers 110
Anemia 23, 57, 58
Angiogenic inhibitory effects 99
ANOVA, two-way 150
Antimicrobial 33, 161, 187, 192, 202, 208
  activity 33, 161, 187, 192
  properties 161, 202, 208
Anti-tumor efficacy 122
Apoptosis 39, 91, 92, 153, 165
Applications 100, 157, 158, 172, 183
  electrocatalysis 183

industrial 172
mechanical 100
medicinal 158
nanomaterial 157
Asparagus racemosus 196
Aspergillus terreus 195
Assay 148, 149, 150, 151,
  chromosome anomalies 148
Atherosclerosis 59, 61
Atomic force microscopy (AFM) 2, 145, 146,
  184
Azadirachta indica 196, 197, 201, 204, 205
Azolla 199
    microphylla 199
    pinnata 199

B

Bacillus 142, 187, 190
    cereus 187
    licheniformis biomass 142
    megaterium 187
    Subtilis 190
Biotechnological processes 190
Blood 6, 57, 58
  disorders 57
  proteins 6
  transfusions 58
Bone 91, 24, 140
  marrow cells 140
  marrow proteins 91
  morphogenic proteins (BMP) 24
Boron 156, 158, 159, 162, 163, 167, 171, 174
  based biomaterials 159
  neutron capture therapy (BNCT) 156, 158,
    162, 163, 167, 171, 174
  NPs for cancer treatment 162
  reagents 174
Boron nitride 156, 168, 167, 169, 170, 171,
  172
  nanotubes (BNNTs) 156, 168, 169, 170,
    171, 172

Wound healing process 165

X

Xanthanolides 152
Xanthine oxidase 74
X-Ray 4, 147, 184
    diffraction (XRD) 147, 184
    emission 4
    photoelectron spectroscopy 147
XRD technique 184